Promising Genomics

Promising Genomics

Iceland and deCODE Genetics in a World of Speculation

Mike Fortun

UNIVERSITY OF CALIFORNIA PRESS

Berkeley / Los Angeles / London

University of California Press, one of the most distinguished university presses in the United States, enriches lives around the world by advancing scholarship in the humanities, social sciences, and natural sciences. Its activities are supported by the UC Press Foundation and by philanthropic contributions from individuals and institutions. For more information, visit www.ucpress.edu.

University of California Press
Berkeley and Los Angeles, California

University of California Press, Ltd.
London, England

Library of Congress Cataloging-in-Publication Data

Fortun, Michael.
    Promising genomics : Iceland and deCODE Genetics in a world of speculation / Mike Fortun.
        p.   cm.
    Includes bibliographical references and index.
    ISBN: 978-0-520-24750-5 (cloth : alk. paper)
    ISBN: 978-0-520-24751-2 (pbk. : alk. paper)
    1. deCODE Genetics, Inc.   2. Genomics—Research—Moral and ethical aspects—Iceland.   3. Genomics—Social aspects—Iceland.
4. Medical records—Access control—Moral and ethical aspects—Iceland.
5. Human genetics—Databases—Moral and ethical aspects—Iceland.
6. Human genetics—Databases—Access control—Iceland.   7. Human genetics—Databases—Law and legislation—Iceland.   8. Medical records—Law and legislation—Iceland.   9. Human population genetics—Moral and ethical appects—Iceland.   10. Privacy, Right of—Iceland.
I. Title.
    [DNLM—   1. deCODE Genetics, Inc.   2. Genetic Research—economics—Iceland.   3. Databases, Genetic—ethics—Iceland.
4. Databases, Genetic—legislation & jurisprudence—Iceland.   5. Genetic Privacy—Iceland.   6. Genetic Research—ethics—Iceland.   7. Genetic Research—legislation & jurisprudence—Iceland.   8. Genetics, Population—Iceland.   QU 450 F745P   2008]

QH438.7.F67   2008
572.8072'04912—dc22   2007044597

Manufactured in the United States of America

17   16   15   14   13   12   11   10   09   08
10   9   8   7   6   5   4   3   2   1

The paper used in this publication meets the minimum requirements of ANSI/NISO Z39.48–1992 (R 1997) (*Permanence of Paper*).

For Kora,
Lena, and Kim

Contents

Acknowledgments

Kim Fortun is first, in so many ways and for so many reasons. Ahead of the now, she has pulled me forward through this book's long writing, and our long life together. Writer of the disaster, extraordinary mother of Kora and Lena, she's the promise that makes me, keeps me. To be promised to her is the greatest gift.

I have tried to thank Skúli Sigurdsson, my friend and advance man, in the book itself, but do so again here just for good measure; his wonderful companion Elvira Scheich was also a wonderful companion to me in Iceland. Einar Árnason, Pétur Hauksson, Tómas Zoëga, Alfred Árnason, Bogi Andersen, Ragnar Adalsteinsson, were all enormously generous with their time, knowledge, and friendship. I also thank Sigurbjörg Ármannsdóttir, Anna Atladóttir, Steindór Erlingsson, Jórunn Erla Eyfjörd, Jón Jóhannes Jónsson, Helga Ögmundsdóttir, Eiríkur Steingrimsson, and all the other Icelanders who helped me over the years. Thanks also to Kitta McPherson, Kristin Philipkoski, and Matt Crenson for their journalistic efforts.

I am indebted to the National Science Foundation for funding my first trip to Iceland in 1998. The Institute for Advanced Study gave me the gift of a fellowship year in 2000–2001, in which this manuscript took shape; my thanks to Joan Scott, Clifford Geertz, Joan Fujimura, Sylvia Schafer, Deborah Keates, Tom Streeter, James Der Derian, Adam Ashforth, and Manuel de Landa for inspiration and many good times.

Elizabeth Wilson read the manuscript at a crucial time, and her encouragement and advice meant the world—a statement which contains

ACKNOWLEDGMENTS

not a shred of hype. My noosphere is continually replenished by Rich Doyle's words of friendship and scholarship. I am also grateful for the support and wisdom of Michael Fischer, David Fortun, Evelynn Hammonds, Stefan Helmreich, Jonathan Kahn, George Marcus, Kaushik Sunder Rajan, Alexandra Shields, and Karen-Sue Taussig.

LavaXLand

Whether we're looking into Iceland, the United States, or another lava land somewhere in between, a book about promising genomics in the latter years of the twentieth century—a book about speculation, capital, DNA, and other volatile, lavalike substances; a book about new technologies and new sciences and new organisms, and the new scientist-celebrities who attempted to turn all these novelties into profitable businesses; a book about volatile combinations of facts and fictions in science and literature; a book about nationalism in an era of globalization; a book about privacy and its shadows, as medical records and genetic information become exchangeable across numerous boundaries; a book about the knowing and unknowing, willing and unwilling participation not only of individuals, but also of *populations* in the making of biomedical futures—such a book about promising genomics in lava land could hardly begin with a more appropriate document than a press release . . .

If you were living in any lava land other than that most famous one, Iceland, the first time you heard about deCODE Genetics might have been on February 2, 1998. Maybe you were one of the many avid online investors who first caught the Internet exuberance and then tried to catch the next big investment wave in biotech, so you subscribed to one of the many e-mail alert services that routinely announced the most promising happenings in the young world of commercial genomics, and you found that day's media release illuminated on your screen: "Roche and DeCode

Genetics Inc. of Iceland collaborate in genetic diseases research." Since the media is a major force not only in the public perception of genomics but also in the genomic economy itself, and since press releases, sound bites, photo ops, celebrity, and the effective but curiously nebulous thing called "hype" will feature prominently in the remainder of this book, the book opens with excerpts from Roche's press release:

Roche and the Icelandic research company DeCode Genetics Inc. are to collaborate in genetic research with the aim of developing new therapeutic and diagnostic products to combat disease.

Based on the unique genetic properties of the Icelandic population DeCode will map and discover genes causing disease. . . .

"DeCode's access to the unique source of genetic information is a huge opportunity to shed new light on the causes of common diseases and to find truly effective ways to diagnose, prevent and treat illness," said Dr. Jonathan Knowles, Head of Global Pharmaceutical Research at Roche. . . .

DeCode is able to base its research on the genetic homogeneity of the Icelandic population whose geographic isolation has left the gene pool little changed for some one thousand years. In addition detailed genealogical and health records going back several generations, a highly educated population and first-class clinical expertise provide excellent preconditions for tracing the genetics of complex diseases.

Dr. Kári Stefánsson, President and CEO of DeCode Genetics Inc. said, "My company is happy about this chance to see the fundamental work it has already done in the field of genetics research bear fruit in collaboration with an experienced partner such as Roche. We are an Icelandic company that together with the government and people of the country is proud to be building up a world class research environment and at the same time contributing to solve some of the medical problems facing mankind."

The five-year collaboration agreement will focus on the discovery of genes with alleles or mutations that predispose people to the development of up to twelve common diseases including four cardiovascular diseases, four neurological/psychiatric diseases and four metabolic diseases.

The agreement could lead to potential payments by Roche in excess of 200 million US dollars over the period of the collaboration, in the form of equity investment, research and milestone payments and royalties. . . .

As part of the agreement and collaboration, Roche will provide the Icelandic people free of charge with pharmaceutical and diagnostics products that emerge from the collaboration.

The agreement has also been welcomed by the Icelandic government. The Prime Minister, Mr. Davíd Oddsson, said he was delighted to see foreign investment in a high technology venture in his country. "I view this agreement as a huge step toward securing high technology industries an important role in the Icelandic economy. The government of Iceland will do its best to assist the two parties in the agreement to achieve the goals of the collaboration."[1]

You had probably never heard of deCODE Genetics, even though you might have already been buzzed about new companies such as Human Genome Sciences Inc. (HGSI), Millennium Pharmaceuticals, and Incyte Pharmaceuticals. These genomic companies were entirely new phenomena, which had emerged in the mid-1990s, in the same accelerated time, high-speed culture, and fast and volatile economy as the Internet and the innumerable dot-coms. Think of them as bio-dot-coms, since they too traded on the promise of information—promising to turn the recent torrent of DNA sequence information, genetic information, and other kinds of bioinformation unleashed by the Human Genome Project into new understandings of disease, new diagnostic tools, and new drugs.

You had *definitely* never seen an agreement of this size between an established transnational life sciences corporation such as Roche and one of the genomic start-ups; a $200 million promise had never been made in the (very brief) history of the genomic economy, even to one of the more "established" companies such as HGSI, Millennium, or Incyte. These were about the only major companies on the genomic map—corporations that had formed in the previous few years to employ new high-throughput sequencing technologies in combination with new database capabilities in business plans that centered mostly on selling scads of promising bioinformation and swarms of promising genetic loci and biosubstances. (This crude but not inaccurate definition of the genomic business will be refined later on.) Incyte Pharmaceuticals (later Incyte Genomics) in Palo Alto had gone public in 1993 with a business plan to sell access to its DNA sequence databases, which had names like LifeSeq and ZooSeq, to major pharmaceutical companies in search of new drug targets. Millennium Pharmaceuticals in Cambridge, Massachusetts, also founded in 1993, had soon built alliances with over a dozen "Big Pharma" corporations. Its slightly different business plan integrated the bioinformatics-intensive, *"in silica"* approach—also pioneered by Incyte—with the "wetter" *in vivo* research programs that were part of more traditional molecular genetics and drug development. Human Genome Sciences Inc. in Rockville, Maryland, was a comparative granddaddy to these young genomic whippersnappers, having been founded in 1992 and having signed a deal in July 1993 that would set the bar for blockbuster promises until the deCODE-Roche agreement: HGSI would get up to $125 million from SmithKline-Beecham in exchange for exclusive access to its biogenetic databases. And there was Celera Genomics, the genomic company whose prominent CEO, Craig Venter (previously with HGSI), became famous for promising to sequence the entire human genome in three years, initiating a race with the more or less public Human Genome Project that would make Venter the genomic guy in the United States that everyone loved to hate. Celera Genomics was, if there is such a thing, probably the only household name in genomics in the United States for those who did not routinely watch the stock prices racing across the bottom of the screen on CNN, and Celera Genomics wasn't even incorporated until May 1998, three months after the deCODE-Roche deal.

It appeared that deCODE Genetics was as big and new as it got, in a territory in which big and new accounted for nearly everything. The deCODE-Roche deal was, like the lizard in the remake of *Godzilla* that was then making its way to Icelandic theaters, the biggest thing to hit the *terra nova* of genomics — that abstract but real territory that we all inhabit, and which this book refers to as lavaXland.

What could account for this surprising debut of deCODE?

Maybe it was what the press release referred to, not once but twice, as the "unique" Icelandic population: "isolated," "little changed," "homogeneous." Such a unique population — and maybe an image of blonde, blue-eyed gorgeous women and handsome men flashed across your cortex as the press release flickered on your computer — would surely make the company unique too. Maybe the word "Vikings" stirred somewhere in your unconscious. Or maybe you were a little more consciously thoughtful, impressed by the "welcome" that the nation-state of Iceland was showing to this private investment in an "Icelandic research company." You'd be hard pressed to remember Bill Clinton or Tony Blair giving such an endorsement to one of "their" genomic companies. Maybe you remembered reading about the country's burgeoning tourism industry as well, with its slogan "Iceland: Next Door to Nature," and how Reykjavík had become a hot spot for the tragically hip. And if you had no idea who this Kári Stefánsson guy was, maybe another Icelander came to mind: *Björk* . . .

If you could have tapped into the future back in February 1998 — and accessing the future is another recurring theme in this book — you would have seen that this one press release that already said a world of things would leverage deCODE Genetics into the pages of the *Wall Street Journal, Forbes, Business Week,* the *New York Times, Time, Der Standard, Der Spiegel,* the *Guardian, Das Magasin,* the *Financial Times,* the *Independent,* and many other popular periodicals in the United States and Europe. Kári (referred to by his first name following the practice of Icelanders) would be profiled almost as frequently as Björk, not only in popular science magazines like *Discover* and *Technology Review,* but in venues like *The New Yorker* as well. And for the next several years, *Science, Nature,* the *British Medical Journal, Nature Biotechnology, The New England Journal of Medicine,* and other major scientific and medical journals would follow the unfolding story of deCODE Genetics. Books with titles like *The Gene Masters* celebrated Kári and deCODE Genetics alongside the likes of Craig Venter and Celera Genomics. James Watson waxed enthusiastic about the Icelandic project in his biggest and most immodestly titled book, *DNA: The Secret of Life.* It would even become the subject of a *60 Minutes* segment.[2]

What happened? How did the deCODE Genetics story go from Roche's Jonathan Knowles's perfunctory niceties about shedding "new light on the causes of common diseases" and finding "truly effective ways to diagnose, prevent and treat illness," to Ed Bradley poking around Iceland with a *60 Minutes* film crew trying to get to the bottom of . . . what?

Let's go slowly, returning briefly to early 1998. In that February's issue of *Scientific American,* a short article appeared whose title alone suggests some of the tumult to come: "Natural-Born Guinea Pigs." This was of course a reference to those Icelanders who were described, as they were in the initial Roche press release and as they would be in numerous articles to come, as "more genetically homogenous than most other industrial societies"—or somewhat more luridly, as "one of the most inbred populations in the world." That quality gave deCODE a competitive edge in the ongoing race to isolate so-called disease-causing genes and to develop drugs from them. Kári was characterized as "one of Iceland's prodigal sons," who nevertheless thinks of himself as somehow genetically marked by his genealogy: "Despite my dislike of the long winter nights, life in Iceland is the experience I was born to live—it fits my genetic background." *Scientific American* wryly commented that "more compelling even than his own genes was the opportunity of mining his compatriots'." The article noted that deCODE claimed to have mapped two genes implicated in different conditions, familial essential tremor and psoriasis, and was "hot on the trail of a major gene for multiple sclerosis." And finally, the article also revealed that "deCODE [was] lobbying Iceland's Parliament to allow the company to supplement its family trees with medical records gathered from the national health service." The resulting database, Kári "hasten[ed] to point out," would protect privacy through secure encryption standards, with the decryption keys "held by local clinics, not by a central authority, to be doubly safe." While such an idea "might incite riots in some countries," *Scientific American* suggested, Iceland's "near-universal literacy has made Icelanders scientifically sophisticated."[3]

While a riot may not have broken out in Iceland, something pretty unruly and multiplicitous certainly did.

It's vitally important to appreciate how the introduction of the Bill on a Health Sector Database (HSD) at the end of March 1998 changed everything. Until then, deCODE had by and large been greeted with either enthusiasm, mild interest, or benign indifference. Muffled disgruntlement or perhaps watchful unease would have been about as extreme a reaction as one got from physicians and scientists not affiliated with the company. While deCODE in its first year or so of operation gave a number of causes for concern, the initial troubling questions were nothing like what would emerge after March 1998 and the introduction of the HSD legislation. Even now, Icelandic physicians and scientists carefully try to separate deCODE the corporation from the government-authorized Health Sector Database when they advance criticisms. As we'll see, this is not always an easy task, and Kári and deCODE—or KáriXdeCODE—did little to make the separation any easier. But it's necessary to remember that an Iceland with a commercial genomic company—or more than one commercial genomic company—does not necessarily entail an Iceland with a Health Sector Database. And it was the introduction of the HSD legislation that caused the nation to erupt.

Article 1 of the HSD bill was succinct and clear—as long as one didn't ask too many questions about what the terms meant: "The objective of this legislation is to authorise the creation and operation of a centralised database of non-personally identifiable health data with the aim of increasing knowledge in order to improve health and health services."[4]

But people in Iceland, particularly in the scientific and medical communities, began asking questions about the apparently straightforward terms. There would be much confusion in subsequent months and years about what people were referring to when they talked about "the database." While nothing is said in Article 1 about a genetic database comprised of DNA information extracted from the blood of participating Icelanders or a database of Icelandic genealogies—two other databases that deCODE said it was constructing—it was often hard to disentangle, legally or practically, these three different databases of genotypes, genealogies, and "health data." Even "health data" itself was a difficult term to disentangle; in this version of the legislation, "health data" was later defined as "information on the health of individuals, including genetic information." So confusion about what "the database" involved is quite understandable.

And what is "non-personally identifiable data"? This is later defined in the legislation as the negative of "personal data." Fine—so what's personal data? "All data on a personally identified or personally identifiable individual. An individual shall be counted as personally identifiable if he can be identified, directly or indirectly, especially by reference to an identity number, or one or more factors specific to his physical, physiological, mental, economic, cultural or social identity." The status of individuals in this database of health data, strictly health data—but that includes genetic information, doesn't it?—would become a major bone of contention in the future that was already coming to Iceland in the summer of 1998. The problem was usually summed up—badly—in the word "privacy." Would the data in this database in fact be "non-personally identifiable"? *Could* it be non-personally identifiable in a nation of Iceland's size (with a population of less than 300,000) and cultural character? Was that the same as "anonymous"—the term that would be used most frequently by advocates of the database?

"The database" was to be created and operated by an entity known simply as "the licensee." "The licensee" would pay a number of fees of an unspecified amount to the government: one fee up front for the granting of the license, an annual operating fee, and a fee to cover the cost of committees, such as the Data Protection Committee, involved in the oversight and operation of the database. In exchange, "the licensee" would have exclusive rights to the database for a period of at least twelve years—although the Icelandic government, as the de facto owner of the database, "shall at all times have access to statistical data from the database in accessible form, so that they will be of use in statistical processing for compiling health reports and planning, policy-making and other projects of the parties specified." "The licensee" was to have a monopoly on "the database" and its contents—whatever they were.

The data were to come from the medical records maintained by the national health care service for decades, as far back as 1915 by some accounts, and from current information generated each time an Icelander walked into a clinic or hospital in search of treatment or advice. This data was, as the notes to the bill proclaimed, "a national resource which should be preserved and used to yield benefits as far as possible." (It will be significant for later discussion that Iceland's fish, too, became subject to a similar conceptual-rhetorical-legal apparatus earlier in the 1990s, designated as a collective national resource that nevertheless only a select few had the right to profit from.) But when it came to placing a value on such a national resource, the language of the bill became slippery:

Health data cannot be evaluated in money terms, because their value consists primarily in the potential for improving health. If this potential is not used, such a collection of data has little value. It clearly increases the value of the data that Icelanders can boast an excellent health care system, good results from various measures to improve public health, and flourishing scientific activity. Due to the nature of the data and their origin they cannot be subject to ownership in the usual sense. Institutions, companies or individuals cannot therefore own the data. They exist primarily due to the treatment of patients. It is, however, both fair and a duty to utilise the data in the interests of the health sciences and to promote public health. This can best be done by the government authorising the creation and operation of a single centralised database, in which these data would be collected and where they would be processed. (Emphasis added)

Allow me to anticipate the way I will summarize and sign these kinds of doubled tangles throughout this book: the Icelandic Parliament says that health data canXcan't be valued, and mustXmustn't be owned. The littleXgreat value of such a resource is a product of collective supportX-private utilization, so the database would have to be a publicXprivate project. Difficult doublings, such as these concerning both the value and the institutional identity of the Health Sector Database, will recur many times in the pages to come. These volatile couplets—marked with an X, for reasons to be explained shortly—are the subject of this book.

For the time being, though, we break from the main stream of the Iceland-deCODE story now that the Althingi—Iceland's Parliament—and its legislation has raised the questions: How does one value a "potential," a capacity for having value? How does one place a value on the future of a commodity, or how does one place a future value on a commodity? What's the price of a promise?

For that matter, what *is* a promise?

XX

deCODE, the Icelandic genomics company, fascinates geneticists in academia and industry. Not only is it one of the fastest growing biotech companies, deCODE also landed the largest genomics deal ever when it sold, last year, the potential rights to 12 genes associated with common complex diseases to Hoffmann-LaRoche for $200 million. deCODE's competitive edge is its alliance with the Icelandic population. Promises of free drugs developed from research on the Icelandic gene pool and free genetic testing for identified susceptibility alleles, as

well as a boost to Icelandic science and economy have led to
wide-spread approval among the 270,000 Icelanders. The
company's corporate summary reads like a gene hunter's
dream, and many experts believe that deCODE's approach
is one of the most promising strategies for dissecting complex
diseases and traits. Consequently, the company provides an
attractive scientific environment to young and ambitious
researchers from Iceland and around the world.

Nature Genetics, "Genome Vikings," 99

What's promising?
A simple question, to be reiterated multiple times in the pages to come.

This opening paragraph from an editorial in a leading scientific journal appeared during the most intense period of the eruption over the
Health Sector Database legislation, in October 1998. We will revisit this
editorial, since it will have more to say about how the international community of scientists who read *Nature Genetics* were asked to think about
these events as they were unfolding. For now, the editorial provides some
sense of the language in which genomics in the late 1990s was—as it *had
to be,* as it *must continue to be*—written about, gossiped about, thought of,
and evaluated: in a language of promising.

The language of promising is a diverse and intricate one, demanding equally diverse and intricate analyses. Starting from J. L. Austin's
exemplary analysis of this exemplary performative speech act, Jacques
Derrida disseminated "promising" all over the place: to write or to speak
at all, about anything, is, for Derrida, to promise. But I'll defer direct
theorization of promising to the scattered notes on the margins of the
main text, and to the chapter "PromisesXPromises" that erupts in the
book's middle. Instead, promising is questioned throughout this text
ethnographically, via its repetitive empirical instantiations in the worlds
of genomics.

What kind of relationship exists, for example, between the promise in
"one of the most promising strategies," in the quote from *Nature Genetics,* and the promise of "promises of free drugs"? Is the relationship as simple a sameness as both of them referring to something that isn't here yet?
Or is it as simple a difference as one promise being a quality ascribed to
a phenomena or object, and the other being some kind of an act, occurring somewhere, put in motion by someone or other, to whom some kind
of responsibility or obligation attaches—or *will have been said to have been*
attached in some future that the promise itself has helped bring about?

Does a promise have to be uttered by an identifiable person, or can it occur by other means—through a press release, for example?

If Austin's influential *How to Do Things with Words* performed the difference between the denotative speech act that describes some state of things present or past—"deCODE is a genomics company in Iceland"—and the performative speech act that exerts some kind of force to effect a future—"we promise free drugs"—*Promising Genomics* promises an ethnography of promising. It keeps this promise by advancing multiple ethnographies—an ethnography of genomics, an ethnography of financial speculation, and an ethnography of Iceland—and interlacing these into an ethnography of promising guided by the overarching questions, *what kinds of statements about the future are made in the territories of genomics, what kinds of force do they exert, and what kinds of effects do these statements have?*

Genomics *must* be analyzed in terms of the promise, because promising is an ineradicable feature of genomics. Where the twentieth-century science of genetics predominantly focused on single genes associated with single disorders—cystic fibrosis and sickle cell anemia are the most frequent examples cited—contemporary genomics is the science, technology, and business of databasing, analyzing, querying, tweaking, and selling not just a gene or two, but *swarms* of them, entire genomes of individuals and even the multiple genomes of entire populations. Speaking very roughly, the timeline connecting scientific work on a gene, or even genes, to the understanding of a condition such as cystic fibrosis will of course be subject to multiple contingencies and uncertainties. But what the whole genome analysis of an individual, or of a complex condition such as schizophrenia, or of the genomic characteristics of a population, will lead to—this can only be promised. "Promised" here, again speaking very roughly, entails a mixture of a high degree of speculation, an avowed commitment stemming from multiple insecure extrapolations, and bets or gambles placed with a combination of care and risk.

Moreover, the contemporary science, technology, and business of genomics is not only about the databasing, analyzing, querying, tweaking, and selling of not only swarms of genes, but also said genes' barely understood interactions with other genes in the swarm *and* with those other entities we might call, for old times' sake, the whole organism and its environment. Out of those multiple interactions among multiple entities on multiple scales emerge those vital entities called "disease" and "health"—and more importantly, one's *future* disease or health status. Genomics promises an understanding of the "predispositions" or "propensities" that an individual harbors that will, at some point—perhaps—

become disease; genomics promises "presymptomatic diagnoses" or "predictive medicine" and the promise of preemptive strikes against disease at both the individual and population level. The genomic corporations like deCODE that emerged in the 1990s were, in effect, banking on the nebulous *futures* of the futural multiplicities that are our bodies, and were promising to produce future products for both today's futures markets and the future's.[5]

Genomics, then, is promissory through and through. I provide readers with an ethnography of genomics' promises as they emerged over the course of the 1990s, from the Human Genome Project in the United States, to the rise of a commercial genomic sector concentrated in the United States but that went global to other locales such as Iceland, Sweden, Estonia, Tonga, Newfoundland, and even more exotic places like the United Kingdom. Or, in the no less interesting and no less philosophical terms of the U.S. Securities and Exchange Commission (SEC), which will occupy us at some length, this will be an ethnography of "forward-looking statements" and their performances in an international political economy. *Promising Genomics* recounts and analyzes events named by a family of terms that cluster around "promising" in that they that also mark places and acts where a future has crossed back—or will have been crossed back—onto the present: forward-looking statements, hype, anticipation, volatility, and perhaps most all, speculations.

"What's value?" is thus another basic empirical question to be pursued along with "What's promising?" Again, the text will shuttle back and forth between the more local circumstances of deCODE Genetics and Iceland to the more global territory of an international political economy in an era now named, retrospectively, a "speculative bubble," blown up by financial institutions like Morgan Stanley (which handled, along with Lehman Brothers, deCODE's initial public offering on NASDAQ in 2000) and by individual investors, many of whom were new to the stock market. In many ways these investors and I shared the same fundamental "What's value?" question, crudely concretized as *how do you tell a real genomic company from a counterfeit one?* It was not easy to answer, especially given the promissory nature of genomics in *any* economy, let alone one as hair-raisingly speculative as the one of the 1990s.

Answering this kind of question became even more difficult for the average investor or the average ethnographer in 1995, when the Private Securities Litigation Reform Act expanded the "safe harbor" for "forward-looking statements." Corporate executives were able to make the most optimistic statements about the future of their enterprises, simply denoting them as "forward-looking statements" and directing people to U.S. Securities and Exchange Commission filings, where one would find not a promise but its apparent antithesis: full disclosure. This ethnography of genomics, value, and promising will thus find itself eventually in the midst of thousands of pages of SEC filings, looking for the right titration of genomic promise and genomic disclosure and finding . . . something else.

Overall, then, *Promising Genomics* diagrams sequences of speculative activity as they operated across a range of global genomic territories in which Iceland was but one particularly "hot spot." This book reads in, across, and between the territories of an informated, networked organism composed of multiple genes and their multiple interactions with each other, with a sea of proteins, and with surrounding biological and social spaces; the territories of an informated, networked genomic industry that grew rapidly in the late 1990s, with a dizzying array of competing as well as collaborating alliances powered by new genomic technologies like the automated DNA sequencer; and the territories of an informated, networked economy of millennial capitalism, in which a growing swarm of investors read more "forward-looking statements" about the promises presented by genes and genomic corporations, listened and watched mostly sunny genomic forecasts on cable television financial channels like CNBC, and eventually participated in all sorts of investing exuberances that seemed to defy the distinction between irrational and rational, perhaps best signed as irXrational.

I opt for a sign like "irXrational" rather than the slightly more popular and slightly less annoying "(ir)rational," or even the almost de rigueur "ir/rational," because this ethnography of promising, genomics, and value is also an ethnography of Iceland, and Iceland demands the X.

XX

Being a hot spot above a mantle plume, Iceland has been piled up through voluminous volcanic material with a much higher production rate per time unit than in any region in the world. It has grown by rifting and crust accretion through volcanism along the axial rift zone, the volcanic zones, which in terms of the plate tectonic framework marks the boundary between the Eurasian and North American plates. Accordingly the western part of Iceland, west of the volcanic zones, belongs to the

North American plate and the eastern part to the Eurasian
plate. . . . The rate of spreading is calculated to be 1 cm in
each direction per year. . . . The best place in the world to
study divergent plate boundaries is Thingvellir, which offers
the possibility of observing, in a graben system, both faults
and tension fissures (gjá) related to the rifting and drifting of
the North American and Eurasian plates away from each other.

Nordal and Kristinsson, Iceland: The Republic, 23

The fissure swarms—this is a precise geological term—run across Iceland
from the southwest to the northeast, diagramming with little black cross-
hatches the volatile zone where the North American tectonic plate separates from the Eurasian. These swarms of fissures—*gjá,* to practice our
first Icelandic word—suggests a country constituted by eruptions, crustal
upheavals, subglacial shifts, lacrustine sedimentations, and other kinds of
multiple flows at various speeds folding into or grinding against each
other, sometimes imperceptibly, sometimes violently.

I'm asking you to take this geo-logic of the fissure very seriously and
very broadly, and to open yourself to its operation in multiple domains
beyond the geological—epistemological, sociological, biological. Coming to understand how each of these domains or territories is fissured—
a stable crust crossed by glowing Xs of erupting liquids and gases—is absolutely necessary for understanding genomics today, for *speculating* on
genomics today.

While most of us do not live in Iceland, when it comes to genomics
we are all inhabitants of lavaXland. The X in lavaXland marks the fissure
out of which emerges both flowing lava and solid land. The figure X marks
the spot of volatility—although it might be better to say that the X marks
the *not.*[6] It marks ·an *and*—lava *and* land—*and* it marks a *not*—not lava,
not land. X marks the place where they are joined, in sameness. It marks
the place where they are separated, in difference. X marks the place of becoming, of unsettling change, of recombination. X marks an event, an
unfolding, a happening. X marks, in a willful contradiction and with a
contradictory will, what can't be marked. X is a figure of difference, divergence, void, interruption, and emergence. X is a necessary and productive (non)concept, but one that has been marginalized in favor of the
more comforting *ground* against which it occurs: identity, stability, presence, continuity, solidity, and perpetuity. X is promising.

Each chapter in this book falls under the sign of the X—not an X, but
the Greek letter *chi,* marking the chiasmus. The chiasmus cleaves a cou-

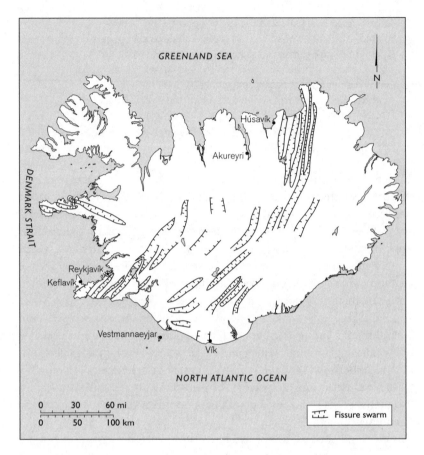

Iceland

plet of terms that are conventionally taken as distinct or even opposed, but that in fact depend on each other, provoke each other, or contribute to each other. Like the geological fissures that swarm across Iceland, making it a volatile lavaXland, chiasma are conceptual fissures that mark the scientific, political, and social landscapes of genomics. Chiasma are *uneasy* relationships: difficult and restless, troubling as well as promising, they resist simple resolution and never quite settle down. By organizing chapters around various chiasma, the book performs its key argument: that new concepts are necessary to better understand and deal with the messy, contradictory complexities of contemporary genomics.

The chiasmus appears in the middle of the analysis here because it is a potent figure both in the field of biology and in the field of rhetoric. In cell biology, the chiasmus is the name given to the site where the two copies of a chromosome are joined, become entwined, and, most importantly and productively, *recombine* in the process of meiotic cell division, rather than simply reproduce or replicate. The chiasma of our chromosomes are sites of chance and an emergent future—sites of volatility, change, and, with luck, evolution.

In rhetoric, the chiasmus plays a similar game. An example can be seen in the phrase a few lines above, "in a willful contradiction and with a contradictory will." The chiasmus joins and distinguishes, combines and reverses two terms. The chiasmus marks a folding of two things into each other that, like any of a number of M. C. Escher prints, never settles down into a *first this, then that* image, statement, or concept. Rhetorically, then, the chiasmus marks the spot where two distinct concepts can't be distinguished from each other, but feed off each other, send silent coded messages between themselves, and set possibilities in motion. The chiasmus is not about the easy interaction between distinct entities (nature and nurture, to cite just one familiar example), but is about unruly, unstable becomings. Volatilities. Emergence-ies.[7]

This should become somewhat more familiar as you read the chapters that follow—unpronounceable *chs*, somewhere between chapters, chromosomes, and chiasma, each headed by the figure of a fissured couplet, joinedXseparated by a chiasmus. Each *ch* is a kind of diagram of a volatile double event, where something unsettling occurs, where two orthogonal forces demand a settlement that can never quite happen.

The ethnographic exploration of genomics in Iceland in the waning years of the twentieth century opened me to the necessity of experimenting with a set of concepts—"promising" above all, but also "speculating," "fissure," "volatility," and "chiasmus"—in the hopes of faring better than we have to date in the expansive territories of genomics. Icelanders have learned to live with geological volatility, with the fact that their land rides precariously on a viscous sea of lava and that apparently foundational groundings are not only more fluid than we habitually assume, but are also always open to rattling, rumbling destruction. It seemed to me there was something worth learning there.

And the more I went there, and the more I learned about Iceland, the more fascinated I became with it, beyond the scope of the deCODE story. I was supposed to be spending that time writing a history of the Human Genome Project in the United States, which I intended to title "Projecting Speed Genomics." I was, as is so often the case, too slow—although some of that material and many of those intents have survived in parts of this book. So I never set out to become an ethnographer of Iceland, but was overtaken by the country and the grist for thought it offered. At the risk of exoticization—and exoticization of Iceland and its history will also be shown to be a powerful force in the deCODE events—it's as though the fissured territory of Iceland fissured everything about the place. I thought Iceland could serve as a general reminder that nature always gets thoroughly crossed with culture—leaving one "perplexed," as a Miss E. J. Oswald told her nineteenth-century readers in her book *By Fell and Fjord,* by a crossing that was "difficult to follow": "Alone in Iceland you are alone indeed and the homeless, undisturbed wilderness gives something of its awful calm to the spirit. It was like listening to noble music, yet perplexed and difficult to follow. If the Italian landscape is like Mozart; if in Switzerland the sublimity and sweetness correspond in art to Beethoven; then we may take Iceland as the type of nature of the music of the moderns—say Schumann at his oddest and wildest."[8]

Now that genomics is part of Iceland's thoroughly modern "nature," perhaps we can tune in to and learn from its odder and wilder effects. And if these overstated claims about nature crossed with culture themselves seem wildly odd, remember that Icelanders enjoy and treasure literature and what the tenth-century hero of his own saga, Egill, called "word-mead." Language is as much about intoxication as it is about information, and a greater appreciation of the crossings of language is, in addition to being simply a pleasure in itself, necessary for living admirably in the territories of genomics.

For many Icelanders, literature is a passion. Kári , founder and CEO of deCODE Genetics, has said that W. H. Auden is his favorite poet, quoting him from memory in one of many interviews.[9] Auden and Louis Mac-Neice traveled to Iceland in 1936 with the intention of writing a kind of travelogue. What they actually produced, separately and together, was a montage of poetry spanning politics, science, travel notes, fragmentary cultural observations, and a hilariously campy account of their horseback trip through the wilds of Iceland, in which they adopt the personae of school-girls on an outing. Auden describes the textual strategy of their *Letters from Iceland* in his "Letter to Lord Byron (Part 1)," which opens the book:

> So it is you who is to get this letter.
>   The experiment may not be a success.
> There's many others who could do it better,
>   But I shall not enjoy myself the less.

Shaw of the Air Force said that happiness
Comes in absorption: he was right, I know it;
Even in scribbling to a long-dead poet.

Every exciting letter has enclosures
    And so shall this—a bunch of photographs
Some out of focus, some with wrong exposures
    Press cuttings, gossip, maps, statistics, graphs;
    I don't intend to do the thing by halves.
I'm going to be very up to date indeed.
It is a collage that you're going to read.

I want a form that's large enough to swim in,
    And talk on any subject that I choose,
From natural scenery to men and women,
    Myself, the arts, the European news:
    And since she's on a holiday, my Muse
Is out to please, find everything delightful
And only now and then be mildly spiteful.[10]

In the following pages I experiment with various crossings of the intox-
icating and the informative. Like Auden and MacNeice, I am above all
"out to please"; I've groped my way through various experimental moments,[11] among multiple voices and multiple subjects, always trying to
provide something delightful enough to keep readers, like one keeps
promises. I, too, found that happiness came in absorption, and I became
more and more absorbed with each brief return trip to Iceland, with each
e-mail exchange, with each Icelandic saga and novel I read, with every
CD of Icelandic music for which I happily paid. And my collage is replete
with my own multiple enclosures: lots of press clippings from media-
intensive genomic discussions, online postings to the Yahoo! finance bulletin board, excerpts from Icelandic novels, letters to *The New England
Journal of Medicine* or the U.S. Securities and Exchange Commission, and
the occasional delicious bit of gossip and rumor. Even the Air Force will
come into play, although while I imagine Auden's Shaw was part of the
Royal Air Force, in this case it will be the U.S. version airlifting a celebrity
whale—an expatriate, like Kári—to its Icelandic "home." There is some
difference, after all, between 1937 and 1998.

Halldór Laxness, Iceland's superb novelist honored with the Nobel
Prize, is an indispensable part of this Icelandic collage. The book contains
numerous excerpts from one of his novels, *The Atom Station*, his 1948 satire
of the "selling of Iceland" to the United States and NATO. But *The Atom
Station* also casts strange Icelandic light—piercing, fleeting, scattered—

on the events described in these pages. I learned a lot about Iceland from Laxness, and I also learned something about ethnography.

"The undersigned" is the nameless narrating protagonist of another of Laxness's novels, *Under the Glacier.* He is also sometimes referred to as Embi, a collapsed sign for "emissary of the bishop." The undersigned is an "inexperienced ignoramus," not unlike an ethnographer, who is charged with producing a report (which is the novel) on the weird goings-on with regard to Christianity at the Snaefells Glacier (where Jules Verne, in another Iceland-based epic, started his heroes on their *Journey to the Center of the Earth*). There might be something wrong at the glacier—the pastor hasn't baptized anyone in years, has boarded up the church, and may have officiated at the burial of someone or something up on the glacier—or there might not be. It's hard to tell, since the bishop has only distant rumors to rely on—which is why he wants a report. "Write in the third person as much as possible," he instructs the undersigned before sending him off. "Be academic, yes, but in moderation. Take a tip from the phonograph."

> *Embi:* Am I not even to say what I think about it, then?
>
> *Bishop:* No no no, my dear man. We don't care in the slightest what you think about it. We want to know what you see and hear, not how the situation strikes you. Do you imagine we're such babies here that people need to think for us and draw conclusions for us and put us on the potty?
>
> *Embi:* But what if they start filling me up with lies?
>
> *Bishop:* I'm paying for the tape. Just so long as they don't lie through you. One must take care not to start lying oneself!
>
> *Embi:* But somehow I've got to verify what they say.
>
> *Bishop:* No verifying! If people tell lies, that's as may be. If they come up with some credo or other, so much the better! Don't forget that few people are likely to tell more than a small part of the truth; no one tells much of the truth, let alone the whole truth. Spoken words are facts in themselves, whether true or false. When people talk they reveal themselves, whether they're lying or telling the truth.[12]

When I first arrived in Iceland in early September 1998, I felt undersigned, all right. Underprepared, underachieved, undermade, underslept, but mostly undersigned. I tried to follow the bishop's advice, just writing things down, taking a tip from the phonograph, writing in small parts rather than whole truths, moderating the academic inclinations. It all seemed sage advice. So the persona of the undersigned will appear repetitively in these pages as the off-balance figure picking his way through a territory as fissured as himself, feeling responsible for producing a report that, despite the insufficiency of the signs at his disposal, he will have to sign for in the future.

Not surprisingly, the undersigned Embi is overtaken by events and, more importantly, slips into a deepening *complicity* with the people he has come to record and investigate. I underwent a similar overtaking, becoming involved not with priests and mystical hippies, but with the Icelandic scientists and physicians who I began to work more closely with as my fieldwork progressed, members of a new Icelandic NGO, Mannvernd.

In a nation where NGOs are far from common, the emergence of Mannvernd (the name means "Human Protection," but the group subtitles itself the Association of Icelanders for Ethics in Science and Medicine) was in many ways as significant a social and political event in Iceland as deCODE was. Mannvernd not only led the organized opposition to the Health Sector Database legislation, but also initiated an education campaign to raise the level of public discussion about genomics, the HSD, and deCODE Genetics. Mannvernd members came to be my main sources of information and perspectives on genomics and other, more established parts of Icelandic culture and politics. I delve into this in "DistanceXComplicity," where I discuss my extended collaboration with Mannvernd, the importance of these kinds of NGOs to technoscientific politics, and the relationship of "complicity" that grew up between Mannvernd and me, as happens so often with ethnographers and those they write about.

XX

Back to Iceland, then.

A letter published in the June 1998 issue of *Nature Biotechnology* would become the first public sign alerting the international scientific community to the deCODE–Health Sector Database eruption. Aptly titled "deCODE Deferred," the letter was signed by four individuals: Jórunn Erla Eyfjörd and Helga M. Ögmundsdóttir, a geneticist and immunologist (respectively) at the Icelandic Cancer Society, who were engaged in world-renowned work on breast cancer; Gudmundur Eggertsson of the Institute of Biology at the University of Iceland, who had first introduced recombinant-DNA techniques to the practices of the life sciences in Iceland in the early 1970s and who had taught the fundamentals of molecular genetics to virtually every practicing biomedical researcher on the island; and Tómas Zoëga, a leading figure in the Icelandic Medical Association and a member of the Department of Psychiatry at the National University Hospital (Landspítalinn). "The bill," wrote this biomedical gang of four, "took the Icelandic medical and scientific establishment completely by surprise. The existence of the bill was unknown to everyone here except the government and leading executives of deCODE until its announcement on March 31. No discussion had thus taken place on the desirability or otherwise of the measures in the proposed bill. It became clear that the government intended to rush the bill through parliament to forestall debate. Following very strong opposition from the medical and scientific community, the bill was postponed to the autumn."[13]

The letter outlined three major concerns: first, it questioned whether the database was "justifiable on scientific, economic, and ethical grounds"— a trifecta whose outcome was exceedingly hard to gamble on. Second, the letter questioned whether such a national and, by extension, public database should become "a commercial asset of a private company." And finally, if such a database were created and commercialized, was it "right to offer a single company legal monopolized control"? (Astute readers will recognize that these three questions and their possible answers are logically distinct; there were multiple ways that genomics could have unfolded in Iceland, including numerous combinations of private and public enterprises.) The letter also cited a concern about access to decades' worth of tissue samples in the Icelandic tissue bank—access that would be governed by a law that had yet to be written.

"*It is to be hoped*," the letter concluded—another sign of the futural, promissory economy, in which hope and hype both have their uneasy place—"*It is to be hoped* that the oldest parliament in Europe does not let democracy slip in order to allow one company the right to order legislation exclusively for its own ends."

Democracy—now *there's* a volatile substance. What exactly is democracy? What might it become? How does it actually take place in specific local circumstances like Iceland in the late twentieth century? How is "democracy" supposed to be applied to or involved in something like genomics or any other science that is supposed to be independent of the political sphere? How does the very word "democracy" order people around with its multiple rhetorical effects? These questions, too, will thread themselves through the following pages. The letter writers' rhetorical reference to the distant founding of Iceland's Althingi in the year 930 under the sign of *hope* suggests that democracy, too, may be best thought of as a kind of promise, the fulfillment of which one still awaits, hopefully—and maybe interminably.[14]

At the very least, one can say in the abstract that trustworthy information will be a vital part of any hoped-for democracy-to-come and its markets-to-come. In the same issue of *Nature Biotechnology* as this "deCODE deferred" letter, an editorial intoned that "biotechnology company executives should convey information to the markets and media in a straightforward manner." However, "inept information management" had recently "left a bad taste in the mouths of some investors and industry commentators," and deCODE was the worst culprit. "Astoundingly, for a company founded on the idea that it will have access to anonymized patient genetic data," the editorial remarked, the HSD act's introduction on March 31 "was the first that the Icelandic medical community knew about it. Some of them, noting the timing, thought it must be an elaborate hoax. It wasn't."[15]

When does a promise evoke the response, Is this some kind of April Fool's joke?

In July 1998, I was in Berlin at a conference called "Post-Genomics?" The conference was the kind of congeries of historians, anthropologists, sociologists, and philosophers of science, as well as molecular biologists, developmental geneticists, and other scientists, that comes together increasingly often these days, when it seems that one can never have too much information and analysis of what's currently passing for the truths of genomics. Whether you're a genomic company, a pharmaceutical corporation, a scientist, or some kind of social science or humanities scholar, you're driven by some compulsion or demand to produce and consume more and more information about genomics—and post-genomics.[16]

There I saw Skúli Sigurdsson for the first time since we had parted ways in graduate school, many years previously. We had each learned how to become historians of science and technology with different sets of materials from different times. I produced a history and sociology of the Human Genome Project in the United States at a time when those events were still unfolding, but many of the principal actors were already narrating and writing their own histories; Skúli's thesis focused on the mathematician Hermann Weyl and the Göttingen school of mathematics and physics that would contribute so much to relativity theory and quantum mechanics in the early decades of the twentieth century. Later, he began to work on a history of the electrification of Iceland, but even this was still some distance from the emergent worlds of genomics—worlds that would come to claim more and more of his time.

During one coffee break at the Berlin conference, a conversation about deCODE was struck up. The Health Sector Database legislation had been withdrawn and was being debated and discussed in the Icelandic Parliament, in the Icelandic media, and everywhere in between. The outcome was unclear, but deCODE and the promised HSD were clearly a unique event in the post-genomic landscape and a harbinger of things to come. In the hallway chatter accompanied by the sporadic clink of coffee cup and saucer, Skúli and I began talking about these events with another Icelander, Halldór Stefánsson, also an anthropologist who at the time was working at the European Molecular Biology Laboratory. Skúli began fulminating about Kári Stefánsson, only to find out that, in this particular case, the shared Icelandic last name was no simple coincidence, as it often is, but in fact pointed to a shared father: Halldór was Kári's brother. Some brief embarrassment ensued, but was apparently unnecessary. There didn't seem to be much love lost between Halldór and Kári, and Skúli is not easily embarrassed by his strong convictions. His use of vitriolic terms to describe Kári continued unabashed. It was simply true, as far as Skúli was concerned, so why not just say so?

The undersigned knew a few things about what was true, but none of them involved the character of a man he had yet to meet or of an enterprise he had read of only in the papers. It was true, I thought, that one must keep an optimism and openness about genomics, and even about genomics in Iceland, as one would keep a promise. It seemed a necessary part of being a true ethnographer. And to be a true ethnographer, to go to work as open as possible to unknown futures and unknown others, was another promise I planned to keep. Promising ethnography is promising to remain undersigned — and to capitalize on it.

It was also true that Skúli was a friend. So when Skúli asked if I would come to Iceland in the not-too-distant future, I could hardly say no. It would be a wonderful opportunity to do the interviewing and fieldwork that any true ethnographer would eagerly undertake — undertake in order to be overtaken, overwhelmed, as is also proper and true to ethnography. And I honestly saw this as a chance to say something *affirmative* about genomics, rather than to replay the constant criticisms I seemed to find myself trapped in whenever I turned to the subject. Going to Iceland promised to be fun and upbeat, or at least offbeat, a kind of vacation from the grind of criticism that genomics in the United States — genetic discrimination! pernicious reductionism! insurance denial! — seemed to so urgently demand.

But there would be a small price to pay for this opportunity to do a little Icelandic data mining of my own—or perhaps a small gift to give in return for the gifts of words I anticipated receiving so gratefully from the Icelanders. I would also be saying yes to Skúli's invitation to give a public lecture—maybe two—on my inquiries into genomics to date. Public talks like that would help, as Skúli saw it, to cultivate a critical literacy about science and genomics in a society and culture for the most part new to the subject.

It was a deal. I made arrangements to go Iceland for two weeks at the beginning of September 1998. I felt well prepared for fieldwork on the genomic front. As for Iceland itself, I ordered two books from Amazon .com: *Egil's Saga,* by a non-personally identifiable medieval Icelander, and Laxness's *The Atom Station.* I dug out an old CD by the Sugarcubes and bought a new CD by the singer who came out of that seminal Icelandic band, Björk. With those few guides and a flight booked, the undersigned left for Iceland . . .

FriendXAdvance Man

The undersigned would wake up early to the sound of a typewriter. I would stumble up the stairs into the small kitchen, casting a brief dreamy look out the window to a modernist metal sculpture that pointed west, out to where the Seltjarnarnes Peninsula stopped being a quiet suburb of Reykjavík and gave on to Faxaflói Bay. The typing continued. I put water and coffee in the espresso pot, put the pot on the electric stove, and went into the dining room. The advance man finished typing out his 3x5 note cards and began the daily briefing for the still undercaffeinated undersigned.

There was the recounting of whatever story about deCODE and things genomic had been broadcast that morning on the daily news from the Icelandic State Radio. There was always a radio story. Then the advance man would go through the newspapers—the conservative daily *Morgunbladid,* the less frequent and leftish *Dagur,* and the tabloidy *DV*—summarizing the news stories, opinion pieces, letters to the editor, or anything else about deCODE. There were always a number of these each day.

We would then go through the freshly typed 3x5 cards, each dated in the upper right-hand corner in a manner that minimized confusion between American and European calendrical habits (08.ix.98). The cards outlined the multiple appointments that the advance man had set up for the undersigned that day: interviews of scientists by the undersigned, interviews of the undersigned by Icelandic print and broadcast journalists, meetings with members of Parliament, coffee dates with visiting journalists, and a host of other appointments. Phone numbers and street addresses were provided. Sometimes there were footnotes. The cards were

usually heavily annotated, clueing the undersigned into familial and social links ("friend of my mother's"; "attended gymnasium with KS [Kári
Stefánsson]") or recent context ("geneticist, wrote anti-deCODE art. in
Mbladid last week"). Explicit advice—"You should ask him about . . ."—
was often offered, and almost as often gratefully accepted. Routes were
drawn on the map of Reykjavík. They arranged to meet or call each other
later in the day in case the advance man had scheduled something new in
the meantime.

By then, the first coffee of the day was ready. The undersigned was not.

XX

Skúli Sigurdsson and I had a brief history of collaboration; the first publication of my academic career was coauthored with Skúli.[1] But two different career paths on the two different tectonic plates that diverge from each
other under Iceland had kept additional layers from sedimenting into the
friendship. So it was really through his work as advance man in September 1998, and on later trips, that Skúli and I became friends.

None of *this*—multiple referents may be substituted—exists without
Skúli's help, involvement, friendship. Skúli tirelessly and even obsessively
set up my meetings, for which those cards served as indispensable guides.
My Icelandic encounters could not have happened without Skúli, and cer-
tainly could not have been so productive, exhausting, and fun without him.
Skúli was always out in front, in advance. My debt to him is incalculable.

It was when Skúli started setting up interviews *of* me by Icelandic journalists that I entered unknown territory—for which I am most grateful.
I had never been interviewed by a reporter in my life, swamped as I was
by the thousandfold dilution that the United States provides over Iceland. But from this point forward it became a routine part of my research
life, both when I was in Iceland and then when I was back in the United
States. My efforts to turn the weird but understandable demand for sound
bites into a more useful genre will be a topic taken up later.

But if I have spent hours on the phone with journalists from the Associated Press, *60 Minutes,* National Public Radio, the *Albany Times-Union,*
the *Newark Star-Ledger,* and elsewhere,[2] it's nothing compared to the time
Skúli has given—*gifted*—to the reporters, social scientists, bioethicists, legal scholars, database experts, undergraduate thesis writers, and other
members of the swarm of curious and concerned writers that has descended on Iceland since 1998—a perverse kind of "genomic hot-spot of

the world!" tourism. Like the other Icelanders who became vocal critics of the database project, Skúli worked tirelessly on these issues, sacrificing time that could have been devoted to more self-directed writing projects, research, and similar marks of civilization that responding to deCODE and the Health Sector Database effectively deterred.[3]

You will have to figure my friendship with Skúli into your assessment of how fairly I respond to the primary iterated question of this text—*How do you tell a genomic company's worth?* In the standard accounting practices applied to social science characterizations of objectivity, my friendship with my advance man—who never wavered from his initial judgment of Kári at that Berlin conference—must figure in the debit column. But perhaps objectivity is not the same as fairness, and friendship a third term to both. Or maybe there is another set of books. We shall see.

For now, all the undersigned can do is *swear*—not exactly a promise, but very, very close—*swear* that in September 1998, on that first trip to Iceland, I thought that deCODE Genetics was an interesting and potentially admirable project. I even said so to the dozen or so physicians, scientists, philosophers, and others—who were already vocal critics of deCODE and the HSD—at a reception that Skúli organized at his house on my first evening in Iceland, where I met many of the people I would later phone for interviews. Or at least I was open to thinking that deCODE was an interesting project. Like many other Icelanders at the time, I was trying to make up my mind.

I stress these paired matters of friendship and objectivity early in this text for several reasons. Other ethnographers of Iceland at this time have suggested that "Iceland is emerging as *the* site of biotech and bioethics," in part as a symptom of "the emerging global market for civic virtue" in which "academic 'capital' is moved from one market sphere to another."[4] The implications are hazy, since such a situation is said to "raise interesting questions of social scientific practice, research ethics, and situated accounts" (94), but such questions, let alone answers, are never stated in any detail. But were I to insert myself into this ethnographic perspective, I might appear as a symbolic capitalist marketing not a "get-rich-quick," but a get-virtuous-quick scheme in a highly speculative ethical hot spot, Iceland, in a globalizing market of bioethics. Such venture virtue-ists, we might say, might "pigeonhole things" and rely on "pre-formed narratives" to produce "partisan accounts" that, while they might sell well and earn handsome returns on one's initial cultural capital, "misses what is actually taking shape, however dangerous, beneficial, or trivial it may turn out to be" (101, 93).

While deferring further discussion of crooked accounts and speculations about ethics to later chapters, I foreshadow the concern here not to "come clean," but to establish a more complex moral economy: my exchanges in the bioethical economy of Iceland, and in civic virtue more globally, were undertaken more out of an ethic of friendship than an ethic of symbolic capital accumulation or portfolio diversification. And while I certainly have my conceptual habits and commitments, I honestly thought deCODE might not fit in any pigeonhole—indeed, this is why I valued the opportunity to learn more about genomics in this other lava land.

So in my first small gesture of return for this gift of learning, I gave the Icelanders a public talk on speed genomics.

FastXFast

The undersigned found himself at the front of a large lecture hall in the Oddi building of the University of Iceland. The advance man had seen that the talk was well advertised. The best translation that Skúli could offer for the Icelandic organization that sponsored the talk (Félag áhugamanna um heimspeki) was the Society of Those Interested in Philosophy. As someone who is interested in philosophy, and since living well in the lavaX-land of genomics requires being interested in philosophy, I couldn't have been more pleased. There were fifty or so well-dressed Icelanders: university professors such as Gísli the anthropologist and the philosophers Magnús and Sigga; Helga and Jón and Alfred and a number of other scientists from the university, the Landspítalinn (the National University Hospital), and the Icelandic Cancer Society; Tómas and Árni and a few other physicians; someone from deCODE; and a number of university students, including one drunk heckler right down front.

The text here is a value-added version of my remarks there, extracted and refined from a rambling set of notes for a talk intended to introduce myself to the Icelanders and to offer my take on the science and business of genomics then coming to Iceland. Since it was a perhaps a unique occasion to do some philosophy of genomics, beginning with an overhead transparency that quoted both the legendary Icelandic band the Sugarcubes (which brought Björk to international attention) and the French Nobel laureate François Jacob, I have taken special care to preserve some of those particular local elements . . .

XX

Like other sciences, biology today has lost many of its illusions.
It is no longer seeking for truth. It is building its own truth.
Reality is seen as an ever-unstable equilibrium.

Jacob, Logic of Life, 16

I began my talk with these words, written not by a much reviled "social constructionist" but by the biologist and Nobel laureate François Jacob (who, with Jacques Monod, first articulated the operon model of the gene in the early 1960s), for two reasons. First, to suggest that we can learn a great deal from life scientists, certainly as much as one can learn from any historian or philosopher of the life sciences. By learning about the truths that are being built *about* organisms and perhaps *into* them, we learn that the widespread view of DNA as the "blueprint" or "code" for organisms such as humans, "programming" them to be sick or smart or shy, is grossly oversimplified. While a number of life scientists are partly responsible for such oversimplifications, many of them know that such simplifications are now unstable and are re-equilibrating around a much more complex set of truths.

Second, this phrase of Jacob's, "ever-unstable equilibrium," is an apropos marker for the variety of phenomena that biologists, sociologists, historians, ethicists, and many others confront in these unstable times. "Ever-unstable equilibrium" is precisely the kind of word concept we need in order to live better within our once seemingly reliable, solid, and stable oppositions—nature and culture, organism and machine, state and individual, public space and corporate economy, science and ethics—and all the other oppositions of the modern era that never fully break down or break up or disappear, but that hang on, quivering, shimmering, haunting specters materialized in new, different, and temporarily (un)stable forms: chiasma, in a word.

We need to be interested in philosophy because language, which allows us to invent concepts that are a little off the chart, is one of the few things that can keep up with the inventions of genomicists. We need new concepts for living in the lavaXland of genomics, and we need them now. Actually, we needed them yesterday, because today's ever-unstable genomic equilibria are very, very fast. And "fast" is a very interesting concept—a very *fast* concept that blinks so rapidly between two meanings that they have to be considered simultaneously:

fast[1] *adj.* faster, fastest. 1. Acting, moving, or capable of acting or moving quickly; swift. 2. Accomplished in relatively little time: *a fast visit.* 3. Indicating a time somewhat ahead of the actual time: *The clock is fast.* 4. Adapted to or suitable for rapid movement: *a fast running track.* 5. Designed for or compatible with a short exposure time: *fast film.* 6.a. Disposed to dissipation; wild: *ran with a fast crowd.* b. Flouting conventional moral standards; sexually promiscuous. 7. Resistant, as to destruction or fading: *fast colors.* 8. Firmly fixed or fastened: *a fast grip.* 9. Fixed firmly in place; secure: *shutters that are fast against the rain.* 10. Firm in loyalty: *fast friends.* 11. Lasting; permanent: *fast rules and regulations.* 12. Deep; sound: *in a fast sleep.* [Middle English, from Old English *fæst,* firm, fixed.][1]

If something like genomics is fast, it moves or changes very rapidly, which can make it elusive and volatile. At the same time, if something is made fast, it has been tightened, secured, fastened. Fast equilibria, you could say, are so fast that they're slow, so unstable that they're extremely stable, so volatile that they're hard to change. When we're dealing with fast genomics, then—whether scientifically in the laboratory, economically in the marketplace, conceptually in our language, or socially and politically in the Althingi or other places of deliberation—when we're dealing with fast genomics, we're dealing with contradictions and doubled meanings. And speed will be the key.

When I can't decide if I should call myself a historian, an anthropologist, or a philosopher, I simply call myself an empiricist. I have spent most of the last fifteen years as an empiricist of what we can call speed genomics. I have read through government hearings and reports, scientific papers, patent applications, and historical accounts by the scientists involved with the creation of the Human Genome Project (HGP). I have interviewed scientists and technicians in university and corporate labs, and I have attended a variety of genomic conferences. I have pondered films, advertisements, and scientific diagrams and images. Mostly, I have focused on the United States, although national borders, as people in Iceland were then relearning, are another ever-unstable equilibrium.

All that activity led me to conclude that, when it comes to genomics, speed is indeed the key. It's also something of a commonplace, as James Gleick has summarized in his popular book *Faster: The Acceleration of Almost Everything,* that speed these days is the key to . . . well, almost everything. But rather than try to summarize almost everything about today's accelerated technoculture, I'll sketch two quick examples.

Writing in *The New Yorker,* John Seabrook called film director George Lucas "a genius of speed." In the article, Seabrook suggests that "perhaps the most memorable single image in 'Star Wars,' is the shot of the Millennium Falcon going into hyperspace for the first time, when the stars blur past the cockpit. Like all the effects in the movie, this works not because it is a cool effect . . . but because it's a powerful graphic distillation of the feeling the whole movie gives you: an image of pure kinetic energy which has become a permanent part of the world's visual imagination. . . . Insofar as a media-induced state of speed has become a condition of modern life, Lucas was anticipating the Zeitgeist in 'Star Wars.'"[2] Lucas had to rely heavily on pacing and editing, says Seabrook, in part because he had little rapport with actors. Harrison Ford told Seabrook that Lucas "had only two directions for the actors. . . . The two directions were 'O.K., same thing, only better,' and 'Faster, more intense'" (40).

As a first, hasty generalization, then, we can say that genomics is the same thing as genetics, only better. Genomics is faster, more intense than genetics. That's it. But that's enough to make a huge difference. Speed is what makes genomics sparkling, irresistible, and surprising. Speed fissures genomics, crashes barriers between disciplines, between nations, and most importantly, between old dualities like nature/nurture or public/private. Which brings us to the next space allusion.

"The Human Genome Project has just entered warp speed."[3] So began an article in the March 1999 issue of *Science* describing the new effort by a recombinant public-private consortium to produce at least a "first draft," 90 percent complete sequence of the human genome by March 2000—approximately five years ahead of projected timetables. The consortium was organized by the U.S. National Institutes of Health (NIH) National Human Genome Research Institute and the United Kingdom's Wellcome Trust, but was funded in large part by such pharmaceutical companies as Bayer, Novartis, Glaxo Wellcome, Pfizer, Roche, and SmithKline Beecham. This quasi-public effort responded to corporate high-speed sequencing initiatives being undertaken by new genomic companies like Celera Genomics (*Celera* from the Latin for "speed") and Incyte Pharmaceuticals, and the likelihood that much of the sequence-based information being produced in those venues would be privatized.

Later we'll take a closer look at the ensuing "race" between the public (but intimately linked to the private sector) consortium and the private genomic companies, particularly Celera. This was just one of the "races" that characterized speed genomics, fueled by many factors, some stated, some unstated: scientists were in a race against a multitude of diseases that were killing people every day; scientists were in races against each other to discover, and patent, particular genes (competition in the cases of cystic fibrosis and the BRCA-1 gene linked to some forms of breast cancer was particularly intense and not particularly nice); James Watson said that he wanted to get the whole sequence read out before he died because that would be a good bookend to a career that started by beating Lines Paling in a race (at least from Watson's perspective) to discover the structure of DNA; the United States in the late 1980s thought it was in a race against Japan, which was supposedly developing DNA sequencing faster than we were.

For now, though, these two examples simply introduce the notion that speed is the key to genomics. By the time I had finished my PhD dissertation in 1993, on the development of the Human Genome Project in the United States, fast science seemed to me the most pertinent and productive way to characterize the HGP, or what I prefer to call "projecting speed genomics": the development of and desire for ever-faster genomic machines, sciences, and economies.[4]

What I'm calling the lavaXland of genomics can be stratified along finer levels of analysis. In the last ten years or so, each of these strata was transformed by acceleration, and understanding these speed transformations is central to understanding what happened in Iceland and in other lavaXlands in the final years of the twentieth century. Figure 1 is a chart that the undersigned presented to the audience in Reykjavík in September 1998.

Probably the least truthful, and certainly the least interesting way to think about the Human Genome Project is in terms of completion. It also happens to be the most popular, since it was the easiest way for both scientists and journalists to convey the grandeur and scope of genomics in the late 1980s and early 1990s, when the HGP was a debatable proposition. It's not that having the complete sequence of the DNA base pairs that constitute the genomes of various organisms hasn't been productive or interesting; quite the contrary. But emphasizing the element of completion directs our attention away from other things that are just as, if not more, important and interesting to think about—namely, the technological, social, and economic conditions through which something like "completion" becomes possible.

And the fact is that even in those years of high debate about what the merits and contours of a "human genome project" were to be, scientists recognized that narratives of completion and arrival were useful fictions (not necessarily untrue), but were not really what was at stake.

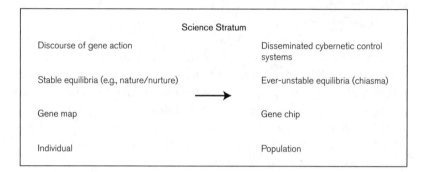

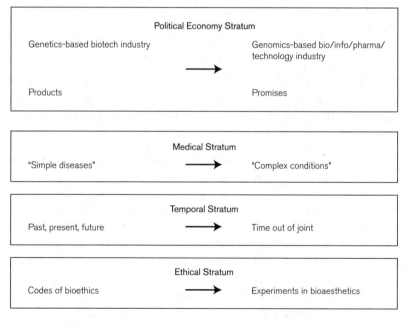

Metascience Stratum

Human Genome Project → Projecting speed genomics

Completion → "Fantastic infrastructure"

Genetics → Genomics

Genomics → Post-genomics

Science Stratum

Discourse of gene action → Disseminated cybernetic control systems

Stable equilibria (e.g., nature/nurture) → Ever-unstable equilibria (chiasma)

Gene map → Gene chip

Individual → Population

Political Economy Stratum

Genetics-based biotech industry → Genomics-based bio/info/pharma/technology industry

Products → Promises

Medical Stratum

"Simple diseases" → "Complex conditions"

Temporal Stratum

Past, present, future → Time out of joint

Ethical Stratum

Codes of bioethics → Experiments in bioaesthetics

FIGURE I. The speed transforms of the genomic plateau, c. 1988–98

As one example, consider the tumultuous session at the 1986 Cold Spring Harbor symposium, "The Genetics of *Homo sapiens*," where the earliest proposals for a "human genome project" were first debated by a large community of geneticists and other researchers. Over the subsequent years of discussions and expert committee meetings, the Human Genome Project would come to be less sequence-centric and more oriented around developing genetic and physical maps, and would also come to be less human-centered in its research scope and more inclusive of genomic studies of other "model" organisms: the fruit fly, yeast, the mouse, and the worm *Caenorhabditis elegans*. But in 1986, when back-of-the-envelope calculations projected that three billion base pairs in the human genome would mean $3 billion in project cost, much of the debate centered around promising that kind of money to the far from certain, simply promising prospect of having every last A, T, C and G transferred from gooey protoplasm to the harder medium of magnetic disk.

At one point in this discussion, a scientist stood up and made a proposal based on the truth that the people gathered were not simply scientists, but were scientistsXpoliticians:

> I'd just like to say that perhaps we should be politicians at this point, and call it sequencing the entire human genome, and spend the money on exactly that thing. I think—[there was laughter in the auditorium and scattered applause]—no, no, no; it's like sending men to the moon. Sending men to the moon was extremely expensive and extremely pointless [more laughter], but it was—because we could have got as much information with half the cost, with machines—scientifically, at least. But if we go and tell Congress we're going to do something like this that the general public can understand, they'll give us the money, as long as we agree among ourselves that what we're actually going to do with it is maybe sequence the one percent of the genome that's interesting and try to develop [laughter], try to develop technologies that in fact will allow us to sequence the human genome in 1999, just in time to meet the deadline [laughter].[5]

Another audience member, more purist than chiasmist in his sensibilities, then argued that the project needed to be defended on its scientific merits alone. To which the initial speaker responded, "Then you're not a politician [huge laughter]. That's the only language those guys understand. Every two years, that's exactly what they do."

Even three years later, when the "human genome project" was still perceived as focused on sequencing, and this was still thought to be a misguided *scientific* strategy, the *political* appeal of such a definition was nevertheless appreciated—even though the scientific and the political were cast as separate spheres, with no X to render things lively and volatile. As human geneticist Arno Motulsky expressed it at a meeting sponsored by the CIBA Foundation in 1989,

From the scientific point of view objections could be raised against a sequencing project for the human genome at this time. On the other hand, if extra funds can be obtained to rally the public around a well-defined project to learn more about the human genome, there may be advantages. It is hard to motivate governmental agencies, or the public at large, to support fundamental work in genetics. However, if we say "Here we have the human genome; by learning everything about its structure and function we shall be able to prevent and cure many diseases and at the same time understand humankind better," we shall interest the relevant agencies and we may obtain additional funds. . . . A special project with a clearcut goal that people can understand has advantages.[6]

The culmination of this joint scientific-political rhetoric of completion—"learning *everything* about its structure and function"!—came years earlier than anticipated, in the 2000 White House ceremony that marked the ritual occasion of the "completion" of the HGP. An ebullient President Clinton played the chiasmus, holding high the hands of both Francis Collins, director of the National Human Genome Research Institute, and Craig Venter of Celera Genomics. ("PublicXPrivate" takes up this volatile chiasmus between Collins and Venter and the "public" and "private" genome sequencing efforts they headed.)

But we have gotten somewhat ahead of ourselves. What transformation does speed effect on this rhetoric of completion? In fast genomics, the complement to completion—the "holy grail" of genetics, in the mythical completion term most repeated—has always been held fast within the same metascientific territory: infrastructure. If completion is all about future, infrastructure is all about a present. Both these rhetorics were intertwined, but the infrastructural present always got the short end of the discursive stick compared to its more understandable, saleable, and enthusiasm-generating partner.

But the infrastructure question was always there, and sometimes even brought into sharp focus. In 1987, Charles DeLisi, one of the earliest and strongest advocates of the HGP in the U.S. Department of Energy (DOE), testified to a U.S. Senate committee that the goal of the HGP was "to develop technologies that would make sequencing . . . a lot quicker than it currently is . . . if you want to sequence a hundred thousand bases [in] twenty people and compare their sequences and understand disease susceptibilities, you can't do that, it's not a clinically viable procedure. We can make that a clinically viable procedure. That's the goal, it's not to sequence the human genome, at least initially."[7]

"Number one," emphasized Leroy Hood, one of the inventors of the automated DNA sequencer, to members of the U.S. Senate in 1990, "the human genome initiative is about developing new technologies. This is the first biological project that has as a major imperative developing new kinds of technologies . . . it is going to create a fantastic infrastructure for biology and medicine which will be centered on the map and the sequence of the human genome."[8]

The Whitehead Institute's Eric Lander also found these rhetorical differences that shaped the metascientific plateau important enough to weigh in, in both congressional testimony and to his scientific colleagues:

I eventually stood up and said, Come on, it's Route One we're talking about. This isn't so fancy. We are talking about building a highway, for god's sake . . . I guess I found it very hard, very troubling that people were cramming this down people's throats as the holy grail. Yes, it's very important, but it's infrastructure, and I thought Route One conveyed better than anything else, a) how you did the project—that you didn't do it in small pieces, but b) that it wasn't such a grandiose thing either. And so it conveyed both of the things, namely . . . people were proposing building this, by everybody go out and build a mile of highway on either side. And that's crazy, because you're going to have too many gaps and things like that. But the other aspect of it is that it somehow demystified the mystique of the human genome, and put it in what I still think is an appropriate context: it's an infrastructure project. It's a very important infrastructure project. You try to build infrastructure [pause] efficiently. And that ought to be our basic metaphor.[9]

Indeed it ought. But let's keep the modifier "fantastic" in our basic metaphor for genomics. A fantastic infrastructure is an "ever-unstable equilibrium," a volatile chiasmus where fantasies, dreams, and visions are meshed and mashed with mundane tools. But where fantasies come and go and dreams give way to the next night's delirium, infrastructure has a habit of sticking around. They are congeries of forces operating at differential speeds: fastXfast. So while we need to pay careful attention to both, the sticky infrastructure merits more of our critical capacities for detail and analysis.

The intended effect of this government biohighway improvement program was far less about holy grails and understanding everything than it was about supporting the U.S. biotechnology industry and "keeping America competitive." As Johnson & Johnson's Jack McConnell, who helped draft early U.S. legislation on the HGP, testified in 1987, "If we want the U.S. to maintain its position as a dominant force in the pharmaceutical industry in the world, I cannot imagine our letting this opportunity pass us by. . . . The group that first gains access to the information from mapping and sequencing the human genome will be in position to dominate the pharmaceutical and biotech industry for decades to come."[10]

Around the time that Lander and Hood were playing their rhetorical moves in 1990, the undersigned began attending genomic conferences—but at this time, genomics was still pretty much genetics. The most frequent images scientists used to illustrate the cutting edge of their science—sometimes with archaic slides or overhead transparencies, before Power-Point—was a linear gene map, representing a chromosome or part of a chromosome, showing where the new gene they had isolated was located in relation to other genes and chromosomal markers that were still fairly sparse. These images were diagrammatic representations that showed where genes were, what the nearby landmarks were, and eventually what letter code existed at those locations.

In October 1990 the hot news story was the isolation of *the* cystic fibrosis gene on chromosome 7; by 1998 several thousand variants had been identified, each deserving the definite article "the." But the 1990 story of the cystic fibrosis gene does say something about the dominant conceptualization or imagination of the HGP endeavor at that time: what was being promised—and it was primarily the state making this promise—was that devoting resources to genomics would fill in these kinds of linear maps, making it easier, cheaper, and faster to discover and characterize individual genes. A small army of researchers and technicians would produce maps like that for the cystic fibrosis gene for the entire genome, placing markers at regular intervals that would help locate specific genes, which could then be sequenced, which would then help cure disease or at least develop diagnostic kits that would let individuals know if they were "at risk" for a particular disorder. The focus was mostly on genes and hardly at all on genomes.

As a further overgeneralization, we can say that the focus was on the so-called simple disorders like cystic fibrosis. Otherwise referred to as "single-gene disorders," they included conditions like Huntington's disease, muscular dystrophy, familial colon polyposis, sickle-cell anemia, beta-thalassemia, hemochromatosis, amyotrophic lateral sclerosis (Lou Gehrig's disease), and many others. They were monogenic disorders, either dominant or recessive, and with the right families (Venezuelan families did the trick for Huntington's) and either a little luck or a lot of time, a researcher could "hunt" down the gene involved—a gene that was usually said to *cause* the disorder, as in the phrase "the gene *for* cystic fibrosis." Proponents and critics of the Human Genome Project both realized that there would be some lag time between our ability to diagnose these genetic conditions, in the sense of identifying a deleterious form of a gene in an individual, and our ability to develop clinical therapies.

The biotechnology industry in the late 1980s and early 1990s was also still entirely based on individual genes. The few biotech drugs developed and sold by companies like Amgen, Biogen, and Genentech that had survived the first die-off of biotech companies in the early 1980s—drugs like interferon, insulin, human growth hormone, tissue plasminogen activase—were based on individual genes that had been laboriously isolated, sequenced, tweaked a bit, and cloned into bacteria for production. Sequencing the gene was often almost an aside; the isolating and cloning were usually the key steps—entirely material steps.

Which is why even Walter Gilbert—Nobel laureate for his part in the invention of DNA sequencing; successful founder of one of those successful biotech companies, Biogen; ardent enthusiast for the Human Genome Project and inventor of the $3 billion price tag, as well as all that "holy grail" schmaltz—even Gilbert couldn't start a "genomic company" that would produce, copyright, and sell human genetic sequence information. Neither the pharmaceutical companies nor the financial community could see how you could get any kind of return on something as immaterial as "genetic information"—or at least not any return soon enough to make it worthwhile. Gilbert's efforts to start such a company in 1987—efforts that would lead to his resignation from one of the government committees then advocating a human genome project, just as he had earlier left Harvard to start Biogen—came to naught.

Less than five years later, it was a whole new situation, thanks in large part to the "fantastic infrastructure" that had been promised and, in part at least, delivered.

XX

"What's the gray powder between an elephant's toes?" asked Mark Edwards of Recombinant Capital (ReCap for short), a San Francisco-based organization that tracks and analyzes the biotechnology industry for biotech corporate executives, venture capitalists, and the occasional ethnographer of genomics. The answer: "slow-moving natives." "Dancing with elephants" was Edwards's metaphor for the interactions between the major pharmaceutical companies ("pharma" for short) and the biotech and genomic start-ups that had appeared by 1997, the year Edwards was writing.

> Biotech alliances with pharma are our "dances," and on this basis we've been dancing together for some time. Yet, at another level, this analogy becomes troubling— perhaps it is really the elephants themselves who are dancing, either individually or with each other, while biotech is simply engaged in the precarious enterprise of inhabiting the elephants' dance floor, moving nimbly around the massive bodies until. . . . Until what? . . . What if new elephants dance differently, or the elephants change their dance? The point of these musings is simply to observe that, for an industry that "dances with elephants," we don't know very much about how, when or why elephants dance. In the past we have relied on our fast reflexes and quick recognition of the relatively few dance steps used by most elephants. Now, however, new elephants have taken the floor and the dance steps are becoming more complicated.[11]

There's an interesting admission of uncertainty and contingency here, especially from a person who makes money by claiming to *know* about biotechnology. Nevertheless, it's safe to say that the genomic dance marathon had become one of the quick and the dead, survival of the fastest in an increasingly complicated and differentiated economy that Walter Gilbert could only dream of in 1987. By 1997 the field was populated by companies like Molecular Dynamics, Molecular Informatics, Darwin Molecular Corporation, Genome Therapeutics, GeneLogic, Digital Gene Technologics, Lexicon Genetics, Ciphergen, Immunex, Hyseq, Clontech, Genaissance Pharmaceuticals, Rosetta Inpharmatics, Exelixis, Affymetrix, Nanogen, and Hexagen. Some of these no longer exist or have been subsumed into larger corporate entities, but the list gives some sense of the eruption that had taken place in the political economy of genomics.

To understand what happened between 1987 and 1997 in the other strata of speed genomics to spur this far more complex political economy, let's consider in brief three of the earliest genomics-based companies, Human Genome Sciences Inc., Incyte Pharmaceuticals (now Incyte Genomics), and Millennium Pharmaceuticals. Each adopted different dance steps with their outsize partners in the pharmaceutical industry, but each participated in a kind of futures market for genomic information that would intensify over the remainder of the 1990s as more genomic companies, including eventually deCODE, stepped onto the dance floor.

When Human Genome Sciences Inc. was established in 1992, near the National Institutes of Health in Maryland, its partnership with one of the fastest animals in the genomic jungle, the nonprofit Institute for Genomic Research (TIGR), laid the foundation for HGSI's large commercial genomic database. TIGR's Craig Venter, who had left the NIH to start this joint nonprofit/commercial venture, had developed enormously generative "high-throughput" production technologies that spewed out genes, gene fragments, mRNA probes, mapping positions, and sequence information. This made HGSI's database among the largest and most useful in the field — and the most proprietary. (See "PublicXPrivate" for more of this story.) In July 1993, HGSI signed an exclusive deal with the pharmaceutical company SmithKline Beecham, in which SmithKline got first rights to develop products based on what it found in the HGSI database. HGSI was promised $125 million, a huge amount of money by the biotech standards of the day. "We were out there ahead of others," said HGSI president William Haseltine, one of the people least likely to end up as gray powder between any elephant's toes. A SmithKline senior vice president also cited speed as one of deal's cementing factors: "We got the data two years ahead of anyone else. . . . We bought HGSI's database to expand our product line, to build our business in the future. . . . We've skimmed the cream that's relevant to our portfolio," and the rest of the information could be resold.[12]

Meanwhile, out in the San Francisco Bay Area, Incyte did a different dance. When it incorporated in 1991, it had a few interesting proteins that seemed to be going nowhere fast. But then came that other signature technology of the 1990s that instantly became part of the fantastic infrastructure of genomics: the Internet. When Incyte went public in 1993, it declared its focus to be genomic databases rather than drug development, dry rather than wet, silicon over carbon. Using relational databases and an interface based on the new Netscape browser, Incyte quickly built several databases — LifeSeq and ZooSeq were two of their most popular. More than just a slew of DNA base pairs, the Incyte databases were the shape of things to come. Sequence searches were just the beginning, and researchers could do far more than just isolate DNA from a sample they were working on, sequence it, and then go look for it in the database. They could compare their sequence to similar sequences in other organisms in the ZooSeq database; they could compare not only the genes, but the messenger-RNA and the proteins from the "knee joint of a 61-year old woman with untreated rheumatoid arthritis, a 53-year old male taking steroids to treat the same disorder, or a 24-year old male with no evidence of disease."[13] Researchers could be instantly connected to other literature published on that particular gene or disease, they could link to a genetic map of markers that showed where their gene was located, they could link to protein databases and protein studies, and on and on.

Incyte sold nonexclusive access to its databases and their interfaces, rather than going the exclusive route that HGSI took. So instead of $125 million from one customer, Incyte took in $15–20 million each from Pfizer, Upjohn, Hoechst, Hoffmann-LaRoche, Glaxo, Johnson & Johnson, and others, each buying access to Incyte's databases for a few years. Incyte's corporate strategy has been described as "more like a software company than a biotechnology firm," and Incyte president and chief scientific officer Randy Scott was himself described as "a product of Silicon Valley, where suing a company in the morning and then inking an alliance with them in the afternoon is just another day in the high-tech fast lane. Valleyites call the attitude 'co-opetition.'"[14]

Finally, let's consider Cambridge, Massachusetts–based Millennium Pharmaceuticals. Millennium was founded in 1993 by, among others, Eric Lander, the mathematician turned genomicist who had already established himself as a leading researcher and policy figure in the federally funded and coordinated Human Genome Project—which, as we've seen, he called "the Route One of genetics." In the years to come, Lander would go on to become an even more leading researcher and policy figure in the HGP, while maintaining dual citizenship (as almost every life scientist does these days) in the private genomic sector with Millennium. Millennium adopted a more "integrated" approach than either HGSI or Incyte did at first. Instead of concentrating almost exclusively on producing, databasing, organizing, and selling DNA sequence and related information, Millennium's research program covered the spectrum from sequence information to gene expression to animal studies to early drug development. By the time Millennium went public in 1996, it had research agreements with multiple pharma pachyderms, including Hoffmann-LaRoche for obesity and type II diabetes, Eli Lilly for atherosclerosis, and Astra for inflammatory respiratory disease (asthma). Millennium called this the "diversified portfolio" approach. The phrase can be applied across multiple genomic strata: multiple corporate alliances, multiple disease interests, multiple laboratory strategies and expertise.

And perhaps most importantly: multiple population resources. Millennium's 1996 SEC registration claimed "that this 'diversified portfolio' approach to human genetics increases the likelihood of rapidly identifying prevalent disease genes and provides a means of independently confirming results found in any single population. For example, in Millennium's type II diabetes program, the Company uses select family collections from homogeneous populations in Scandinavia and Israel and from heterogeneous populations in the United States."[15]

XX

What can we learn from these three examples about the speed transforms of genomics?

The first thing that changed in the field was the size, type, and connectability of biodatabases. In 1987, the U.S. Department of Energy's GenBank was pretty much the only database of genetic information around, and this publicly funded and publicly accessible database was already months behind in entering sequence data from journal publications. The ever-faster automated DNA sequencers and other pieces of genomics' fantastic infrastructure only sped up the data production rates into the early 1990s. By then, the logic behind the feds' speed genomics infrastructure development, that these tools would be privatized to support the U.S. biotech industry, had begun to make sense to pharma and start-ups alike. The genomic start-ups used the high-throughput tools of the fantastic infrastructure to build rich, diverse, and proprietary databases that, thanks to the Internet, could be easily searched and linked by virtually anyone—anyone that paid the access fees. Everyone else—university researchers, NIH, and DOE scientists—could use the public ones.

The disease targets transformed as well. The genetics approach that had yielded the single genes (and their variants) implicated in "simple disorders" like Huntington's and cystic fibrosis had become a genomic approach addressed to "complex conditions" like those targeted by Millennium: heart disease, asthma, obesity. The monogenic conditions were the most amenable to the tools, techniques, and maps available in the early stages of the genomic infrastructure. But from both a commercial and a public health perspective, they held limited interest. There are only about thirty thousand people with cystic fibrosis in the United States, and even if you expand to identifying and counseling the "carriers" of this recessive gene, the disease remains a narrow field of interest and action—although not, of course, to the individuals and families affected by it. But if you're a dancing genomic start-up or a pachydermal pharma company, by the mid-1990s you had shifted your gaze to the complex conditions that were once thought to be intractable from a genetics perspective: most forms of cancer, heart disease, hypertension, schizophrenia, depression, migraines, and a long list of other ills.

These are conditions that affect entire *populations,* and this is the other transformation wrought by the fantastic infrastructure of speed genomics. In a genetics approach, researchers focused on individuals and families. Even if you drew your subjects from that favorite group for geneticists, the Mormons, your work and your attention was organized around families and the individuals who constituted them. You went to them for blood samples, you got them to involve their relatives, you hoped to go back to them personally with positive results, showing how the gene or marker you had discovered "ran in" their family. When Millennium offered its stock to that diverse population known as "the public," it described its access to "homogeneous" as well as "heterogeneous" populations from Scandinavia, Israel, and the United States. While we will have to ask some questions about how researchers arrive at these characterizations, the fundamental point remains: the unit of analysis shifted to the populations that manifest, and suffer from, complex conditions. Access to a well-defined "population" for a particular research program became, from here on out, an important enough asset that it merited disclosure to potential investors.

And with a population now on the research-input end, you can bet that there will be a population on the receiving end, notwithstanding all the fine talk about "individualized medicine." Or to put it another way: the family is concerned with the individual, but it's the state that's most concerned with populations.

The genomic start-ups are also providing something different than their ancestors like Biogen and Genentech. If the earlier generation survived by making products, however unsurely and slowly, the genomic start-ups survive by making promises. When the new companies' databases began, they were loaded with promising information produced by high-throughput genomic technologies. The phrase "drinking out of a fire hose" became popular at this time, as researchers searched these exploding data sets to establish potential drug candidates or to find genes to be tweaked or even just studied further. Pharma promised "milestone payments" to its genomic allies when they provided, say, ten gene candidates that appeared to be associated with obesity, or three new proteins that looked like they were involved in the biochemical pathways associated with asthma. If the vast majority of these leads never went anywhere, that surprised no one. You simply returned to the fire hose and drank again. Success for a genomic company came to be oriented around its infrastructural capacity to make good promises.

None of this in itself is a disparagement of the industry. Promises may be a lot of things, and promises may be subject to all kinds of contingencies and volatilities that together make up "the future," all of which I hope will be seen in the future of this book. But for now, keep in mind that it is possible to make good promises, even if ultimately one is unable to make good on those promises.

Finally, to end discussion of the transformations in the genomic political economy, let's return to François Jacob's phrase, "ever-unstable" equilibria. HGSI, Incyte, and Millennium are ever-unstable equilibria. They are corporate entities whose technological component is always becoming something else, whose research programs shift over time, and that constantly recombine with other corporate entities—all at differential, fastXfast speeds. Even if some companies make single alliances, like HGSI did with SmithKline (which would later agglomerate into GlaxoSmithKline), the "portfolio approach" became the most popular strategy for genomic companies. What else is a poor, ever-unstable equilibrium supposed to do but multiply its partners, multiply its research angles, multiply its capacities to produce promising information and substances? And as another ever-unstable equilibrium, the entire political economy of genomics was also beginning to quiver more violently under the cumulative effects of the growing multiplicity of investors in the stock market.

The genomic sector seethed with activity, much of it characterized by that unstable phrase applied to Incyte, "co-opetition." Alliances shifted and multiplied: in 1997 Incyte and SmithKline formed a joint venture diagnostic company called diaDexus, from the Greek *diadexus,* meaning "presaging good fortune, in anticipation of future discoveries." The announcement that Incyte had teamed up with SmithKline, which was partnered at the time with Incyte's rival HGSI, was called a "shake-up" in the genomic world, but the term presumed something stable to begin with. There was no shake-up; there was only the ongoing unfolding of an ever-unstable equilibrium. And it was rattling across this unstable sector.

HGSI and TIGR, the nonprofit research institute, announced their split on June 24, 1997. The parting saved HGSI from a future obligation of $38 million to SmithKline over the next five years. In a press release, Craig Venter commented on his delinking, along with TIGR's, from the profit-making HGSI that he had helped start a few years previously: "Our discoveries have proceeded at a pace beyond our expectations. . . . That is why it is important for TIGR to be accessible to all those interested in research for new data in a way that allows us to respond to as many as possible as rapidly as possible."[16] This makes a good mantra for genomics generally: as many as possible as rapidly as possible. On June 25, "a day after winning freedom from its commercial partner," as *Business Today* cast it, TIGR released sequence and other data on over twenty thousand genes from eleven species of microbes, on a Web site set up by the NIH's National Center for Biotechnology Information.[17] We are going to have to invent ways of speaking about the ever-unstable equilibria that publicX-private databases in fact are.

The funny thing is that in the early days of genomics something similar was happening at the level of the organism as well. The fantastic infrastructure of genomics brought science to the point where it had to invent ways of speaking about the ever-unstable equilibria that organisms in fact are.

XX

The historian of the life sciences Evelyn Fox Keller has written about the "funny thing [that] happened on the way to the holy grail." Keller traces what she calls the "discourse of gene action"—in which the gene is synecdochically abstracted from the organism and granted legislative authority—back to the split between embryology and genetics effected by T. H. Morgan. "Even in the early days of genetics," she writes, "when the gene was still merely an abstract concept and the necessity of nuclear-cytoplasmic interactions was clearly understood, geneticists of Morgan's school tended to assume that these hypothetical particles, the genes, must somehow lie at the root of development."[18] Morgan made a kind of promise: the future will be one of material genes, and they will be the controlling element of an organism. Keller emphasizes the productivity of such a move: "But in introducing this particular way of talking, the first generation of American geneticists provided a conceptual framework that was critically important for the future course of biological research. . . . It enabled geneticists to get on with their work without worrying about the lack of information about the nature of such action—to a considerable degree, it even obscured the need for such information" (10–11).

The discourse of gene action has allowed geneticists to leverage a future without a full guarantee from a grounding past. Even in its incompleteness and promissory aspect, it provided "powerful rationales and incentives for mobilizing resources, for identifying particular research agendas, for focusing our scientific energies and attention in particular directions. . . . And it would be foolhardy to pretend it has not worked well. The history of twentieth-century biology is a history of extraordinary success; genetics—first classical, then molecular—has yielded some of the greatest triumphs of modern science" (21–22).

But something "funny" has begun to happen within this discourse, argues Keller, especially with its intensification through the Human Genome Project. The "extraordinary progress" we have made with our capacity for manipulating genes "has become less and less describable within the discourse that fostered it":

The dogmatic focus on gene action called forth a dazzling armamentarium of new techniques for analyzing the behavior of distinct gene segments, and the information yielded by those techniques is now radically subverting the doctrine of the gene as sole (or even primary) agent. . . . Current research invites (ever more insistently) a shift in locution in which the cytoplasm is just as likely as the genome to be cast as the locus of control. . . . As we learn more about how genes actually work in complex organisms, talk about "gene action" subtly transmutes into talk about "gene activation," with the locus of control shifting from genes themselves to the complex biochemical dynamics . . . of cells in constant communication with each other. (22, 25, 28)

The fantastic infrastructure of genomics—embodying a discourse that says genes are the primal code, the foundational control agent—instead of stabilizing the gene, gives us the subversive, ever-unstable equilibrium of geneXcell, where control is disseminated across the elements of a complex system.

What does it mean for us to have received this unexpected gift, born, like all gifts, of excess and extravagance?

Genomic corporations are not promising a fuller, more adequate "representation" of what an organism, human or otherwise, is. That supposedly traditional goal of the sciences is rapidly becoming a quaint relic. "Biology today," to remind ourselves of Jacob's dictum, "is no longer seeking for truth. It is building its own truth." Or perhaps we can simply say: it is building. Genomics isn't promising to reveal the "full picture" of "what it means to be human" from little bits and bytes of the organism. Genomics is building new zones of intensities, places in and between the laboratory, the corporation, the experimental assemblages, and the biochemical multiplicities of our bodies, where differences are created, become different from themselves, and recombine with other differences. The successful scientists and corporations will be those who can continually rearrange software, hardware, wetware, and infoware into hybrid combinations that create new intensities, perform new biological effects—and who can do so ever more quickly. Not quite the "pure kinetic energy" announced by Lucas's *Star Wars,* but certainly the ever-hotter pursuit of more, and more intense, productive linkages between virtualities and materialities. Completion isn't promised by genomics; future becomings are.

XX

The undersigned came to the end of the talk. It was too much and not enough—as usual. I hadn't even reached—directly, anyway—the temporal and ethical strata, and I've deferred them here again. I hoped that both the excesses and the gaps would provoke some new effects.

In closing, I was deciding between two quotations, the first from Donna Haraway:

The cyborg is . . . a figure that names the fact that, like it or not, we are constructed historically in places we don't choose. Nobody chose to be a cyborg. . . . Choice is such a weak concept for who we are historically. So little in our lives has to do with choice, despite centuries of liberal theory. . . . The cyborg is a reminder, and it's not a friendly reminder, that there wasn't much choice about this. Historically, discursively, physically (the discourse is physical, the theory is corporeal, it's literal in an extraordinary sense), we are embodied in locations that have nothing to do with choice.[19]

I thought it might be important for the Icelanders, in this time when they appeared to face such a momentous choice, to be reminded of the limits of that discourse. But I couldn't think of a way to make those contradictions play out productively, and I figured Donna Haraway wasn't exactly a household name in Reykjavík. Plus, the quote was long. So I went with Margaret Mead in *Time* magazine, 1954: "There are too many complaints about society having to move too fast to keep up with the machine. There

is great advantage in moving fast if you move completely, if social, educational, and recreational changes keep pace."[20]

It's Mead's last category that I'm particularly interested in, if by recreational we mean those activities designed to renew, revitalize, refresh, and
re-create, particularly when it comes to the creational substance called
DNA. Philosophy is re-creational, and the philosophical re-creating of
concepts is one of the few things that might be able to match the recre-
ations of speed genomics. That's my hope anyway, or that's the experiment that I think it would be interesting to get up and running.

CH 4

CounterfeitXMoney

If a dollar bill is "a written promissory note issued by the United States Treasury to an unnamed bearer," notes mathematician/semiotician Brian Rotman in his book *Signifying Nothing,* then the next logical question is, promising what? Until 1973, "the dollar's promise" was to oblige the treasury to turn over "absent but potentially recoverable specie," in the form of gold, to this non-personally identifiable bearer. After 1973, "the U.S. government cancelled its self-imposed obligation to deliver specie," making the dollar a "currency with no intrinsic internal value whose extrinsic value with respect to other currencies was allowed to float in accordance with market forces." "As a promissory note," continues Rotman, the dollar became "a tautological void."[1] The dollar was worth what the dollar was worth, and the treasury was obliged to continue being obliged. It keeps keeping the promise.

This void or fissure at the heart of our currency was always there and has only become more noticeable, more volatile. Whether we're talking about dollars, cotton cloth, or microchunks of sequenced DNA, value is always "phantasmagoric," to use Marx's word, or "spooky," to use Derrida's favored wording in his channelings of *Specters of Marx.* If Marx thought these phantasms or voids of value might be exorcised and fetishism overcome, Derrida argues that "the limits of phantasmagorisation can no longer be controlled or fixed by the simple opposition of presence and absence, actuality and inactuality, sensuous and supersensible." Thus "another approach to differences must structure . . . the field that has thus been re-opened. Far from effacing differences and analytic determinations, this other logic calls for other concepts."[2]

49

George Soros has offered "reflexivity" as an "other concept"—"a two-way feedback mechanism in which reality helps shape the participants' thinking and the participants' thinking helps shape reality in an unending process in which thinking and reality may come to approach each other but can never become identical. . . . The key element is the lack of correspondence, the inherent divergence, between the participants' views and the actual state of affairs."[3] Close enough to a chiasmus for me.

"The future" might be another name for this divergence. For Soros, "financial markets cannot possibly discount the future correctly because they do not merely discount the future; they help to shape it." How then does one evaluate or, more directly, *value* something that isn't present yet, that will in part come into being as a result of your valuing act?

How does a genomic company like deCODE Genetics put a price on the rights to future discoveries that might be wrought from the gathered blood of the Icelandic population? The question is even more perplexing when you consider the exact wording of such deals: how does a genomic company sell the "potential rights" to future discoveries, since even if a gene of interest were to be isolated from Icelanders, it might already have been patented or otherwise claimed by a rival company? Or perhaps said gene is in the public domain or some other contingency obviates future rights.

Just how much, to rephrase, would you be willing to pay for such a promise?

If "you" is a conglomerate like Hoffmann-LaRoche, how do you decide that $200 million is a fair price to pay—no, *to promise* to pay for *potential* rights to the biomedical potential that *might* lie in twelve genes that *might* exist somewhere and *might* be developed into a therapy that *might* work for some percentage of customers who *might* be in a position to pay in a future where higher-priced drugs are a near-certainty? And how do you do this when, in 1998, no other conglomerate has ever promised anything approaching that amount to any other genomic company such as Human Genome Sciences or Celera or Millennium—none of which had existed as a corporate entity for more than five years?

How do you *structure* a deal like this, when it involves, in such multiply involuted ways, such spectral entities and events? You—Hoffmann-LaRoche—can set up "research milestones" for your partner deCODE to mark waypoints during this long, uncertain, and costly process toward a therapeutic drug or diagnostic test: Isolate some small fragment of DNA shared by a significant portion of people with arthritis, trigger a small milestone payment. Characterize the protein produced by that DNA segment, trigger the next milestone payment. And so on.

This structure was hardly unique to deCODE. In the genomic economy that spun itself out so rapidly in the 1990s—a largely U.S.-centered genomic sector whose future "dominance" in a competitive global bioeconomy was one of the principle rationales for federal spending on the Human Genome Project—Human Genome Sciences, Incyte, Millennium, GenSet, and other companies began working and trading on the promises of forward-looking genetic information, and pretty much *only* on the promises. What else was there? No one had secure knowledge of what would pan out over what period of time: how many genes there were, what kinds of uses could be made of how many of them, what proteins would be good "drug targets" and which would veer wide of the mark, what the long-term prospects were for genetic sequence databases, and so many other contingencies. Every genomic company had to promise to play the game

But deCODE was unique in another respect: for its first years of existence, it had only this single major promise from and to Hoffmann-LaRoche. Most genomic companies thrive on multiple alliances with multiple pharmaceutical companies, biotech start-ups, and sometimes specifically with other genomic companies. The pharmaceutical companies, in turn, forged multiple bonds with multiple genomic companies. Together they all pursue multiple technological strategies—new search strategies for databases, combinatorial chemistry, rational drug design through molecular modeling, monoclonal antibodies, and many others—since it's not clear which one of these promising "technology platforms" will cash out, most likely some ensemble and not any particular one.

Such are the volatilities of promising that in the final analysis there seem only to be "rules of thumb" for valuing futures, and the Big Pharma company surely heeded the strategic advice offered to the individual investor in genomics: "It's a rule of thumb among biotech investors that for every 10 stocks, one or two may succeed, two or three will be marginally successful and the rest will fail."[4]

XX

While it's tempting to ask, "How do you tell a counterfeit genomic company from a real genomic company?" the chiasmus or reflexive two-way feedback mechanism at the voided heart of value makes a definitive decision impossible. "How do you tell a counterfeit telling from a real telling?" is only the first question to come screaming out of this fissure, and from there you're hard pressed to fend off vertigo. What we seem to need are some "rules of thumb" or another kind of "telling." Perhaps a telling that works through a novel, rather than by way of UV light or watermarks or threads of precious metals, might allow the vertiginous X itself to remain in the telling. As I did in that first September 1998 trip to Iceland, I now open an extended engagement with Halldór Laxness's 1948 novel, *The Atom Station*.

The Atom Station is set in Iceland at the end of World War II and during the early years of the Cold War, when debates raged over whether U.S. forces should be stationed in the small island country. But it is not simply a novel about the "selling" of Iceland to foreign interests; it is also about the role of romanticism in the construction of an Icelandic nation for sale just after it had become independent from Denmark in 1944, and about the problem of legitimating illegitimate reproduction. Its protagonist is a young woman, Ugla, the "wise owl" from the rural north who has come to the big city of Reykjavík to be a maid in the household of an Althingi member. (The affable, powerful, and somewhat inscrutable minister and his three children will be met later.)

In her free time Ugla takes organ lessons from . . . "the organist" is the only name given to this bohemian/saint figure. In Ugla's first visit to the organist's house, she is introduced to two other men, Brilliantine and the Atom Poet, who also have the feel of protobeatniks, but without the saintly part, even though they are often referred to as "gods." They arrive in a Cadillac. The evening of music and conversation goes on for a long time, as many such gatherings of Icelanders seem to do, with the organist performing a kind of musical/dance number, with Brilliantine strumming on some twine strung across a salted fish. This culminates in a minipotlatch in which the organist pulls out "vast sums of money" from his pockets and, "in a sudden fit," begins tearing them up, crumpling them, throwing the torn and folded pieces on the floor "and grinding them down like a man killing an insect. Then he sat down and lit himself a cigarette."[5]

On the walk home, Ugla queries Brilliantine (who will eventually show himself to indeed be oily, shiny, and superficial):

When we had walked for a while along the road I could not restrain myself from asking, "Was that real money, or was it fake?"

"There is no such thing as real money," he said. "All money is fake. We gods spit on money."

"But the Atom Poet must surely be well off to be driving such a car."

"All those who know how to steal are well off," said the god. "All those who don't know how to steal are badly off. The problem is to know how to steal."

I wanted to know where and how that little poet had stolen that huge car. (22–23)

Soon after Ugla and Brilliantine finish their conversation, the organist comes running after them, out of breath, asking to borrow a single króna coin. Brilliantine has nothing; Ugla fishes a króna from her pocket and gives it to the organist. He thanks her and promises to repay her. "You see," he explains, "I need to buy myself fifty grams of boiled sweets tomorrow morning."

XX

Ugla will later find out how the poet managed to steal the car. It involves paper, money, the prime minister, and a joint U.S.-Icelandic corporation, as if these things can be spoken of separately. This early excerpt is only to introduce some of the characters and the questions of value and worth that will be threaded through the rest of the novel, and this book. It's too slick, Laxness is telling us, to say that "all money is fake." But neither is money simply "real" or "genuine." The "monetary copula," as ethnographer of value Bill Maurer puts it—X is worth Y—is a fantasy that draws attention away from the "lateral reasoning" that in fact makes value happen in systems as diverse as Islamic banking and "Ithaca Hours," those productively worthless pieces of paper exchanged in upstate New York.[6]

Maybe living in a cracked landscape gave Laxness a genius for keeping volatile tensions in play and in view, for letting contradictions and double-binds do their thing. Laxness's advice to wise girls and other readers would seem to be the same as that offered by ethnographers like Maurer: trace the exchanges, map the desires, gauge the effects. And don't forget about the excesses—the sweets that have no use value, the vaporous smoke and ash that are the remainders of all expenditure. These are the terms of a different telling of a more general economy that does not revolve exclusively around the opposition of counterfeit and true.

KáriXdeCODE

If the distinction between the promised Health Sector Database and the corporate entity deCODE Genetics was a fine one, that between deCODE and its CEO Kári Stefánsson was practically fissureless. This near conflation between CEO and corporation was not unusual in the 1990s. One need only think of Michael Dell and Dell Computers, Jeff Bezos and Amazon.com, Larry Ellison and Oracle, Bill Gates and Microsoft.

While Kári and deCODE didn't share popular appeal that these Internet and computer CEOXcorporations did, the fortunes of the bioinformatics-intensive genomic companies of the late 1990s could be just as tightly bound to the celebrity status of their CEOs as the more generic informatics-intensive companies. Millennium Pharmaceutical's CEO Mark Levin didn't make the cover of *Rolling Stone*, but he did become a temporary icon of *Worth* for the genomic sector, the "next wealth machine" that was supposed to have "more upside than the Internet." But in the United States, the CEO who was the most celebrated, the most notorious, and the most twinned to the fortunes of the genomic company he "headed," was Craig Venter.

Long before he founded and became president of Celera, Craig Venter appreciated the main goal and underlying logic of the Human Genome Project: not to fully sequence the genomes of humans and other organisms, but to create an infrastructure of faster, more efficient genomic technologies that promised to inject power into the engines of the U.S. biotechnology industry. Working within the U.S. National Institutes of Health in 1991, at the time when the Human Genome Project was just officially getting underway, Venter was already developing and advocating high-throughput technological strategies. Venter leap-frogged seemingly endless discussions about the most appropriate strategy for sequencing generic stretch after generic stretch of DNA by assembling and automating a variety of technologies that used messenger-RNA (mRNA) to focus on expressed genes. In this method, you don't know and you don't care what particular genes are involved. In the body, this mRNA is eventually transformed into proteins; in the genomic lab, the mRNA is converted into the complementary DNA (cDNA), which matches it. More importantly, the cDNA also complements at least part of the original, unknown gene that first expressed the mRNA. So the cDNA—a "man-made" substance and not "natural," and therefore patentable—can be used as a tool to "fish out" unknown genes that might prove interesting and important in the future. As a genomic tool, in other words, cDNAs are used to locate promising genes for a genomic science and business for which promises are almost everything.

Venter's lab at the NIH began churning out large quantities of cDNA fragments, only working out just enough sequence information to "tag" them (hence the name for the overall technology, "expressed-sequence tags," or ESTs) and render them useful.[1] It was a stroke of technological and scientific brilliance on Venter's part, although more than a few scientists considered it rather mechanical and base. When the NIH in 1991 applied for patents on thousands of Venter's gene fragments, with practically no understanding of their biological function, but for their utility as basic tools for further genomic research, many biologists lined up behind HGP director James Watson in their outrage, lambasting the patenting as "mindless," a "land grab," "unscientific," "monkey business," and a "Gold Rush."[2]

Venter had already moved on, however. Along with most of his laboratory staff, he left the NIH in July 1991 to begin a venture straddling the public-private divide, the hybrid operations known as The Institute for Genomic Research and Human Genome Sciences Inc. The high-throughput sequencing technologies and faster search algorithms that Venter's group developed at the NIH did double duty in the double TIGR-HGSI: producing loads of sequence data on a panoply of organisms from bacteria to fruit flies at the nonprofit TIGR, and producing loads of potential human gene candidates and drug targets exclusively for HGSI (which in turn had an exclusive arrangement with the pharmaceutical company Smith-Kline Beecham). As one commentator put it, creating a mental image of Venter as living chiasmus, "Venter had one foot in the world of pure science and one foot in a bucket of money."[3]

In early 1998, Applied Biosystem's Michael Hunkapillar showed a prototype of the ABI Prism 3700 to Venter. Within the right context, Venter realized, a few hundred of these representatives of the next generation of automated DNA sequencers could sequence and assemble any large genome in a few years. In May 1998, the PE Corporation (now Applera) was formed, a parent company with Applied Biosystems and Celera as squalling twins: one for building, selling, and servicing sequencers to all customers, "private" and "public" alike, and one for sequencing, databasing, annotating, and patenting genomes. Celera announced its intention to fully sequence the human genome in three years, far ahead of the public project's timetables; everyone else, it was suggested, could do the mouse.

The public consortium responded immediately and vehemently. With the prodding of John Sulston of its Sanger Centre, the Wellcome Trust in the United Kingdom dramatically raised its funding levels for human genome sequencing by a hundred million pounds. At the behest of National Human Genome Research Institute director Francis Collins and ex-director James Watson, the U.S. government also pumped money into the sequencing side of its efforts. Reorganization occurred, and a few large labs (including the Sanger Centre, the Whitehead Institute, Baylor College of Medicine, and Washington University) received the lion's share of the money, along with responsibility for large-scale production and quality control; other labs that had been sequencing saw their funding evaporate. The international public consortium announced it would complete a "working draft" sequence of the human genome by spring 2001.

But all that is in this book's future. For the time being, our concern is only with the ways that value in the genomic sector is bound up with some form of status that attaches to a human organism—biocelebrity.[4] Venter-XCelera became vastly successful and wealthy, although *how* and *why* would be difficult to say—maybe even impossible, some maintained. As Hamilton O. Smith, one of Celera's top scientists, watching the value of his own Celera stock track up in December 1999, said, "This defies common sense. It's really impossible to put a value on this company."[5]

Smith might be exaggerating when he says "impossible," since all you would have to do is call a stockbroker and ask the value of Celera at that very moment, and the stockbroker would say exactly how much cash you would need to exchange for a share in the company. Value is that simple. But there is indeed something impossible about value, as the previous chapter suggested and later ones will echo.

Smith's comments about value defying common sense were made to Richard Preston, who profiled Venter as "The Genome Warrior" in *The*

New Yorker. As Preston tells the story, sometime in the early spring of 2000, in its race with the public consortium to the "complete" sequence of the human genome, Celera began assembling the human DNA sequences it had been churning out from multiple shotgunned fragments—"a pretty boring" job, according to Venter. This could explain why the moment had to be amped up with a little ritual:

Minutes later, one of [Greg] Myers's people, a computer scientist named Knut Reinert, hurried in, and told him that the first assembled human-genome sequence had just come out of the computers. Myers put the 'Ride of the Valkyries' on the boom box, and fifteen people tried to crowd into Reinert's cubicle.

Myers bent over Reinert's shoulder and said, "We got it! We got the first one! This is the first assembled human sequence we've gotten out of nature! . . .

They talked about it for a few minutes, and then everyone drifted back to work. That day, Celera's stock dropped another twenty percent. (83)

Here in the lava land of genomics, all roads seem to lead to Iceland. An oblique path follows the dramatic Germanic musical purveyance of old Norse myths of supernatural women swooping over battlefields to gather dead Viking heroes (or maybe just their DNA) and resurrect them in (virtual) Valhalla. A slightly more direct route threads through *The New Yorker* again, which in the 1990s seemed to be running weekly articles on bioscientists and their corporate ventures, or on why sociobiology wasn't as stupid a theory as was thought in the 1970s. A year before Venter and Celera were lionized in *The New Yorker,* Michael Specter profiled that other celebrated genomic amalgam, KáriXdeCODE.

XX

If I seem preoccupied today that is because my enemies have deposited the usual lies and half-truths in the newspapers again. They are saying that if we go forward with genetic research in this country, if I am allowed to prepare the database that will help solve so many medical mysteries and make heroes of the people here, then Iceland will be stigmatized and the people will become pariahs in the world. What a horrendous crock of shit.

Kári Stefánsson, quoted in Specter, "Decoding Iceland," 43

Kári confessed to being out in front of himself, preoccupied, when he spoke these words to *New Yorker* writer Michael Specter in November

1998, so he may indeed have believed that his yet-to-be-delivered promise regarding solutions to medical mysteries and the lionization (and even Valhallification) of all Icelanders was, by way of opposition, shit-free full truth. After all, he "seems incapable of humility," as Specter went on to note, a quality Kári no doubt shared with Craig Venter and who knows how many other CEOs of genomic companies; some collecting and analysis of blood samples might yield promising results.

Specter also noted that Kári "treats his intellectual combatants with contempt," allowing the man to speak for himself: "'Now it has become like the Sturla period in Iceland again. I am besieged by little people. This is a fascinating controversy and I understand it well. But these few people, opponents'—he spat the word out as if it were a rusty nail—'are scared of change and unwilling to lose their standing in the scientific community. But remember one thing while you are ingesting their propaganda: those who are opposed to what we are trying to do are a small group. They are not important. And they will lose."[6] Another promise from this man who "plays basketball regularly, and 'with an extreme and sometimes ugly need to win,' according to one of his colleagues" (45). Another gaming reference appeared in the Icelandic newspaper *DV* around this time, this one offered by the psychiatrist Ernir Snorrason, a cofounder of deCODE who had parted ways with Kári and the company and become a vocal critic of the Health Sector Database. Despite the parting, Ernir said of Kári, "we are good friends and will remain so. . . . But let me tell you a parable: A little more than twenty years ago I played a game of chess with Kári. He was an aggressive and intense player. Gradually the game turned in my favour. When his position was hopeless Kári rose and upturned the chessboard. He was no longer interested in the game."[7]

Specter was visiting Iceland and writing at a time when the Althingi had yet to have its final debate and vote on the HSD legislation, and his article would not appear until January 1999, after the vote occurred. The outcome of that game was as yet unclear in November 1998 to writers like Specter, and to the other journalists who had swarmed to the island to learn and write about Kári and deCODE. But Kári's character was coming into focus.

XX

"Have you met him yet?" the Swiss journalist Christoph Keller asked the undersigned as we sat in a café in Reykjavík's city center, drinking coffee and occasionally glancing at the nearby Parliament building across the square.[8]

"No, I go on Thursday," I replied, "the day the interview with me comes out in *Dagur,* which makes me a little nervous. I have no idea what I said to that reporter. What did you think of him?"

"He is very . . . imposing."

Keller's hesitation prompted me to ask for the German word he was apparently translating. *Eindrucksvoll.* Formidable, grandiose, impressive, spectacular, striking, or commanding. "Imposing" worked for me.

I often found myself following in the footsteps of foreign journalists like Keller that September. I envied them their jobs, or what I imagined their jobs to be like: talk to people, write the story, get a couple of good quotes, meet the deadline, don't get distracted and go flowing all over the place. I imagined some crusty editor at the home office giving them advice: "Keep a lid on the magma, kid, and you'll be all right."

The journalists were all calling the same people, like the signatories to the *Nature Biotechnology* letter that had first brought Kári's "enemies" and the whole subsequent mess to an international public. Some of this stampede was because Skúli made sure that all the writers, and not just his undersigned friend, had the phone number of and background on every critic of standing. Skúli also encouraged meetings among the information gatherers. He and I met with John Hodgson, the reporter for *Nature Biotechnology* whose coverage of the ongoing eruption was as careful as it was critical.[9] Skúli harangued Hodgson for over an hour in the lobby of the Hótel Esja, and I couldn't get a word in edgewise.

I had little room to complain, however. My advance man had done so much for me already, including arranging the interview with the *Dagur* reporter that I was anxiously worrying about in these days before I met with Kári. That reporter was a young Icelandic woman studying art and aesthetics in France, home for the summer and earning some extra krónur by writing for this leftish newspaper. Sharp as she was, this was a small sign of the undeveloped state of science journalism in a na′ ∪n that was making a serious decision about its science-based future.

We met at the Hótel Borg, on that same downtown square a stone's throw from the Althingi building where I would meet with Keller. I was unnerved by my first experience on the other side of the tape recorder. The interview was a blur. I was sweating from a combination of nervousness and the eight cups of coffee that had powered my own crammed schedule of interviews that morning. I talked about why I was interested in genomics, about my dissertation at Harvard on the Human Genome

Project. (I shamelessly played the Harvard card, since the media was already playing it with Kári, whose budding biocelebrity persona was augmented by repeated references to him as "a former Harvard professor"; "a University of Chicago professor," where he had in fact spent the bulk of his career in the United States did not have the same ring.) In the interview, I led with the part of me that was most enthusiastic and optimistic about genomics in general, and even genomics in Iceland. I tried to be as indirect as possible when asked about the legislation, hedging my words like the careful wagers they were.

The interview was published the day before I went to see KáriXde-CODE. Unable to read a speck of Icelandic, I had no idea what I had said. Skúli told me it was very good and relatively neutral; the headline read "The Debate Comes Too Late." Innocuous enough, yet open to a more critical reading. It was clear that my ethnographer self was indeed in an "experimental moment," having entered the frame of the culture and story that, by the canons of ethnographic tradition, I was supposed to be outside of. One more chiasmus to mix things up.

Driving out to the eastern suburbs of Reykjavík the following day, on my way to deCODE, I tried to think through the implications of this media frenzy for the country's "democratic debate" as well as for my own practices of scholarship. The radio played a mix of music that would never be thrown together in the United States: an old Janet Jackson tune followed by a B-side track from the Pixies, which segued into some unfamiliar Europop. The announcer came on and began a long-winded commentary, and through the opaque floe of Icelandic came names in a sequence that was all too easy to decode, no matter how severely undersigned I might be: *Kári Stefánsson* gjá gjá gjá *Josef Mengele* gjá gjá gjá *Hermann Göring* gjá gjá gjá *Idi Amin* . . . I felt a brief flash of sympathy for Kári as I turned off the main highway.

XX

At the time, deCODE Genetics (Íslensk erfdagreining in Icelandic, although it remains to be seen if these are one and the same corporate entity) was in an industrial-park-type setting that could easily make you forget what country you were in. I couldn't begin to imagine how many sets of driving directions to how many start-up corporations like deCODE in how many peripheries of global capitalism included the instruction "turn left at the Coca-Cola plant." Except here, Mount Esja hulked on the horizon, dusted with the first snow of the season. DeCODE was in what used to be the Kodak film-processing plant, gone defunct with the rise of in-store, one-hour developing machines. The big open space, with its great ventilation system, was ideal for this new wave of imaging technology. Family photographs seem quaint when you can have your relatives' DNA splayed across gels and downloaded into a centralized database. *Here's Grampa, strong as an ox, and Uncle Jökull, not looking too well—and me, the spitting image of . . .*

In the small lobby sat two women wearing headsets and seemingly speaking into the air; a photograph of President Ólafur Ragnar Gríms-son and his wife, looking like royalty, oversaw this multitasking envi-ronment. I was whisked away and given a quick tour of the place, which was still literally under construction: workers with tool belts slung under their bellies carried battered slabs of metal through the heavily trafficked hallways, new desks stood on end in half-finished offices, carpeting was still being laid in some sections. In front of the scanner at each door, my escort flashed his ID card; when the light turned green, as I imagined it must in every country, we passed through.

First stop, main lab, a huge open space crammed with roboticized in-struments for large-scale, high-speed production and analysis of DNA—a common sight in the commercial genomic world. There are a number of instrument suppliers to genomic companies, but the leader at this time was Applied Biosystems, or ABI (in 1998, still unjoined to Celera Ge-nomics). Lined up in rows were twenty-two ABI 877s, which amplified the DNA samples using the polymerase chain reaction and automatically parceled them out into the microtiter grids. Load 'em up in the morning and again at night, and the machines churn out scads of DNA with min-imal supervision. The amplified samples were then transferred to the next rows of robots, the ABI Prism 3700s, the top-of-the-line automated DNA sequencer. The place was literally humming with the high-pitched white noise of nucleic acids, extracted from the cells of Icelanders, being pushed and squeezed through expensive machinery at what, in the talk of the trade, is called a very "high-throughput" pace. Eventually, all of this body gunk was shot through some silicon and converted into nice clean bytes on magnetic media, housed on various computers in floor-to-ceiling shelves—a Sun Microsystems computer, a slew of desktops, a Hewlett-Packard jukebox tower of cartridges that can be grabbed and played—in a large, silent closet of a room.

I was taken upstairs to an office and given a quick demonstration of the genealogy program. I know from conversations with other journalists that I got the same show as everyone. DeCODE pointed out with pride that its database of genealogies was perhaps the most extensive in existence, going back to the first settlements in the tenth century. These genealogies contribute to the exoticization of Iceland, as Kári's comments make clear: "People were huddled on mountains in the howling wind. For eleven hundred years, everything in Iceland has always been about the lists of names. It's what we all have in common. Without those links we really have no heritage."[10]

I then got a few moments to myself, waiting in the hallway for my appointed meeting with Kári, to ponder a few favorite questions of ethnographers in experimental moments: *What the . . . ? Is it a good or bad thing that beneath my feet the blood of Icelanders is being fragmented, amplified, transduced into charges on magnetic media and finely networked with multiple other data sets? Is it a good or bad thing that we have such clumsy categories of good and bad? What difference does it make that the undersigned is so underdetached by standard social science accounting practices? But Skúli said that interview with me that appeared in* Dagur *today sounded balanced, or open— which I still am. I think. And my talk last night at the university—no harm there, I stayed away from the legislation business. Still, it's not like it's not obvious to everyone, including Kári, that I'm staying with Skúli, one of the most visible and vocal critics of the whole business. I'm glad I agreed when they asked me if they should invite him to lunch too. He could use a real face-to-face dose of Kári—might break up some of his antigenomic certainties . . .*

Kári emerged from his office. He looked at me sitting there. I looked at him.

Undersigned, rising: "We recognize each other from our photos in the papers."

Kári, shaking hands: "Your interview suggests that you're quite enthusiastic about all this."

I think "all this" refers to genomics generally, and not necessarily to deCODE's part of the game, but I'm relieved in any case. "I like to try to be."

There were a few awkward minutes of small talk, body and limb shuffling, as we settled in to Kári's office. Skúli arrived and was introduced; it was the first time they had really met.

While the slices of smoked lamb on thin squares of dense, dark bread remain firmly fixed in my memory, most of the conversation has slipped through the ever-widening mesh of my neural net. Kári occasionally went to the newsprint pad on the easel in the corner and scribbled a few phrases or crude diagrams. The conversation was untaped, off the record. The content resembled another script then circulating in Iceland, the "Non-Confidential Corporate Summary" dated July 5, 1998, and excerpts from that document are better signs of the KáriXdeCODE plan than anything I could reconstruct:

deCODE Genetics is a population-based genomics company that is founded on the assumption that the scarce resource in human genetics as an industrial endeavor is a population that can yield the genetics of common diseases. . . . deCODE is taking a revolutionary approach to genetic research by supplementing leading edge technology with instant access to an ideal population. . . . deCODE takes pride in its ability to create genetics programs that are tailored to individual partner needs—from gene identification and clinical trials to disease management. . . .

deCODE Genetics can decide to work on a disease without concern over whether it can find and secure an appropriate patient population. If a partner expresses a desire to collaborate with deCODE Genetics on a particular disease, the Company can act quickly. . . .

Genotyping that is done on patients for a particular disease, has value for all subsequent diseases that deCODE Genetics studies because of the size of the population and extensive genealogy of the nation. . . .

This database will contain an unprecedented amount of integrated information that could be used to design comprehensive approaches to the management of patients with a particular disease or constellation of diseases. . . . It is important to keep in mind that although *disease management* is the buzzword today, it is likely that in the near future the emphasis will shift to the management of health rather than disease. When this occurs the flagship of the health care system will be preventive medicine. . . . The . . . database will provide an excellent opportunity to design approaches to preventive health care that are based on detailed phenotypic, genotypic, and genealogical information. Furthermore, it will allow for the design of approaches to cost cutting in the management of health and disease.

deCODE Genetics will be in a position to offer its corporate partners access to the Icelandic population for clinical trials of drug candidates that are based on information obtained through its work on genetics of diseases in Iceland. In the case of complex diseases, it may be necessary to have access to the population that yields the genetics to perform some aspects of clinical trials.[11]

Sketchy notes scrawled between bites of food indicate that Skúli and I asked some questions addressing dominant concerns at the time. Why, for example, did deCODE need a twelve-year exclusive license to the database they were proposing to construct? The ability to model health care systems, for "preventive medicine" as well as cost cutting, was the real payoff, in this presentation. And since no one had tried to sell anything like that before, argued Kári—which was certainly true, given that we were all in the anticipated, futural, speculative markets of genomics—and since building an initial database would cost far more than building any subsequent databases, the innovators would have to be guaranteed some sort of security. What about the prospect of clinical trials, a part of deCODE's plan that was receiving little attention and discussion in comparison to other issues like exclusivity and privacy? He didn't write the clinical trials part of the plan, Kári said, so that wasn't as clear as the other parts, but in any case, pharmaceutical companies were moving away from clinical trials and pharmacogenomics and more toward modeling both diseases and entire health systems *in silico,* which was deCODE's ultimate goal.

Every response, every gesture was very smooth. There were no flashes of anger or impatience, no hint of contempt, as other journalists had described. The luncheon ended as it began, in an exchange of pleasantries. *Skúli, we must agree to keep meeting. I know we don't agree but I enjoy talking to you. I don't often get a chance to talk like this.* I told Kári about the Mengele-Göring-Amin-Stefánsson rant I'd heard on the radio, and, recalling the bishop's advice to his emissary in *Under the Glacier*—"One should simply say and do as little as possible. Talk about the weather. Ask what sort of summer they had last year, and the year before that. . . . Not reform anything or anyone. Let them talk, not argue with them"[12]—Kári shifted into a quick riff on Keiko, the killer whale better known as Free Willy, who was then being returned to his native Iceland. *Keiko is my offensive linesman,* Kári said with a laugh, *running interference for me. He's kept me out of the papers for a while.*

The meeting over, I asked for and received a couple of deCODE T-shirts; ethnography and tourism have historically enjoyed a chiasmic relationship. Kári invited me to fly to Húsavík on Saturday, on the north coast of Iceland, with a deCODE delegation. They were going to speak to the hospital workers there and to a town meeting, to present their case for the database. Would I like to come along and see what happened? A generous offer and I, like any ethnographer and tourist would be, was glad to accept.

DogXWhale

Iceland may be roughly characterized as a big block built up by
eruptive masses, broken up by vertical and horizontal crust and
subcrust movements, and moulded by erosion, abrasion, frost
action and other denuding agencies. Geologically speaking, the
country is still very young and bears many signs of still being in
the making.

Nordal and Kristinsson, Iceland: The Republic, 30

I was early, as usual, so I sat in the nearly deserted Reykjavík airport early
on a Saturday morning, waiting for the deCODE team to arrive for the
flight to Húsavík. P. arrived first: PhD in computer science, the chief informatics guy. Then came the lawyer O., looking unenthusiastic about the
early hour, followed by the psychiatrist E. Kári walked in a bit later and,
as was almost always the case, became the tallest person in the room by a
good head. Brown camel hair coat, dark steely gray suit, white shirt, hair
a bit mussed, carrying only a large sketchbook—"in case I get nervous,"
he joked. I can't imagine Kári nervous about anything, but then I'm sure
Kári wants me and everyone else in the world to think exactly that. There
was a lot of fidgety waiting as Íslandsflug airline switched our party to a
big plane, an eighteen seater, instead of the little one as planned. Finally
J., Kári's administrative assistant, arrived, and we were off.

The flight took us over Thingvellir, symbolic site of Iceland's democracy—and what better symbolism for democracy than to found it in a place
split down the middle by a huge, dramatic fault. Here, along this *gjá*, the

Althingi first met in 930; and here, the European and North American tectonic plates continue to withdraw from each other. As the flight continued northeast into the interior of Iceland, I could see only the marks of ancient and recent flows, striations, eruptions, tumbles, strewn glacial deposits, upheavals, cataracts, rifts, gullies, canyons, ridges, pockmarks, and other geological excrescences and strains—a skewed world.

P. read a review article, "Issues on Searching Molecular Sequence Databases." I flipped through a magazine, grasping only the pictures and the fact that in Iceland, like in so many other places, "nature" is convertible into tourist dollars. *Should I go back and talk to Kári, who is deep in conversation with the lawyer and psychiatrist? What's an undersigned ethnographer supposed to do in a situation like this? I've got a report to write, after all.* I continued to gaze out the window, dozed a bit.

We landed in Húsavík, on the north coast of Iceland, where it was cold and drizzly. There was some discussion with the pilots about when to expect them back; the English phrase "bring your own" was thrown with a laugh into the otherwise incomprehensible conversation. The dentist who invited Kári to come speak—"I don't know if he's for or against us," Kári had told me, and I had no way of judging the veracity of such a statement—took the main deCODE team away. J. and I got a ride with a woman who appeared to work at the airport; she took us and the pilots into the town of Húsavík, just a few kilometers away. She dropped J. and me off at the small local hospital, where we met up again with the deCODE team.

Kári and the deCODE team were presenting their plans, wants, needs, wishes, demands to a group of about fifteen physicians, nurses, and administrators. In this milieu I was not just undersigned; I was at a sign nadir, clueless as to what was being said. But Kári was smooth, working the floor, speaking softly and confidently, pausing at the overhead projector to point to one of the few simple Icelandic phrases on the PowerPoint transparency. There was some questioning, but it was easy to tell that everyone seemed pleased, especially the deCODErs.

We were then hustled off to the dentist's house in the country for lunch. The dentist's wife engaged Kári in conversation, and I milled around with the rest of the deCODErs. A small dog scurried up to me, and I crouched down to pet it.

Dentist: "This is a typical Icelandic dog."
Undersigned: "What kind of dog is it?"
Dentist: "It's an Icelandic dog."
Undersigned: "Yes, but what *kind* of dog is it?"

Dentist, brow a bit furrowed: "It's an Icelandic dog."

I felt as though I'd entered an Icelandic Abottsson and Costellosson skit. The dog was put outside for a while, but soon began barking at the floor-to-ceiling window in the back. The dentist's wife shouted something in Icelandic and motioned toward the front door. The dog bolted and reappeared through the front door.

"Sheesh," I quipped to J., "the dog understands more Icelandic than I do."

J., laughing, "How does that make you feel, Mike?"

"Well, to be fair to myself, she did use some body language, too, and that kind of sign I understand as well as any dog. Most dogs, anyway."

Lunch was a delightful affair, with everyone talking and laughing as we ate a light seafood soup—tiny scallops and shrimps, still memorable years later—various cold cuts, cheeses, breads, and eventually cake with berries and *skyr*, Iceland's alternative to yogurt. Coffee made its inevitable rounds. We all thanked our hosts and headed back for the main event: a town meeting in the whaling museum turned civic center.

From a town of 2,500 there were about 45 people there, seated at four long tables. There would have been more, I was told, if it weren't for the annual sheep round-up, which included much singing and drinking. I had the predictable if misplaced nostalgia for the good old days of anthropology. A shrunken and bent old man in a worn but clean suit pulled out an old camera and snapped a photo of Kári sitting at the deCODE table just before the meeting started. Everyone understands celebrity.

Kári gave the same presentation as at the hospital, as far as I could tell. Six hours of undecipherable words was beginning to wear on me. I watched Kári perform again, watched the Húsavíkings watching Kári, though again about sheep and drinking. I left when the lawyer's turn came around again, ducking out the back and down the stairs. I ran into a young woman standing just outside the door. She spoke to me, and I apologized in English for not speaking Icelandic. She quickly switched tongues.

"Would you mind telling me when you come back up if my baby is awake or asleep?" She gestured to the blue baby carriage parked by the wall.

"Not at all. I'm just going to take a quick walk through town."

There was no one on the street or wharf on that dim day. Down near the water was a kind of whale center, offering tours and a few exhibits—probably the ones that used to be in the meeting hall—but it was closed. I walked back to the meeting hall. The baby carriage was still outside, zipped tight against the wind and rain and cold, but otherwise unattended.

The child was awake, quietly staring up at the gray sky. I walked back up to the meeting and told the mother her child was awake but happy. She sat listening for a few more minutes and then went out.

I had returned in time for the coffee break, which included horn-shaped morsels of fried dough spiced with cardamom. I ate about seventeen. washing them down with dup after cup of local coffee, following the local custom

The meeting reconvened. A few people stood up, asking lengthy questions or making long comments, I couldn't tell which. Nor could I tell if they were critical or supportive, either. But even after all my undersigned hours that day, I could still admire the sheer speechifying, the stamina for words these Icelanders displayed in meeting halls or living rooms. After a good half hour, someone made a suggestion that sent a ripple through the room. He was a young guy, big, with big hair—1970s big, not 1960s big. There was some buzz and some laughs around the deCODE table, but I could make out only the whispered English words "Pink Floyd," which were enough. He was asking for a vote, I was informed, an expression of confidence in what deCODE was attempting, support for the legislation, so that the Althingi would know that Húsavík was with Kári. (Húsavík, I was later told by several people, is in the former home district of Kári's father, who had been a member of Parliament.) Someone asked if this was actually legal, or in any other way significantly binding. Whatever. Symbolic was good enough. All in favor? All raised their hands. Opposed? Not a soul.

Walking out of the hall, Kári turned to me: "See? There's enormous support out there for us."

"Yeah. Uh, democracy's an amazing thing." Stupid, but even after ten years of replaying the scene in my head, I still haven't thought of a better response.

Riding back to the airfield, the deCODE team was ebullient. I was generously called "a real Icelandic hero" for sitting patiently through it all. On the plane ride back everyone more or less crashed, and I had plenty of time to ruminate about the day's events. A tangle of images, mostly, with one in particular continually resurfacing. Up in a corner of the meeting hall, on the wall near the ceiling, there were two fading words written in neat script—a lingering trace from the museum days: *uppruni hvala*. With my less-Icelandic-than-a-dog brain offline, my eyes had been drawn to this phrase, and I simply wrote it down and forgot about it. When I got back to Reykjavík, Skúli translated for me: "origin of whales." As in

The Origin of Species. The meeting room had once been an exhibit on whale evolution.

Which was funny, and would become funnier, since the only other word—aside from "Pink Floyd"—that I had grasped that day was uttered by the local doctor who introduced Kári. As the doctor expounded at great length, one word swam recognizably toward me from the ocean of Icelandic: *Keiko.* All the Icelanders laughed.

I began to think that should be taking these whale jokes more seriously.

HistoryXFable

One of the literary effects produced by the fabulous Icelandic sagas is quite close to the one I seek with this ethnography—an effect lucidly described by Robert Kellogg:

> The saga never tells us what it "means," but its thought resides instead in the narration of events and in the particularities of character and event. We are not told that such-and-such a thing will always happen, or even that it will ever happen again, but rather that this is a case in which serious and responsible people of goodwill landed in a conflict that tested their characters and abilities, as well as the social structure of the nation. And it usually sounds true enough to what we know about people that we believe it and remember it.[1]

The production of that literary effect required a different kind of author than the ones who wrote the great medieval poetry of Europe, says Kellogg, a more anonymous author (few if any of the sagas can be confidently ascribed to an individual). The saga author's "persona is that of the historian," who "derives his authority not from the originality of his style or story but from his fidelity to events, or to others' accounts of them and their judgments on those who were involved—in other words, to what has been *said*" (xxiv).

True enough. But I have to say that I gave up reading the sagas after finishing *Egil's Saga*, which I read because Kári (along with practically everyone else on the island) proudly claimed direct descent from this head-banging, vomit-spewing, tenth-century hero-poet. I became more inclined toward the novels of Halldór Laxness, who understood that language constantly exceeded its descriptive function—what's *said*. In *Under the Glacier,* you'll recall from the opening chapter, the bishop's undersigned emissary, Embi, has been sent to the area around Snaefells Glacier to investigate the deviations from the faith rumored to be practiced by the pastor there, Jón. One of their conversations, taped by the Embi as he gathers signs for his report, turns to the matter of language. Like the figure of the organist in Laxness's *The Atom Station,* Pastor Jón is a bemused quasi-saint whose logic follows a nonordinary chain, when not a non sequitur altogether.

> *Pastor Jón:* It's a pity we don't whistle at one another, like birds. Words are misleading. I am always trying to forget words. That is why I contemplate the lily-flowers of the meadow, but in particular the glacier. If one looks at the glacier for long enough, words cease to have any meaning on God's earth.
>
> *Embi:* Doesn't the dazzle cause paralysis of the parasympathetic nervous system?
>
> *Pastor Jón:* I once had a dog which was a stray for so long that he had forgotten his name. He didn't respond when I called him. When I barked he came to me, right enough, but he didn't know me. I am a little like that dog.[2]

The Embi doesn't buy the analogy and thinks the pastor is more like "[one] of those blissful people in religious paintings—the ones who smile while they are being hacked to pieces." To which Pastor Jón can only reply: "Sometimes I feel it's too early to use words until the world has been created."

> *Embi:* Hasn't the world been created, then?
>
> *Pastor Jón:* I thought the creation was still going on. Have you heard that it's been completed?
>
> *Embi:* Whether the world has been created or is still in the process of being created, must we not, since we are here, whistle at one another in that strange dissonance called human speech? Or should we be silent? (88)

No, the pastor responds, he's not advocating silence. He just thinks "that words, words, words and the creation of the world are two different things; two incompatible things." He expounds a bit on history, which "is always entirely different to what has happened," and on the difference between a historian and a novelist:

> *Pastor Jón:* The difference between a novelist and a historian is this, that the former tells lies deliberately and for the fun of it; the historian tells lies in his simplicity and imagines he is telling the truth.

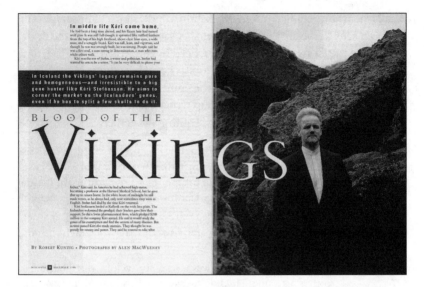

FIGURE 2. Photograph of Kári by Alen MacWeeney, from Robert Kunzig's article "Blood of the Vikings," *Discover* magazine, December 1998. Reprinted with permission.

> *Embi:*   I set down, then, that all history, including the history of the world, is a fable.
>
> *Pastor Jón:*   Everything which is subject to the laws of fable is a fable. (89)

XX

In the deCODE mass media stories, no one leveraged the saga effect better than Robert Kunzig in his December 1998 piece in *Discover,* "Blood of the Vikings." The issue was on U.S. newsstands as the Althingi sped and slogged to its final vote on the Health Sector Database legislation. "In middle life Kári came home," the article begins next to a photo of Kári, severe against jagged, lichened black lava (figure 2).

He had been a long time abroad, and his flaxen hair had turned wolf gray . . . Kári was tall, lean, and vigorous, and though he was not strongly built, he was strong. People said he was a fire-soul, a man strong in determination, a man who runs while others walk. . . .
   Kári Stefánsson landed at Keflavík on the wide lava plain. The Icelanders welcomed the prodigal; their leaders gave him their support. So did a Swiss phar-

maceutical firm, which pledged $200 million to the company Kári started. . . .
But as time passed Kári also made enemies. They thought he was greedy for money
and power. They said he wanted to take what was rightly the nation's heritage
and make it his own. . . .

Kári rose before dawn one day and, rounding up all his supporters, rode down
Miklabraut in Reykjavík to the edge of the marsh, where his enemies lived. He
and his men fell upon them while they were still turning on their computers and
PCR machines. Kári laid about him with his sword, hacking and thrusting. His
men saw his courage and tried to match it. Soon the laboratories were littered
with corpses. . . .

But probably the saga won't end like this.[3]

Not literally, anyway.

The passage works by pushing the incongruous congruencies of a time
out of joint to their limit, reterritorializing an eleventh-century sword into
the territorial battles of twentieth-century biosciences, where the opposition is not so much unarmed or unprepared, but unplugged.

Many other articles on deCODE deployed an exoticized Icelandic history and culture in this way, although not with nearly as much style. Skúli
never liked what he called "sagamongering," spoken with the same sneer
as when he talked about deCODE's business plan as "genemongering."
And the two mongerings were indeed entwined, vitalizing each other.
Every reference to sagas and Vikings exoticized, idealized, and heroized
the events then occurring in Iceland. Not that some dose of fable wasn't
advisable or, at any rate, unavoidable when sounding the name of these
events. But Skúli thought the fictions of someone like Franz Kafka much
more appropriate for talking and writing about bloodletting not by sword,
but by needle and test tube, in clinics with a genealogy and not just a
mythology, regulated by an intricate state bureaucracy that would have
confused, frustrated, and utterly disarmed someone like Egill.

There's no question that deCODE Genetics, genomics, the 1990s, and
Iceland are all subject to the laws of fable, even if such laws should turn
out to be unruly, unwritten, or unreadable; Kafka would indeed be
profitably consulted on this score. Speculation is surely one element of
the unruly laws of fable. Speculation involutes a future into the present,
complementing the mythic foldings of past into present, generating
anticipation—the excitement, thrill, and risk of awaiting the arrival of what
might, or might not, come.

Ever slow on the uptake, I learned about how fable crosses with history
not from the deCODE events themselves, but from the fable of another expat who returned to Iceland at the same time as Kári: Keiko, a.k.a. Free Willy.

KeikoXK.Co.

Keiko, the killer whale known to millions as Free Willy, was liberated from a sea-theme park in Mexico to the freedom of . . . well, an aquarium in Oregon. But then he was liberated from the Oregon aquarium in 1998 to the freedom of . . . well, an elaborate sea pen with feeding platform and underwater cameras connected to the Internet. But at least Keiko was "home," back in the Vestmannaeyjar—the Westman Islands off Iceland's southern coast.

For a long time I saw Keiko only as an amusing, distracting Icelandic pop cultural event that happened to be going on at the same time as the deCODE–Health Sector Database eruption. For example, a member of the Icelandic Parliament cut short a conversation we were having about database anonymity and the importance of public funding of science in addition to private investment. The MP had to leave early because, as a veterinarian, he was flying to the Westman Islands to inspect Keiko's sea pen in preparation for the arrival of the herring eater (oh, how Icelandic fishermen hate the less famous killer whales). Every day on the rear page of *Morgunbladid:* Keiko and deCODE. Every day on the television and radio: deCODE and Keiko. Stories told of Keiko's imminent heroic return "home," just like the expat Kári had returned triumphantly, promising to make Iceland a great genomic power. Editorials, opinion pieces, letters, photos, ads. You could buy inflatable Keikos and stuffed Keikos at all the bookstores and tourist shops. Keikomania. Keikophony.

But it wasn't until the town meeting in Húsavík, when the convener joked about Keiko being the only thing able to keep Kári off the rear page, that the possibility suddenly swarmed over me: Keiko and Kári were somehow kin. I thought that they must share something like 90 percent of their genomes, although the precise homology studies that would back up such a claim have yet to be done. So eventually I got it through my thick ethnographic skull that Keiko was another significant biocultural eruption, a product of the same bio-tele-geo-politico-economic magma field that was throwing up deCODE Genetics. Keiko and K.Co. seemed to be enmeshed in similar nets or to be components in equally crazy and elaborate machines rigged by a wild-eyed engineer just off stage, for vague ends that can only be speculated on. So a bit of Keiko analysis might also offer insights into the strange and multiple effects of celebrity, money, nationalism, and technology on genomics, in Iceland as well as in the United States.

XX

The fable begins in indetermination: Keiko was born somewhere in the Atlantic Ocean near Iceland, in 1977 or 1978. This particular and as yet unnamed DNA-protein-seawater emergent assemblage was captured in 1979 by those other DNA-protein-seawater emergent assemblages known as Icelanders and did some time in an Icelandic aquarium before being bought by Marineland in Ontario, Canada, in 1982. Marineland turned around and sold him to the Mexico City amusement park Reino Aventura in 1985 for the pre-NAFTA price of $350,000. Keiko performed routines routinely there for the next seven years.

A film crew from the media conglomerate Warner Brothers arrived on the scene in 1992 to begin filming *Free Willy,* a movie about a killer whale performing routines routinely in an amusement park who is befriended and eventually freed by a boy. It may have been the film's unexpected success that intensified the latent irony in this situation enough to fuel a popular movement. Or Keiko defenders may have needed the story published by *Life* magazine in November 1993, depicting the whale's chronic health problems despite what were said to be the best efforts of the park owners. An "avalanche" of fan letters and inquiries set in motion months of "confidential negotiations" between Reino Aventura, the Earth Island Institute (a San Francisco–based environmental and marine advocacy group), the film directors from Warner Brothers, and a few unknown marine-oriented facilities, as they tried to find somewhere for Keiko to go.[1] Eventually an agreement was reached with the newcomer Oregon Coast Aquarium, which could promise good facilities and, most importantly, no routine performing demands.

An anonymous donor appeared, and in November 1994 the Free Willy–Keiko Foundation was formed with $4 million in donations. Half of that came from the anonymous donor, later revealed as Craig and Wendy Mc-Caw, who made their whale-sized fortune the 1990s way, propagating first electrons and later electromagnetic waves. Craig McCaw began his career by building a local cable television franchise into the twentieth-largest cable operator in the United States and then became chairman and CEO of Mc-Caw Cellular Communications, a huge wireless communications company bought by AT&T in 1994. McCaw founded Teledesic in Kirkland, Washington, in 1994, planning to make it a telecommunications company that was going to use satellites to build a "global, broadband Internet-in-the-Sky™."

By early 1995 a deal was made: Keiko would be donated to the Oregon aquarium, provided it built what was termed a "$7.3 million rehabilitation facility." This may seem like a lot of money to spend on a sea mammal that, in other circumstances, an Icelander (or someone from Norway or Japan) would have hunted for culinary or, since 1986, "scientific" purposes.[2] But not even personal telecommunications wealth plus entertainment conglomerate capital was enough to keep the Keiko machine going. The U.S. Humane Society chipped in a cool million. Still more was necessary. Another kind of "avalanche" in addition to fan letters needed to be produced and tapped.

In July 1995 Warner Brothers released *Free Willy 2: The Adventure Home.* Gala benefits were held. A swarm of schoolchildren collected coins, sold baked goods. In November, six million video tapes of *Free Willy 2* were released in the mother of all marketing avalanches, the Christmas rush. Each bore a message from one of the movie's cast members, urging assistance. The Discover Channel began planning a special on the whale move.

In January 1996, Keiko was delivered to the Oregon Coast Aquarium by United Parcel Service. You might imagine some nice man or woman in brown shorts and shirt, getting an aquarium representative to sign one of those clunky but business-like electronic clipboards—"Have a good one." "Thanks, you too." You would not have an overactive imagination, as we'll see.

Over the next year Keiko put on a thousand pounds, then another thousand, eating a steady diet of dead fish, since the natural-born killer whale couldn't kill a meal to save his life. His skin cleared up as the virus that had colonized him in Mexico slowly lost numbers and territory. Keiko's adventure began to resemble a weird NAFTA success story.

But even though in *Free Willy 2* the real and/or cinematic whale is supposed to journey or adventure home, the $7.3 million rehabilitation facility in Oregon was never meant as more than a way station, a rest stop, rehab. "Home" was still in the future, in Iceland. The next stage, which could have been called Free Willy 2.1, would require the assistance of the U.S. Air Force. And UPS again.

XX

These goings on were completely unknown to me at the time of my first trip to Iceland in September 1998. Even on board Icelandair—the country's dominant air carrier, like deCODE was trying to be the country's dominant gene carrier—with Keiko gazing off the cover of the in-flight magazine directly into my eyes (figure 3), I couldn't be bothered to pay attention to some corporate welfare whale.

The Free Willy–Keiko Foundation—which by 1998 had enlarged its corporate partner pool to include Mattel, Nextel, and Time-Warner—arranged for Keiko to be flown to the Westman Islands. The U.S. Air Force C-17 Globemaster III ($180 million per plane) was the only aircraft that could fly nonstop from Oregon to Iceland (with two in-flight refuelings), *and* carry a 4.5-ton whale plus life support equipment (for a total of 81,000 pounds), *and* land on a runway as short as the one in the Westman Islands, which usually handles only the small Íslandsflug prop planes from Reykjavík. This entire episode was called, with maybe an unconscious nod to the Berlin airlift of the Cold War in which Iceland occupied a strategic position, "Operation Keiko Lift."

UPS took Keiko from the Oregon Coast Aquarium to the airport, where he was turned over to the air force crew. Technical Sergeant Lono Kollars captured the moment on camera, a picture later posted on the Operation Keiko Lift Web pages (figure 4). The original caption read in part, "Master Sgt. Bill Couture and Staff Sgt. John Gallo sign for their United Parcel Service package, Keiko, the whale star of 'Free Willie' movies."[3] So you see, I imagined only the shorts.

The flight itself was a dense amalgam of military mission, corporate

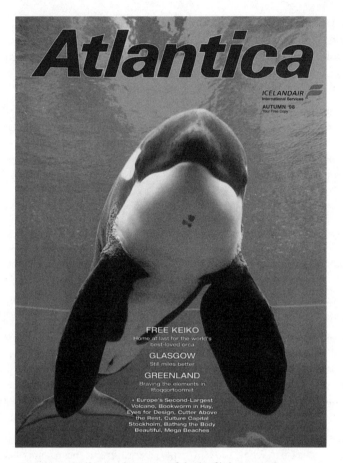

FIGURE 3. Keiko on the cover of the in-flight magazine
of Icelandair, Autumn 1998. Reprinted with permission.

venture, and media sideshow. The Air Force Communications Agency
has a special unit, called the Hammer Adaptive Communications Element (ACE). In describing Hammer ACE's capabilities, the *Air Force
News* suggests something about the global, flexible role played by the U.S.
military:

Hammer ACE is the Air Force's special purpose, quick reaction communications
unit supporting worldwide emergency and disaster response forces, aircraft and
nuclear mishaps/investigations, civil disaster relief operations and military exer-
cises and communications equipment testing/evaluation. . . .
    When Hammer ACE technicians deploy, they take with them some of the

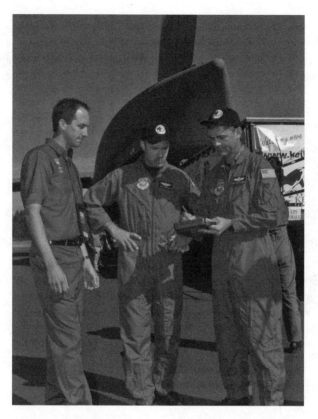

FIGURE 4. Signing for the whale. Photo by Tech. Sgt.
Lono Kollars, U.S. Air Force. Reprinted with permission.

latest communications equipment. These experts and their gear respond to situations as small, fast-moving, flexible teams. They can adapt to any situation's
communications needs with cellular telephones, facsimiles, land mobile radios,
message traffic support, air-to-ground communications, satellite communications
and still-frame photography.[4]

The Hammer ACE team of Master Sergeant Michael D. Riley and
Staff Sergeant Sam Moore, continued *Air Force News,* "worked in conjunction with Ericcson Inc., and RealNetworks and provided near real-
time video documentation of Keiko's 'Flight to Freedom' via the Internet. Internet viewers tuned in to the Free Willy Keiko Foundation web
site at www.keiko.org/webcast/ to watch 30-minute video updates of the
event." It was, the air force said, the first time something like this had

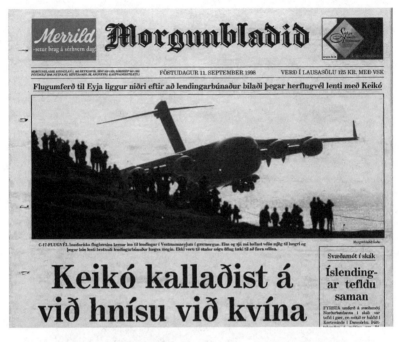

FIGURE 5. Rear page of *Morgunbladid,* September 11, 1998, showing U.S.
Air Force plane delivering Keiko to Iceland. Photo by Ásdís Ásgeirsdóttir.
Reprinted with permission.

been attempted in-flight. Total cost of the mission: $370,000, which, the
air force was at pains to point out, was reimbursed to them by the Free
Willy–Keiko Foundation.

The Icelandic daily *Morgunbladid* carried a rear-page photo on September 11, 1998, showing the C-17 Globemaster III looming over a gag-
gle of reporters and other observers on a cliff of the Westman Islands
(figure 5). The technowhale landed safely, but the plane's landing gear
suffered damage that left the C-17 hulking on the modest runway for a
few days, temporarily stranding the media.

Keiko entered his new football-field-sized floating sea pen designed
to "allow Keiko to be introduced gently to his native environment. . . .
Foam-filled pipes keep the enclosure afloat, which includes, among other
things, a medical pool, food preparation area, dive locker and generator
room, not forgetting sixteen underwater cameras that will allow the rest
of the world to follow Keiko's progress." *Keiko's progress.* Whales, too,
have become pilgrims, embarked on a technoscientific becoming, sam-

pled and monitored in the name of a baroque combination of preservation and evolution.

Keiko stayed in his Westman Islands pen for the next several years, trying to learn again to be "wild." You could watch his progress on the Web site www.keiko.org, where I used to go every once in a while to check out the Keiko Cam live updates that provided images of this movie star orca to kids of all ages around the world. Stories began claiming that Keiko needed finally to learn how to survive on his own, and not from a private foundation's handouts of herring, so he could be truly free to roam the Icelandic seas. Local entrepreneurs also wanted to turn the valuable harbor space occupied by Keiko's sea pen into a commercial fish farm, which generally require the absence of orcas. Keiko's monthly bill, after all, came to about $360,000.[5]

Keiko's progress was beginning to look a little dubious, and there were no further avalanches of attention to be generated. The "live-fish" training went agonizingly slowly, as Keiko continued to prefer eating dead ones. He called out to passing orca kin, and even ventured out of his pen a few times, but never strayed too far and always returned. One day I went to the Keiko.org Web site, only to find an "error—page not found" message. I had a brief moment of panic, until I discovered that I could still find Keiko on the Web, albeit in "Keiko's Corner," part of Jean-Michel Cousteau's Ocean Futures Society. I couldn't tell if this was a step up—I loved watching Jacques Cousteau's television programs as a kid—or if the oblivion of forgetfulness was the next stop after being placed in the corner.

I was surprised again when Keiko left his pen on July 17, 2002. His travels were "monitored closely" via satellite. A month later, he was tracked to about eighty miles north of the Faroe Islands, swimming with other whales, but a spokesperson for the Keiko Association said it was "still too early to assert that Keiko has left his human caretakers and begun to find his own food."[6] But soon after, the whale's progress seems to have recapitulated the migratory pattern of many Icelanders, in reverse: Keiko was in a Norwegian fjord. One Norwegian, not very impressed by celebrity, suggested that the orca be "put down."

TrustXGullibility

> The King of Denmark has paid a visit and I watched him
> come out of the prime minister's house accompanied by
> distinguished citizens. I know top-hats and frock coats don't
> make people look their best, but on their appearance alone
> I wouldn't have trusted one of them with the spoons.
>
> Auden and MacNeice, *Letters from Iceland*, 107

W. H. Auden went to Iceland intending, he said, to escape politics. But soon after he arrived, the Spanish Civil War broke out; Auden would later join (briefly and without much satisfaction, it seems) the International Brigades.

Seeking the isolation that Iceland was supposed to offer, Auden instead found new and renewed connections, ties, and feelings of commitment that would come to shape his work of the next few years. Sometimes he was casual about encounters he was supposed to be avoiding. "I saw Goering['s brother] for a moment at breakfast the next morning," Auden notes nonchalantly in the 1937 *Letters from Iceland*, "and we exchanged politenesses. He didn't look in the least like his brother, but rather academic."[1] Far from being remote and shut off from the world, modern Iceland has long been a place of meetings, crossings, chiasma—a place of politics.

I, too, had looked to Iceland as an opportunity to step outside the inescapable politics of genomics and the Human Genome Project in the United States that I had been immersed in researching since 1989. The politics of genomics were and are, of course, multiple. In the period between

1985 and 1989, there were often intense and sharp disagreements between life scientists of different generations, with different disciplinary specialties, committed to different research organisms from yeast to human, with different institutional affiliations, as to how much money to sink into what strands of technoscientific research and development in how many centers, how fast, with which federal agency, the National Institutes of Health or the U.S. Department of Energy, holding the purse strings. Nobel laureates testified before admiring senators and representatives. Expert panels were convened by the NIH, the DOE, the National Academy of Sciences, and—may it rest in peace—the Office of Technology Assessment of the U.S. Congress. Options were weighed, arms were twisted, promises were made. Many, many promises were made—to heal people, to advance basic science, to encourage new corporate development, to ensure that the United States would dominate a global pharmaceutical industry. Billions of dollars were to be invested in order to fulfill those promises as quickly as possible. *Tax* dollars, it's worth remembering—although worth, remember, is a difficult thing to establish. Simply put: no state, no genomics. Or, saying yes to genomics meant saying yes to the state—at least it did in the United States in the 1980s, and one would be well advised to look for the visible or invisible hand of the state in other states and other times as well.

On top of these politics internal to the state-science assemblage, there were the incessant demands made on scholars like myself to "be political" by commenting on the politics of genetic screening, the perils of genetic reductionism, the specters of eugenics and genetic discrimination—the fissure swarm just goes on and on. Many of these kinds of critiques demanded careful thought and commentary and I found them not only exhausting, but also soul chilling. Nothing like constant suspicion and criticism, however well reasoned and necessary, to dampen the fires of enthusiasm. In September 1998 I still maintained my hope that the Iceland case could offer some fuel for those fires.[2]

Any fantasy that I had of fueling enthusiasm while avoiding politics in Iceland, however, quickly proved unsustainable. The long summer and autumn months of 1998 would later be extolled by many—Kári included—as a most commendable time of "democratic debate." As evidence of democracy, many fingers would point to the hundreds of newspaper, radio, and television stories that appeared in Iceland in 1998, in which deCODE and the Health Sector Database were presented and discussed—as well as town meetings like the one I attended in Húsavík.[3] In this book democracy will come up for review again and again, since this is what democracy is supposed to do. We start here with the intersection of democracy and the media in Iceland—a heavily trafficked intersection where I sometimes feared for my safety.

I was becoming convinced, through my advance man's tireless efforts, that more media opportunities were better than fewer. I agreed to all that Skúli arranged. If this was not without its elements of pride and vanity, it was also not without its elements of honestly felt intellectual responsibility. It was also a hoot. I got to see the lobby of the state radio broadcasting agency (established in 1930), where the display of large old phonographs and Telefunken radios summoned fleeting fuzzy images of invisible electromagnetic waves lapping at the Western Fjords for decades, weaving woolened Icelanders crouched around radios in one-window turf houses into family and nation. I was there to be interviewed by one of the station's regular commentators. This radio personality tended toward the old reliable "should we be playing god?" and "aren't these things unnatural?" questions, with the predictable figures of Frankenstein and Jeremy Rifkin making appearances. I leaned into the microphone to offer a few kind words for the monster and a few unkind ones for Rifkin. Better a lurching, sutured, nature-culture assemblage with a bone to pick with his maker than a preaching purist. Besides, I added, hadn't we already become somewhat monstrous in our creation of and affection for unnatural things like radio technology? What mattered more than big abstractions like god and nature were specific, concrete arrangements and making thoughtful decisions about creating and deploying them—assuming for the moment that there were decisions to make and that it was possible to make them. The interviewer asked my opinion of the Health Sector Database bill; I demurred.

Another time, Skúli and I had coffee and a chat with a senior editor at the *Morgunbladid* newspaper, who in the made-for-TV-movie version of these events will be played by the hastily manufactured clone of Ed Asner. Charmingly crusty, one arm slung over the back of his chair as he regaled his visitors with frank stories carefully designated as off the record, he admitted to being somewhat tired of the whole damn issue, as well as disappointed with the lack of subtlety and nuance that had come to characterize the endless public debate about the HSD and deCODE. *Morgunbladid* nevertheless continued to feature the most unsubtle, glowing articles about deCODE, salted by the most occasional expression of skepticism.

Those were the easy, fun times. Occasionally, though, these encounters with the media took on frenzied, disorienting proportions. In the hour before my third public lecture—the dreaded one on "bioethics"—I was photographed for one newspaper, interviewed by another reporter for Icelandic State Radio, and interviewed in front of a video camera outside in the stiff wind by a fairly witless but certifiably handsome television personality. In these and all my other media ops, I was always asked for my opinion on the HSD legislation. And although I knew I could not avoid politics any more than Auden could, I did my best to sidestep any direct answer. "There are already a lot of very strong opinions on the legislation," I tried to say, "and I don't know enough about Icelandic politics to add anything of value." And then I would try to inject something more indirect: that the issues were complicated and required long, patient analysis and discussion; that like all ecological systems, the biomedical research ecology needed diversity, and the government would have to increase funding for the national hospital and university systems, *especially* if Iceland developed a strong private biotech sector; that difference and disagreement were good and should be heard and respected rather than pathologized and trivialized.

I was all too aware that I was treading that fine fissure between the cool, detached data-gathering mode of ethnographic fieldwork as usually conceived and some yet-to-congeal ethic and method of magma ethnography—hot, viscous, unpredictable, and well worth keeping an alert eye on. In chapter 11, I discuss this as a process of becoming complicit, where complicity is a matter of folds, *pli*. I did pay careful attention to these kinds of folds, in which the languages and demands of the generic ethnographic Other—whether a state broadcasting network, a politician, or a scientist—get folded into the ethnographer's thoughts and acts like beaten egg whites into a chocolaty liquid. It's a delicate operation: folding that is too vigorous or that goes on for too long produces unappealing results; too little is just as much a mistake.

A year or so later, when comparing my soufflé of ethnographic complicity to the recipes advanced by other professionals, I asked one of my interlocutors, an Icelandic scientist working in the United States, for his own reading of my Icelandic media persona. Had I overstepped the bounds of neutrality? Had I taken sides too soon, or too visibly? I cared about the answer to these unbelievably traditional questions. Since I had no recollection of what I had said to the artist/*Dagur* reporter, was incapable of reading the printed article, and could trust Skúli only for a strong-willed opinion, I asked for a reading by a third party: "Thank you very much for your letter. I had already read the Dagur interview. You come across, if anything, as pro deCODE. The journalist is asking you very specific questions, trying to make you take a stand on the debate, and you seem to be making efforts to wiggle yourself out of it."[4] Wiggling, as any child of two can tell you, is exhausting, and you don't always end up with the freedom you were trying to achieve.

Several hours after the above-mentioned frenzy of photos and interviews, I sat with Skúli in his car and listened to the state radio news; in the few hours while I delivered my third public talk on ethics, the reporter had put her story together for broadcast. It followed another story about the release of a legal report (written by Jón Steinar Gunnlaugsson and Karl Axelsson) favoring the database legislation; Skúli translated, adding that they failed to mention that the report had been commissioned by deCODE. The next story appeared to present "the other side." Within the Icelandic floe, I heard one English sound bite in a voice I eventually recognized as mine: "The absolutely wrong way to go about these things is fast."

All the complexities and subtleties of speed, its contradictions and attractions and dangers, that I had tried to convey in my first talk, had been reduced to this simple message: Slow down, Iceland! The half hour I had spent talking to this reporter had been boiled down to this one liner, which included a word that I hardly ever employed consciously, "absolutely." Ridiculous, futile, wrong. Skúli was very pleased; I was near despair.

XX

From another angle, the public discussion about the HSD legislation was nothing less than glacial. And from that other angle, a glacial pace was absolutely appropriate to the complexity of the proposal and the number of details and their interactions that had to be considered—not to mention their spectral future possibilities. By this time (September 1998), various expert organizations had taken the necessary time to produce their own analyses and recommendations about the HSD. The majority of these were negative.

My sound bite, I realized later, echoed one of the main themes sounded by the Ethics Council of the Icelandic Medical Association (IMA) in their analysis:

It is obvious from the public debate that it is impracticable to deal with a bill like this in only a few months. There are simply too many unclear points. It is unclear what information is to go into the database. It is unclear how the information in the database is to be linked to other databases, such as the genetics and genealogical databases or biological specimen banks. It has not been convincingly shown that it is necessary to collect data in the fashion provided for by the bill. No estimate exists as to whether it is possible to deliver on the promises which, directly or indirectly, have been made. No argument has been produced to show that the main objectives of the bill cannot be attained by linking distributed databases. Therefore the possible advantages of the database are uncertain.[5]

Here the Ethics Council recognizes that promises do not have to be made directly—"I promise you that . . ."—but can also occur through a more indirect modality, although the IMA's Ethics Council does not directly state what might qualify as such an indirect promise. We can only remind ourselves again of the questions: *how are promises made, kept, and/or delivered?*

But if evaluating or "estimating" promises is an uncertain procedure, unclear on multiple scores, people still do it all the time. When Sigurdur Gudmundsson, who became director general of public health of Iceland in the fall of 1998 (succeeding Ólafur Ólafsson, who had been critical of the HSD), was asked questions about privacy issues and the kinds of discrimination that might arise from the Icelandic database in the future, he began by acknowledging the formal undecidability of the promise:

None of these questions can be answered. I have done loops in the air all year long. And it has been painful. Of course there are serious dangers. Is it scary? Very. But we have to find a way to make this happen. The benefits just outweigh the problems. It doesn't mean there are no doubts. We are walking into a new world. But I don't think it is wild to say this may turn out to be a tool like none other. And I don't think this country can just sit here and say, Nope, sorry, we are going to stand on rules that existed in a different era for a different world.[6]

It's unclear what happens between the statement "None of these questions can be answered" and the statement "The benefits just outweigh the problems." How was such an impossible weighing undertaken? How does one transition from doing painful loops through the substanceless air of speculation to the apparent ground of "a tool like none other," which the HSD *may* turn out to be? How, in the impossible evaluation of an (in)direct promise, does one discriminate between the "wild" and the sober? How does one know that old rules don't apply in a genuinely new world?

There were many old rules, laws, and regulations that the HSD was being weighed against. These included international regulations regarding the exchange of data within the European Economic Community (EEC) and similar EEC and European Free Trade Area (EFTA) regulations to which Iceland was supposed to be subject. The IMA's Ethics Council gestured to some of these, and also to previous legislation passed in Iceland with which the HSD legislation seemed to be in conflict, before concluding with a promise of its own in the form of a threat:

The committee of ECIMA considers that the draft bill on a health sector database is in breach of art. 10 of the law on the rights of patients from 1997 and paragraph 4 of art. 2 of the same concerning consent to scientific research. The committee of ECIMA also considers that the bill is in breach of the Council of Europe's rules on bioethics.

The committee of ECIMA considers that discussion of the draft bill is still in its early stages and that many questions remain unanswered concerning personal privacy. The committee is completely opposed to the present bill and will advise Icelandic physicians not to participate in the setting up of the database.[7]

The exclusive twelve-year license was another major boulder in this glacial floe of opinions, along with privacy and informed consent. Consider the report of the University of Iceland Medical School's Committee on Medical Databases:

The committee's majority advises against permitting construction of a centralised medical database. . . . Such a database would violate basic principles of science ethics as it would contain coded but not anonymous information on individuals. Scientific research by exclusive licensee for the database, including linking together comprehensive data on individual medical history, genealogy and genetics, would not be subject to review and approval by the National Bioethics Committee or other public supervising agencies such as the Data Protection Committee. Conducting genetic research on individuals without their knowledge or informed consent addressing whether and how results will be communicated to the participants, will never be approved by the international science community. If Iceland decides on such a system it will meet with widespread international opposition and contempt.

The centralised database will first and foremost serve the interests of the exclusive licensee at the expense of all others. It is the opinion of the committee's majority that a centralised medical database, if approved by law, will greatly limit the ability of Icelandic medical doctors and scientists to conduct research and participate in international collaborations, in addition to creating unacceptable legal quandaries.

The majority concludes that decentralised databases are superior to a centralised one and that the construction of a centralised database cannot be justified based on its potential for scientific research. . . . Creation of a centralised database will transfer very valuable information from the healthcare system to the proprietor of the database. It has not been demonstrated that a centralised database is the best option for further development of biotechnology in Iceland. On the contrary, it will hamper biotechnological industries because of the proprietor's in effect monopoly on medical research.[8]

The IMA and the University of Iceland Medical School represent only a few of the Icelandic institutions that commented on the second draft of the HSD legislation, released in July of 1998. The director general of public health (before he left office), the Science Ethics Committee, the Data Protection Committee, the Icelandic Cancer Society, the Icelandic

Mental Health Alliance, the Icelandic Medical Association, the Icelandic Consumers Association, the Center for Genetics of the University of Iceland, the Medical Faculty of the University of Iceland, the Blood Bank and even the sponsoring Ministry of Health's own Ethics Committee all registered a position of "strongly against." Other organizations like the Ethics Research Center of the University of Iceland, the Competition Authority, the Icelandic Nurses Association, and the Icelandic Research Council held that the legislation raised "serious concerns."[9]

The various positions were summed up by a nongovernmental organization that constituted itself in October 1998, Mannvernd (Icelandic for "human protection"), the Association of Icelanders for Ethics in Science and Medicine. This grassroots group of "scientists, physicians, and other concerned citizens" will be discussed in more detail later. In the fall of 1998, they began documenting the controversy on their Web site, which became an invaluable source of information and opinion to multiple international communities. Mannvernd produced a chart (compiled by Tómas Helgason) of the main bones of contention in the HSD legislation and compiled opinions from organizations and individuals (figure 6).

At the end of November 1998, the Althingi's Health Committee concluded its examination of the legislation. Some revisions were made to the summer's second draft of the legislation, but the main provisions were still there and, according to Mannvernd, still problematic:

The main criticism against the bill has not been taken into account and an exclusive license to a single operator is still being proposed. Essentially, sensitive health information covering the whole Icelandic population, will be donated to a private American company, without seeking the consent of individuals. "Presumed consent" instead of "informed consent" is still the ethical basis of the database. The bill has no provision regarding the rights of those unable to deny registration, i.e., children, the mentally disabled or demented, or the deceased through their living relatives. Death, therefore, will deprive Icelanders of their rights and dignity.[10]

In early December, the Icelandic newspaper *DV* reported that about one-third of the nation's general practitioners had signed a letter to members of Parliament, informing them that they would not send information about their patients into the proposed central database unless they got a written request from the patient.[11] The more conservative *Morgunbladid* published an opinion piece the same day by engineer Páll Pálsson, said to be a member of Prime Minister Davíd Oddsson's "inner circle" of informal advisors. Pálsson criticized the monopoly provision: "Individuals who believe in

Legend: ▓ Opposed/negative ☐ Opinion not clear ▒ Agrees/positive

Association/individual	The bill/central database	Patient consent	Scientific freedom	Exclusive license	Nature of data entered
The Blood Bank	Opposed	Opposed	Opposed	Opposed	Opposed
Dr. Bogi Andersen	Opposed	Opposed	Opposed	Opposed	Not clear
Federation of State and Municipal Employees	Opposed	Opposed	Opposed	Opposed	Not clear
Genetical Committee of the Univ. of Iceland	Opposed	Opposed	Opposed	Opposed	Opposed
Dr. Ernir Snorrason	Opposed	Not clear	Opposed	Opposed	Not clear
Icelandic Podiatrist Association	Not clear	Not clear	Not clear	Not clear	Not clear
Icelandic Nurses Association	Agrees	Opposed	Opposed	Opposed	Opposed
Félag íslenskra sjúkrathjálfara	Not clear	Opposed	Opposed	Opposed	Opposed
Félag læknaritara	Opposed	Opposed	Not clear	Not clear	Opposed
Icelandic Mental Health Alliance	Opposed	Not clear	Opposed	Opposed	Opposed
Mental Health Association	Opposed	Opposed	Opposed	Opposed	Opposed
Western District Chief Physician	Not clear	Opposed	Opposed	Not clear	Not clear
The Icelandic Heart Association	Not clear	Not clear	Not clear	Not clear	Not clear
Dr. Jóhann Malmquist	Opposed	Not clear	Not clear	Not clear	Not clear
The Icelandic Cancer Society	Opposed	Opposed	Opposed	Opposed	Not clear
Icelandic Directorate of Health	Opposed	Not clear	Opposed	Opposed	Opposed
Federation of Icelandic Health Care Centers	Not clear	Not clear	Opposed	Not clear	Opposed
Federation of Icelandic Hospitals	Not clear	Opposed	Not clear	Not clear	Opposed
Univ. of Iceland Department of Pharmacy	Not clear	Opposed	Opposed	Not clear	Opposed
Univ. of Iceland Faculty of Medicine	Opposed	Opposed	Opposed	Opposed	Opposed
Univ. of Iceland Faculty of Medicine (minority)	Agrees	Opposed	Opposed	Agrees	Opposed
Icelandic Medical Association	Opposed	Opposed	Opposed	Opposed	Opposed
Reykjavík Medical Association	Opposed	Opposed	Opposed	Opposed	Not clear
The Medical Board of Reykjavík Hospital	Opposed	Opposed	Opposed	Opposed	Not clear
Icelandic Human Rights Center	Opposed	Opposed	Not clear	Not clear	Not clear
Mannvernd	Opposed	Opposed	Opposed	Opposed	Opposed
Center of Genetics, Univ. of Iceland	Opposed	Opposed	Opposed	Opposed	Opposed
The Icelandic MS Society	Agrees	Agrees	Agrees	Agrees	Agrees
Department of Nursing, Univ. of Iceland	Opposed	Opposed	Opposed	Opposed	Opposed
Consumer Association	Opposed	Opposed	Opposed	Opposed	Not clear

FIGURE 6. The NGO Mannvernd summarized opinions on the Health Sector Database legislation in this chart and gave it to the Health Committee of the Althingi. Adapted with permission from Mannvernd, www.mannvernd.is/english/.

Association/individual	The bill/central database	Patient consent	Scientific freedom	Exclusive license	Nature of data entered
Fifteen full and assoc. professors, Faculty of Medicine, Univ. of Iceland					
The Icelandic Research Council					
Faculty of Natural Sciences, Univ. of Iceland					
State Trading Center					
National Univ. Hospitals–Council of Cooperating Hospitals					
Dr. Ross Andersen					
Competition and Fair Trade Authority					
Federation of Icel. Industries–Federation of Software Companies					
The Ethical Committee of the Directorate of Health					
Ethical Committee, Icelandic Medical Association					
Center for Ethical Studies, Univ. of Iceland					
The Icelandic Accident Prevention Council					
National Union of Icelandic Pharmacologists					
Board of Directors, Reykjavík Hospital					
Faculty of Odontology, Univ. of Iceland					
Data Protection Committee					
European Data Protection Commission (Peter J. Hustinx)					
National Bioethics Committee					
National Federation for the Handicapped					
Opposed/negative	67%	73%	63%	59%	51%
Opinion not clear	18%	20%	35%	31%	47%
Agrees/positive	14%	6%	2%	10%	2%

Opinions from deCODE employees or individuals paid by deCODE

Association/individual	The bill/central database	Patient consent	Scientific freedom	Exclusive license	Nature of data entered
Hákon Gudbjartsson (deCODE employee)					
Högni Óskarsson (deCODE associate)					
Jón L. Arnalds (lawyer paid by deCODE)					
Jón Steinar Gunnlaugsson (lawyer paid by deCODE)					
The Law Institute, Univ. of Iceland (an opinion from three institute lawyers paid by deCODE)					

market economy, who have put their faith on individual freedom and the power of competition have difficulty accepting that at a time when monopolies and special licenses are being done away with in many fields in our society people are thinking of introducing this very ideology into biotechnology, one of the most important knowledge bases of the future, and thereby disturb the development of the market in a field which perhaps will be very important in our economy in the decades to come."[12]

In December 1998, nine months after these issues had first been sprung on the physicians, scientists, and other "concerned citizens" of Iceland, the disagreements were, if anything, more pronounced. The Althingi vote loomed.

XX

The conservative Independence Party had effectively controlled the Althingi since 1991, when Davíd Oddsson became prime minister and his Independence Party (Sjálfstaedisflokkurinn) formed a coalition first with the Social Democrats and then, in 1995, with the Centrist Party (Framsóknarflokkurinn). Oddsson had attended the same secondary school as Kári, although each maintained that the history was immaterial.

Pens, however, are definitely material. And it was Prime Minister Davíd Oddsson who, in February 1998, in a public ceremony held in the restaurant in the futuristic Perlan dome atop the geothermal tanks that store surplus hot water for Reykjavík, passed the pen between Kári and the representative of Hoffmann-LaRoche as they signed the potential $200 million promise. It was Oddsson who, in this role of statesman and middleman, said "I view this agreement as a huge step toward securing high technology industries an important role in the Icelandic economy. The government of Iceland will do its best to assist the two parties in the agreement to achieve the goals of the collaboration."[13]

Oddsson never seemed to entertain the uncertainties about the HSD that the director general of public health, personal advisors, and others did. Like them, however, Oddsson had to acknowledge the difficult demands presented by a future that remained promised. He summed up his sentiments and beliefs to *The New Yorker*'s Michael Specter in 1998:

Obviously, this is all about trust. In Iceland, trust is everything. I once saw a documentary about a famous defense attorney. He was asked, "How do you choose a jury?" He said, "First, I take out all the people who wear bow ties—because they are not likely to be part of a team. Then I get rid of everyone of Northern European descent. They are too trusting and they all believe in authority. When the police testify, Northern Europeans and Scandinavians tend to believe they are telling the truth." At first I was outraged and considered it a complete stereotype. But I sat there and thought about it for five minutes and I realized he was completely right. I happen to be proud of that quality and I think it says something about why we are willing to put ourselves forward and make this database work.[14]

Leave aside any question of the validity of the ethnic characterization, and assume that Oddsson is right. Oddsson opens up the whole domain of government, founded on the law as much as an organism is founded on its DNA, to the operations or demands of strategy and expediency. He confirms for us that juries are *made,* not found or founded—they are strategized for particular hoped-for effects. Decisions are engineered— not completely, maybe not even sufficiently, but the attempt is made. In the midst of an "open debate" in Icelandic society, the prime minister relates a story, under the heading of trust, about engineering decisions.

He also expresses his admiration for "that quality," but the referent is slippery: Trust? Or "belief in authority"? Are these the same thing? Would Oddsson have been comfortable saying about the HSD legislation, "Obviously, this is all about belief in authority; in Iceland, belief in authority is everything"? Are there limits to trust, or does one trust *anyone* who makes *any* promise? How would such limits be established and tested? What gives a promise enough authority to be trusted?

XX

I had returned home long before mid-October 1998, when the vote on the second version of the Health Sector Database Act was scheduled to occur in the Althingi. Much of the action had shifted behind the doors of Parliament by that time, and the action went on longer than anyone had thought or planned. November came and went, and while the bill was revised again all those individuals and organizations who were critical of the legislation remained so.

Hjörleifur Guttormsson of the People's Alliance political party was one of the leaders of opposition to the bill. He had a long-standing interest in things biological, having an early 1960s degree in biology from Leipzig, and he followed biotechnology and genetics as part of his civic role. "Genetics was a new area for most of the people in Iceland, including the politicians, who did not know much about genetics," he told me in an interview in 2001. "What helped me in this, and what made me voice such strong views even at the beginning, was that I had followed developments in this field since 1985—scientifically, as well as the practical steps being taken for genetics in biotechnology. I was part of the Nordic Council, following issues in Scandinavia. Also through contacts in Brussels, I was working for my party on issues related to the European Economic Area [EEA] and European Free Trade Association [EFTA], which was another big issue in the last decade. So this close watch helped me form my views on the database bill."

Hjörleifur struck me as someone I *would* trust with the spoons, contrary to Auden's blanket observation about top-hatted and frock-coated Icelandic politicians. Hjörleifur had long been involved in Icelandic politics, joining the Youth Movement of the Centrist Party as a boy of twelve growing up in eastern Iceland and eventually being elected to the Althingi as a member of the People's Alliance. When I characterized the People's Alliance as a "splinter group" of the Communist Party, based on what I had read in a cursory history of Iceland, Hjörleifur gently corrected me:

In Iceland there existed a Communist Party only in the period 1930–1938, being a member of the Comintern International. From this party and a group of left Social Democrats there was formed the United Socialist party, which was on the stage from 1938 until 1956. Then a new electoral platform of socialists and left Social Democrats was formed, named the People's Alliance, and this alliance became a regular political party in 1968, keeping the same name. The political opponents of the Socialist Party and later of the People's Alliance tried to stamp both those parties as Communist organizations, especially in the rhetoric abroad.

While the HSD legislation was being debated and revised, the People's Alliance was undergoing its own revision. Most of its members voted to form a new, larger party by combining with the Social Democrats and the Women's Party, two other left-of-center political parties in Iceland, in the hopes of constituting a serious challenge to the conservative coalition that had been in power for nearly a decade. Hjörleifur, a twenty-year veteran of the Althingi by that time, respectfully disagreed with this strategy and instead helped establish an entirely new party, the Left-Green Party, with like-minded people from the People's Alliance and the Women's Party. Power based on size was not an issue for him. "I have never believed in participation in government as an aim as such. I believe that a minority has an important role—not just as part of a coalition government. The Left-Green Party would join a coalition of course, but that is not the aim as such. The real aim is to influence the electorate, and change politics indirectly as a result." The party's four chief planks were "conservation of the environment," "equality and social justice," "fair and prosperous economy," and "independent foreign policy." It continued to oppose NATO and any other military installations in Iceland, and rejected participation in the European Union (EU).

"This is of course a very big issue in Iceland," Hjörleifur took time to remind me in the midst of our discussion about the territory that most interested me, the lava land of genomics. But he highlighted the geographical aspect to the EU issue as well: "The Left-Green Party is quite clear on this: we don't think it is good for Iceland to become a member of the EU. We will try to keep Iceland out of the big power blocs in the east and west, but with good ties to the U.S., to the U.K., Scandinavia, and other parts of the world. To use Iceland's unique geographical position to be independent, but a good partner to the outside world."

But all that reshuffling and strategizing of political geography was still in the future in the autumn of 1998. We returned to the subject of the HSD legislation. "I know that the first version of the HSD legislation was written very badly," I said. "Surely Oddsson and his health minister and the rest didn't actually think it was going to pass through so quickly and easily in the spring?" Hjörleifur replied:

That was the clear intention, to pass the legislation as it was written in March 1998. The first sign that you saw that something was happening was the signing of the agreement between deCODE and Hoffmann-LaRoche. You have maybe seen it on video? That was very, very interesting to see the prime minister of Iceland in that position between those two. I wonder how close he was in the preparation of the legislation, or what part of this big project he understood, I'm not sure. What he understood at least, and a big part of the motivation as I understand it, was to get foreign capital directly or indirectly into the country, a new firm in a new field with the prospect of a lot of people working there, especially scientists. All these positive things . . .

There was no mention of a centralized database around this event, as far as I can remember. Maybe you could find something in March, that there was something going on in the Ministry of Health. But it wasn't until the last days of March that you heard that a new bill was being worked on in the Ministry. And then it was presented on 31 March, and the first discussion was on 7 April. And declared by the minister of health [Ingibjörg Pálmadóttir] to the media, before the discussion began in Parliament, that this would be passed by the end of the session, in the first week of May. She was quite firm on this, that it would be passed.

But after the first reading, many questions were raised in Parliament. And the bill went to the Committee on Health and didn't come out to the plenary again in April. And the science community woke up in those days, and it created a big debate in the media, as you know. And of course this influenced the process dramatically. I cannot say what would have happened if it was only up to the parliamentarians, but I stress that the debate outside had a very big influence on what happened at the end of April: that the minister of health accepted that she would not press the bill becoming a law, and made a "contract" with the chairman of the committee [Össur Skarphéðinsson], being a member of the opposition—the first time that the opposition got a chair of a committee—I think I can say a "private contract," with quotation marks. It was not taken up by the committee in any way, it was between him and the minister—that the ministry would take the bill back, work on it over the summer, present it at the beginning of the autumn session in October, and that it should be passed within three weeks of the beginning of the session. That would mean 21 October or so.

I criticized this move by the chairman, and made it public in the media and in Parliament, that this was not a wise move by Parliament. The committee should keep the bill and work on it during summer, and present its view to Parliament at the beginning of the next session, instead of handing it back to the ministry, keeping silent, doing nothing during summer, and meeting a new version presented by the Ministry during autumn.

We are not in the abstract territory of "democracy" and "democratic debate" here, despite repeated references to these bloodless terms in subsequent narrations of these events. We are in the same territory that Oddsson unwittingly described when he discussed the strategies of decision making by jury making, a territory where "private contracts" are in play.

Over the summer of 1998, Hjörleifur compiled an extensive set of documents and analyses related to the HSD legislation. He introduced these as another formal part of the parliamentary discussion in addition to the act itself.

One issue that I stressed was the aspect of the health registers [medical records]. The Law on the Rights of Patients was passed in May 1997. And a very interesting change took place in the parliamentary work on that bill, concerning the ownership of health registers.

In the bill presented by government, the health institutions—hospitals, etc.—were declared to be the owner of the records. This was taken out by the Parliament, and nothing was clearly stated or decided as to who owns the register, not to mention who owns the information in the register. Not to talk about who was the owner of the information. And I presented the view that the patient himself or herself is the owner of the information given to the register, so it is illegal and unethical to take that information without informed consent. And I view this as one of the central issues to be taken to court. I think the answer could fall in favor of the patient, and not in favor of the institution. This has not been taken up by the doctors, I don't know why.

Despite some last-minute difficulties, as we'll see, it was becoming clear that the majority in Parliament was going to pass the legislation. By early December, there was only one more thing for Hjörleifur to try: the filibuster. Or, as he preferred to call it, gently chiding me for employing a word with such vulgar connotations, "a very long speech." Unlike a filibuster, his speeches were substantive, he said, with the serious intent of "demonstrating to the Parliament and the public that this is a big issue."

>   *Mike:*   OK, so you didn't filibuster but gave a very long substantive speech. But how long are we talking about? I've been to enough Icelandic meetings to know that there's a different speech culture here. Even at a birthday party I was at, there was a speech that lasted nearly an hour! In the U.S. we sing "Happy Birthday" for about thirty seconds and get on with it. So how long was it? And do you do that kind of thing often?

>   *Hjörleifur:*   On three other occasions I have held long speeches in Parliament— I mean speeches taking longer than two hours. One was when I was minister of industry in 1983; this was on the issue of transfer pricing and AluSuisse, the aluminum company with the smelter here. We took on AluSuisse, and we had very strong arguments that they had been cheating the Icelanders on transfer pricing on bauxite from Australia to Iceland. They increased the value at sea; the term "increase at sea" became part of the vocabulary of Icelanders at this time. The parliamentary coalition I was part of was dissolving just before the election. The government had been pressing on this case for two years, and it was a very hot potato in Parliament, and I was the focal point as minister. And I together with my fellow minister from the People's Alliance met a proposal initiated by the Conservative Party for a vote of no confidence on me—I met it with a long speech. It was clear they couldn't pass it.

Another occasion for a very long speech also involved aluminum (smelting it requires huge amounts of electric power, and Iceland's "unique geographical location" gives it plenty), in that case the construction of a new smelting facility. And the third came in a debate over Iceland's participation in the European Economic Area: "There were a lot of people opposing it, so I didn't have to speak too long—two or three hours." But Hjörleifur outdid himself, even by the Icelandic system of speech measurement, in the final hours before the database vote in mid-December 1998:

>   *Hjörleifur:*   I was informed during the night that the presidency had promised not to continue the session past 1:00 A.M. or so. This was said to me. I got the word after midnight, and my information

was that maybe in one hour it would stop. As this didn't happen, I continued.

Mike: What time did you stop?

Hjörleifur: At five o'clock in the morning.

Mike: Does everybody have to stay?

Hjörleifur: No, no. But I had some people up on the balcony. It was refreshing.

XX

Halldór Laxness may not have employed the term "increase at sea," but don't think that he didn't understand the operation or that the Icelandic economy wasn't sufficiently "global" in 1948.

When we last saw Ugla in *The Atom Station,* she was discussing the status of counterfeit money with the beatnik Brilliantine, who reduced money to nothing and economic activity to stealing. Ugla asked him from whom he had stolen his Cadillac.

"From whom but our master, Pliers?" said the god. "What, you haven't heard of Pliers? Two Hundred Thousand Pliers? F.F.F.? The man who sits in New York and fakes the figures for the joint-stock company Snorredda and the rest? And wrote an article in the papers about the next world and built a church in the north?"

"You must forgive me if I'm a little slow in the uptake," I said. "I'm from the country."

"There's no difficulty in understanding it," he said. "F.F.F.: in English, the Federation of Fulminating Fish, New York; in Icelandic, the Figures-Faking-Federation. One button costs half an eyrir over there in the west, but you have a company in New York, the F.F.F., which sells you the button at two krónur and writes on the invoice: button, two krónur. You make a profit of four thousand percent. After a month you're a millionaire. You can understand that?"[15]

Ugla asks the minister in whose home she works about Pliers. The minister relates some of Pliers's history and expresses some hopes for his future:

While he was a straightforward drunkard and businessman, newly arrived from the north, he bought two pliers and five anvils for every single Icelander; hair nets, six for each and every person; an unlimited quantity of boiled American water in cans, to use in soups; ten-year-old sardines from Portugal; and enough baking powder to blow up the whole country. . . . Finally, he had resolved to buy up all the raisins in the world and import them to Iceland, but by that time he had also lost his voice except that he continually screeched the vowel A. The Snorredda company saved him. We adore idiots. We are hoping that Two Hundred Thousand Pliers can become a Minister. (59)

Meanwhile, the negotiations over building a base in Iceland for global atomic warfare are heating up. The "nice Americans" come to the minister's house around midnight, but they don't stay long. After they leave, the politicians come, talk through most of the night, and leave "remarkably sober." But every day after these "clandestine but dignified" meetings at the minister's house, a more public crowd appears at the other end of the street, at the prime minister's house. These crowds go by different names, but they all deliver addresses and petitions "not to sell the country; not to hand over their sovereignty; not to let foreigners build themselves an atom station here for use in an atomic war; Youth Fellowships, schools, the University Citizens' Association, the Road-Sweepers' Association, the Women's Guild, the Office-Workers' Association, the Artists' Association, the Equestrian Association" (66).

There is great "unrest in the town," and plenty of speeches are given about "this one thing" on which the nation obsessively fixated:

You can impose on us limitless taxes; you can have companies that add many thousand per cent to the prices of foreign goods we buy off you; you can buy two pliers and ten anvils a head, and buy Portuguese sardines for all the nation's currency; you can devalue the krona as much as you like when you have managed to make it worthless; you can make us starve; you can make us stop living in houses—our forefathers did not live in houses, only turf hovels, and they were yet men; everything, everything, everything, except only this, this, this: do not hand over the sovereignty which we have battled for seven hundred years to regain, we charge you, Sir, in the name of everything that is sacred to this nation, do not make our young republic a mere appendage to a foreign atom station; only that, only that; and nothing but that. (66–67)

Over time, the crowds in the streets swell and the speeches become more vehement. The Althingi meets in secret session. The "pressure of the throng" eventually bursts open the Parliament doors, and people stream in and sing the patriotic song "Our Fjord-Riven Fatherland." Soon the prime minister appears on a balcony, lifts three fingers on the air, and makes an oath, a promise: "I swear—swear—swear: by everything which is and has been sacred to this nation from the beginning: Iceland shall not be sold" (67).

XX

I defer to Mannvernd, the NGO that was formed in these shortening Icelandic days and that will be discussed in more detail later, to describe the final scenes:

The 3rd discussion in Parliament was temporarily postponed at 2 AM this morning in the middle of the speech by MP Jóhanna Sigurdardóttir. The 3rd discussion will resume at 12 noon today Wednesday 16 December with Jóhanna continuing her speech which she said would be shorter than the speech she was prepared to hold into the late hours last night. The Speaker agreed to this. The opposition is thus using delaying tactics to the full extent of Parliamentary procedures. How much longer they can hold out is doubtful, so the vote will come later today or tomorrow. The delaying is important because public awareness is slowly being raised that something fishy is going on. The more public awareness the better Mannvernd will stand in the job ahead when the bill has been passed: to educate the public and to oppose the creation and operation of the database using legal action to the full extent of the law.

Miss Vigdís Finnbogadóttir, former President of Iceland [1980–1996], is reported to have resigned from the board of deCODE Genetics, Inc., according to the Icelandic State Radio reported at 5 o'clock newshour Tuesday 15 December. According to deCODE spokesman the reasons for Miss Vigdís's decision for stepping down from the board is that sitting on the board of a biotechnology company is in conflict with her role as head of a UNESCO Committee on Ethics in Science and Technology. . . .

The bill was then sent back to the Health Committee. The Committee called in the Data Protection Committee and deCODE representative today, Friday 11 December. The committee refused requests from several bodies, including the National Bioethics Committee and Mannvernd . . . to express their views.

At this moment it seems only a miracle can bring the Icelandic government to its senses. A miracle is considered rather unlikely. A battle is lost but the fight goes on. Pragmatists are therefore already considering next steps in the fight: legal action and civil disobedience are being considered. Condemnation from abroad is welcomed. Please write to the government of Iceland and express your disgust/ happiness with the legislation. Flood them with mail.[16]

The final vote came on December 17, 1998: 37 in favor, 20 against, 6 abstaining. The Health Sector Database Act was law. An unnamed future licensee of the future government database—the suspense was surely killing people: would it be deCODE?—would enjoy a twelve-year exclusive license to the health records of the nation; and the 275,000 Icelanders then living immediately found themselves in the curious position of having given their consent—although *given* is actually a misnomer, since the consent was simply *presumed,* and the HSD Act required no actual act of giving—to have their health records included in the future database. But if getting a new past in which you've consented to be included in a future database seems weird, consider the far stranger ontological fissure that opened around the ghosts of Icelanders past: their consent to be in the database was also presumed. Suddenly, somehow, these spirits were *there* on December 17, made present by an altered past and promised future.

PromisesXPromises

You can only pay so much for promises.

Motley Fool

Genomics is real. In the end, I am sure its promise will materialize.

Jürgen Drews, former president for
global research at Hoffmann-LaRoche

"Biotech valuations in Germany are not built on anything fundamental," says Michael Sistenich, a fund manager at DWS. He says chief executives promise more than they can deliver to build up their valuations.

Financial Times

Linkage analysis and positional cloning have had a remarkable track record in leading to the identification of the genes for many mendelian diseases, all within the time span of the past two decades. Several of these genes account for an uncommon subset of generally more common disorders such as breast cancer (BRCA-1 and -2), colon cancer (familial adenomatous polyposis [FAP] and hereditary non-polyposis colorectal cancer [HNPCC]), Alzheimer's disease (β-amyloid precursor protein [APP] and presinilin-1 and -2) and diabetes (maturity-onset diabetes of youth [MODY]-1, -2, and -3). These successes have generated a strong sense of optimism in the genetics community that the same approach holds great promise for identifying genes for a range of common, familial disorders, including those without clear mendelian inheritance patterns. But so far the promise has largely been unfulfilled, as numerous such diseases have proven refractive to positional cloning.

Neil Risch, population geneticist

As I've said in the past, [Genentech] has a promising pipeline and room to grow based on its cancer and cardiovascular drugs. . . . The potential for IDEC [Pharmaceuticals] will get better as the company's promising compound Zevalin comes to market. . . . With that in mind, the outlook for the remainder of 2000 is quite promising.

WorldlyInvestor.com

DeCODE promises that Icelanders will get any drugs or diagnostics based on their genes for free during the patent period—a promise [Jórunn] Eyfjörd calls "a joke. . . . How many drugs do you think are going to be developed, and how many people will really benefit from that?"

Science

A promise was made somewhere.

Member of the Althingi (Icelandic Parliament), on how the Health Sector Database Act came to pass

Promises, promises. The colloquialism exposes the always doubled and usually even more multiple qualities of promises. And like the doubled "yeah, yeah" that fissures the most basic truth statement through a mere doubling, "promises, promises" establishes the instability that should rightfully inhere to the simultaneously admirable, commendable, disconcerting, and in any case unavoidable event of promising.

The epigraphs above span genres, contexts, nations, and domains of activity in their multiple instantiations of promising's multiplicity. They cover the territory through which this book is wandering: a complex landscape comprising fissured zones of biotechnological research, economic predictions, bets in the most speculative economy we've witnessed, political deal making, and personal oath taking. Each zone itself is in turn layered with the others, begging for some hyper–geographical information system interface to help us visualize the spectral superimpositions. Sometimes promising's zone is hard if not impossible to map—"a promise was made somewhere"—but unlocalizability does not negate the force of promising.

While promising has been theorized most often in terms of the performative utterance that begins "I promise . . . ," locating it in a more or less intentional subject (e.g., a groom) in a more or less secure context (e.g., a wedding ceremony), this does not delimit promising's work. The few statements quoted above make it clear that molecules are promising, the sciences of those molecules are promising, outlooks are promising, markets are promising, and, yes, people in particular contexts are promising. The differences—swearings, speculatings, vowings, hopings, anticipatings, sheer happenings—are as important as what all promisings appear to share: a volatility so radical that promising "never takes place but has always already occurred or is always about to occur. The place of the promise is not here and its time is not now."[1]

Promising occupies the place of the X: not—yet . . . something's coming, on its way, just down the road or pipeline. You can sense it, even if you can't see it. You can bet on it, should you want to gamble on it.

You *should* want to gamble on promising.

You *have* to, anyway, so any exhortation is excessive.

I have preferred, throughout this text, to defer direct theorizing of promising, relying instead on the inferences that ethnographic empiricism offers, or at least promises. I have no doubt tried some readers' patience, and arguing that trials of patience are in fact what the act of promising is about would be impertinent, however truthful. But while we may not need, or indeed be capable of, a full theory of promising, some promise of theory may be productive here in the chiasmic middle of the text. So here I gather *some* promising effects that have been treated by J. L. Austin, Jacques Derrida, and Shoshana Felman, to help us further tune in to the disparate and disjointed ways in which promising manifests itself in genomics.

XX

It's no exaggeration to say that everything in Shoshana Felman's book on promising in *Don Juan* and in the philosophical writings of J. L. Austin is inscribed in its main title, *The Scandal of the Speaking Body:* promising is always an event involving, and evolving from, an amalgam of language and matter. When the matter is flesh, a human body, we are in the familiar world of weddings and similar events involving the performatives analyzed, albeit in different ways, by all speech act theorists since Austin. But there is no reason why the category "speaking body" should not encompass, say, a molecule, or a segment of a chromosome ("human" and "nonhuman" would lose their distinction here) implicated as one (possibly powerful) force in the developmental event we name a "condition":

osteoporosis, obesity, schizophrenia, to give only a few names to the volatile but patterned unfoldings that deCODE, like other genomic companies, promises to pursue, if not catch.

Isn't it the case that when genomicists speak, as they so frequently do, of the "genetic predispositions" or "propensities" to which we are all given, that this can be translated (with all the infelicities to which that act is prone) as: your flesh harbors promises; your flesh is bound to promise; your flesh is made flesh, becomes flesh, in its vast and only partially traceable *entrelacements* with the promising forces of words, speech, discourse?[2] Actual fleshy promisings that, as promised, are nevertheless "not here, not now"?

In other words . . . we've gotten ahead of ourselves.

In his inaugural analysis of speech acts, the 1952 *How to Do Things with Words,* J. L. Austin accomplished many things. One of these was to diagram, not the *distinction* between constative and performative statements, but their zones of entanglement. Austin not only "dislocated" any and every easy distinction between the two, but, as Felman so beautifully demonstrates, *took pleasure* in doing so. Far from locating a lack in philosophy, language, or in the world, a lack that would then provoke or produce an effect of mourning, Austin diagrammed the devilish, seductive, scandalous, and above all hilarious "misfires," overreaches, and slips produced as the plenitudes of both flesh and language slid and smacked and sloshed against each other, and within each other.

Felman uses Austin to pursue Nietzsche's question of the problem of the promising animal (see the final *ch*) and takes "the very logic of promising"—a logic of "a paradox, a problem"—as "a sign of a fundamental contradiction which is precisely the contradiction of the human."[3] Being promising, in other words, is a fundamental aspect of the being of that favorite model organism of genomicists, a human. And this fundamental aspect is fundamentally paradoxical and contradictory

If these connections between promising, humor, scandal, paradox, and the human seem too hastily drawn, I would only point out that Felman also demonstrates how promising is "tied to a time of speed and urgency"— what the French psychoanalyst Jacques Lacan called in another context "the haste function" that stems from "the assertion of anticipated certainty" (Felman, 32). The haste function, as I hope to have shown, certainly operates within the science and business of genomics—economies that compel my complicity just as Mannvernd does: genomics puts *everyone* in a hurry. So I will continue to try to make these fast connections, established by and between the doubled acts of promising animals, hold fast.

To continue attuning ourselves to promising's qualities and effects, we should take into account some of Austin's other analytic achievements. First is his dislocation of the act of promising from the intentional subject:

> Surely the words must be spoken 'seriously' and so as to be taken 'seriously'? This is, though vague, true enough in general—it is an important commonplace in discussing the purport of any utterance whatsoever. . . . Thus 'I promise to . . .' obliges me—puts on record my spiritual assumption of a spiritual shackle.
>
> It is gratifying to observe in this very example how excess of profundity, or rather solemnity, at once paves the way for immorality. For one who says 'promising is not merely a matter of uttering words! It is an inward and spiritual act!' is apt to appear as a solid moralist standing out against a generation of superficial theorizers: we see him as he sees himself, surveying the invisible depths of ethical space, with all the distinction of a specialist in the *sui generis*. Yet he provides Hippolytus with a let-out, the bigamist with an excuse for his 'I do' and the welsher with a defence for his 'I bet.' Accuracy and morality alike are on the side of the plain saying that *our word is our deed*.[4]

Again, let's not miss how Austin savors perverting the "vague, true enough" "commonplaces" that we hold as knowledge of promising. It's clear that he relishes—or at least, in that understated British way, finds "gratifying"—the way our model organism's zeal for the profound, the nonsuperficial, and the moral sets the stage, in the event of promising at least, for the corrosion of these very ideals. When we attempt to ground ethics in an interior of intentionality, we open a fissure in that very ground. If promising counts only when a human *really truly* intends it to, then some variation on the classic comeback of kids everywhere is always possible: I had my fingers crossed. Which makes you a jerk, but not a promise breaker.

To the extent that promising can or should be located at all, locating promising in language has the doubled advantage of having ethical enforceability—you said it, you did it—while at the same time being an "accurate" account of things. Promising, after Austin, does not require intentionality; saying will do.

Derrida ratchets the analysis of promising up another notch. Over numerous essays, he has articulated how promising is disseminated throughout language, rather than being the exclusive quality or effect of a particular subset of speech acts, those Austin called "commissives." Derrida thus dislocates promising not only from any intentional subject, but from any localizability in a particular set of speech acts. He dislocates the location of promising entirely, making promising occur as a kind of general feature of language—although that's not the most promising way of putting it:

> Each time I open my mouth, each time I speak or write, I *promise*. Whether I like it or not: here, the fatal precipitation of the promise must be dissociated from the values of the will, intention, or meaning-to-say that are reasonably attached to it. The performative of this promise is not one speech act among others. It is implied by any other performative, and this promise heralds the uniqueness of a language to come.[5]

> An immanent structure of promise or desire, an expectation without a horizon of expectation, informs all speech. As soon as I speak, before even formulating a promise, an expectation, or a desire *as such,* and when I still do not know what will happen to me or what awaits me at the end of a sentence, neither *who* nor *what* awaits whom or what, I am within this promise or this threat—which, from then on, gathers the language together, the promised or threatened language, promising all the way to the point of threatening and *vice versa,* thus gathered together in its very dissemination. (21–22)

I suggest we trust him on this for now. Derrida's assessment indicates several things for future analyses of promising like this one. First, promising occurs everywhere in language, which is never sufficiently present to itself to fully guarantee all its workings or capacities. Language runs on credit, if you like—which is not to say, as you surely know, that bills don't fall due. Second, the fact that promising occurs everywhere in language means it is also at work, or in play, within the analytic language that produces such a statement as "promising occurs everywhere in language." *Et voilà:* promising turns threatening—and just as quickly turns back again. The promiseXthreat of language is its poisonXgift. Really.

And third: the promise and the decision, "which is to say responsibility, owe their possibility to the ordeal of undecidability which will always remain their condition."[6] Which could be shortened without too much violence to: no chiasmus, no promise.

It's vital to stress the "ordeal of undecidability," which is decidedly different than something like "the ordeal of uncertainty." When a representative of Hoffmann-LaRoche, for example, says the promise of genomics will materialize, this is not a statement marked by simple uncertainty: maybe he's wrong, maybe he's right, we just don't have enough information to know for sure, so we'll have to take a chance with our money. Statements of promise are undecidable, and that's much more of an ordeal than uncertainty: nothing you can do will quell this volatility that arises not within knowledge, but *beyond* it. Uncertainty mobilizes efforts in knowing, which can ameliorate the condition, and even cure it. Undecidability calls for promising, and there's no resolution in sight— only a responsibility for a decision, a responsibility shared in different ways by promissor and promissee.

To better understand the important difference, consider Hannah Arendt's treatment of the promise in *The Human Condition*. Starting from Nietzsche's groundbreaking discussion of promising from *On the Genealogy of Morals,* Arendt justly emphasizes the centrality of promising to our conceptions of the political. But Arendt gives Nietzsche's promise a rather banal reading, reducing the promise to a human assertion that establishes "an island of certainty" in a future marked by radical uncertainty.[7] Vague, I can almost hear Austin saying, and "true enough in general," but it misses something crucial. Arendt's promise seeks to anchor an uncertain future through a willing that establishes some certainty.

My promise, as it were, opens a channel to a volatile future that promising itself helps to bring about, a future that *will have provided* the only underwriting the originary promise can be said to have ever had.

That's twisted, you say—and you're right. But my understanding of promising coincides with that of Federal Reserve chairman Alan Greenspan's. Looking back on the frothy times of the late 1990s, the political-cultural economy in which infotech and biotech companies bubbled up together, Greenspan reflected on the undecidability of promising, rather than its mere uncertainty, and thus its unmanageability. "The struggle to understand developments in the economy and financial markets since the mid-1990s," Greenspan said in an August 30, 2002, speech,

> has been particularly challenging for monetary policymakers. We were confronted with forces that none of us had personally experienced. Aside from the then recent experience of Japan, only history books and musty archives gave us clues to the appropriate stance for policy. We at the Federal Reserve considered a number of issues related to asset bubbles—that is, surges in prices of assets to unsustainable levels. As events evolved, we recognized that, despite our suspicions, it was very difficult to definitively identify a bubble until after the fact—that is, when its bursting confirmed its existence.
>
> Moreover, it was far from obvious that bubbles, even if identified early, could be preempted short of the central bank inducing a substantial contraction in economic activity—the very outcome we would be seeking to avoid.[8]

In other words, you can't tell you're in a speculative bubble until after it has burst. It only becomes the case that there was nothing underwriting the promise in the future, which the promise helps establish but can't define. And even if you could *predict* the emptiness of the promise, you can't *preempt* its effects. And that truly is twisted.

XX

There are a few more things we can come to appreciate about promising and its forces, even if it escapes our predictive and preemptive capacities.

Beyond or outside of an epistemological economy, promising "*engages* desire and pleasure," Felman's analysis of *Don Juan* via Austin tells us.[9] Promising works on the level of affect, in the field of the body. If a new molecule, a new gene association, or some other experimental results seem "promising" to a scientist, it's because the result has *engaged* something other than the scientist's cognitive capacities. The power of that engagement, its force, needs to be respected, even if it can't be justified or proved. And the rules of engagement have their own logics, even if those logics are not those of what we traditionally call "scientific rationality." No scientist or science would ever flourish on such a restricted diet, even if scientists risk being misled by these *supra*rational forces that push and pull their work and ideas.

Promising comes, therefore, to be associated with the quotidian, the singular, the field of practice, rather than with the theoretically generalizable:

With Austin as with psychoanalysis, the irreducible triviality of the idiosyncratic is that of a *practice* of the singular.

Of a practice, that is, of what belongs to the order of *doing*. For unlike saying, doing is always trivial: it is that which, by definition, cannot be generalized. . . . Thus true History, belonging to the order of acts or of practice, is always—however grandiose it may be—made up of trivialities.

The same is true of writing. (69)

Analyzing promising, then—or coming to appreciate its forcefulness—is a job for history, ethnography, or other practices that find the trivial important—literature or literary theory, for example.

Lastly, promising is indissolubly linked to scandal. The reasons for this are complex, as are the linkages themselves, and it's important to plumb some of this complexity to keep from falling into a moralism in which "scandalous" is simply equated with "sinful" or "shameful."

Both Austin and Don Juan, Felman shows, take pleasure in "playing the devil," whether that play engages women or the rational, natural distinctions that logic prides itself on. And to "play the devil" is "above all to renounce playing God; that means . . . not believing in the promise of Heaven as the power that underwrites the promising animal; not believing, by the same token, in the promise of the promising animal, even if that animal is oneself" (110). Here is where promising becomes threatening, and threatening to itself in particular:

The devil, in other words, does not take himself for God. With Austin, at the very least, the devil's chief characteristic is precisely that he *does not know* whether he is playing seriously or not, whether he is or is not in the process of playing or joking. That is the truly diabolical question inherent in joking, or in play: Is it a joke? Is it simply a game? The distinguishing feature of the Austinian performance is not that it turns "seriousness" against "unseriousness," but rather that it *blurs* the boundary between the two. (96)

This is the "*scandal* of infelicity" that John Searle, Emile Benveniste, and so many other "followers" of Austin in the analytic philosophy tradition can't assimilate, because it unsettles every analysis, rattles every solid structure. By playing the devil with philosophy, Felman is arguing, Austin ends up tapping into the "radical force of negativity itself," the undermining of *every* underwriting. Like the "plague" that Freud brought to America in the form of psychoanalysis, this radical negativity is extremely contagious and virulent.

Usually the negative "has always been understood as what is reducible, what is to be eliminated, that is, as what by definition is opposed, is referred, is *subordinated* to the 'normal' or to the 'positive.'" The plague, in other words, is almost always thought to be curable. In still other words, the chiasmus is thought to be dis-entangle-able. "The logic of acts," says Felman, "thus becomes . . . a *normative* logic" (101). The normative desire is to rid disclosure of all promise, for example, or to rigorously distinguish between trust and gullibility, to cure speculative mania with a solid dose of fundamentals, and so on.

"Now in all these theories (psychoanalysis, the performative, Nietzschean philosophy), radical negativity, as the original thinker understood and grasped it, *cannot* be reduced to a negative that is the simple—symmetrical—contrary of the 'positive,' to a reducible negative, caught up in a normative system," Felman contends. And now the threat—*However will we make judgments?!*—turns back into the promise:

Now if the Austinian negative does not aim simply to treat the negative as a function of the positive, neither does it aim—it aims still less—simply to reduce the positive to the negative. Even though the term "positive" is in the last analysis undone, the defeat of the positive does not involve any nihilistic complacency. . . .

"For the sake of folly,' says Nietzsche, "wisdom is mixed in all things. A little wisdom is indeed possible." If negativity resides, in Don Juan's case, in the *lack of satisfaction,* Don Juan, in fact, is *never* satisfied, not even—especially not—with negation. If the devil, in other words, refuses above all to play God, it is especially not in order to *believe* in negativity. The "fallible" is not itself infallible; in a world that is fundamentally without guarantees, one cannot be sure of anything at all, not even infelicity. . . .

Thus negativity, fundamentally fecund and affirmative, and yet without positive reference, is above all *that which escapes the negative/positive alternative.* . . .

Radical negativity . . . belongs neither to *negation,* nor to *opposition,* nor to *correction* ("normalization"), nor to *contradiction* (of positive and negative, normal and abnormal, "serious" and "nonserious," "clarity" and "obscurity")—it belongs precisely to *scandal:* to the scandal of their nonopposition. (101–4)

This "scandal of the *outside of the alternative,* of a negativity that *is* neither negative nor positive," is "what history cannot assimilate" but is "nevertheless the *cornerstone* of History" (105, 107). Or in my terms: the chiasmus is outside the alternatives that it crosses and cannot be assimilated by historical or ethnographic understanding, but the operations of chiasma—their admixtures, their volatility, their eruptive flows—are nevertheless what constitute historical and ethnographic understanding. "The scandal, in other words, is always in a certain way the scandal of the promise of love, the scandal of the *untenable,* that is, still and always, the scandal—Don Juanian in the extreme—of the promising animal, incapable of keeping his promise, incapable of not making it, powerless both to fulfill the commitment and to avoid *committing* himself—to avoid playing beyond his means, playing, indeed, the devil: the scandal of the speaking body, which in failing itself and others makes an act of that failure, and makes history" (111).

XX

Why do I give you these excesses, perhaps trying your patience in a time and territory where delimited, practical, *normative* actions seem so urgent? Because promisingXgenomics in lavaXland *is* a matter of excess. An organism like you, me, or a zebra fish, exceeds its genetic "code." It exceeds its "nature" or genes, it exceeds its "nurture" or environment (which in turn is always exceeding itself and changing), it exceeds every wonderful technoscientific tool that has ever been invented and that ever will be invented to grasp the truths of it. More, more, more: that's why we and zebra fish and every other genomic-proteomic-culturomic enterprise *develop*. We become, along with everything not-we. Organisms, illnesses, events, politics, ethics, technological development—all of these are matters of excess that happen without our full understanding or control, as the cumulative, emergent effect of a multiplicity of forces. *We* happen our way into a future without our full understanding or control, and that's something for which we should rejoice and be glad.

It's the "inability" of any given present or any given thing to coincide with itself—or to identify fully with its opposite partner, or to fully differentiate itself from its partner—that underwrites the possibility of its becoming something else. The unquiet remains are our promise; the excess that bursts forth geyserlike from every chiasmus is our guarantee. No, not our guarantee—our stake.

Because of these excesses, the genomic fissureXlandscape is not something that is going to be *solved*, after which we will all live ethically ever after. The genomic fissureXlandscape is not something that is going to be *controlled*, through a more exact science, a more representative politics, or a more humanistic ethics. The genomic fissureXlandscape is where we live, and like Iceland, it is a harshXbeautiful world. We may not live in Iceland, but we do all live, now, in lavaXland. And even if such a territory is too volatile to be fully solved or controlled, the lavaXland of genomics can be inhabited more or less carefully, more or less thoughtfully, more or less justly, more or less admirably. My hope is that these *chs*, for all their fissuredness and excesses, agglomerate into an ethnographic mapping of some of the main streams flowing through the lavaXlands of genomics today, to be used as a guide that might improve our odds for having more of the *more* and less of the *less*.

That's why the body of this text allegorizes those structures of the body that resonate with particular intensity today: chromosomes/chapters are rendered as a series of undecidable *chs*, which also happen to be chiasma. If the chromosomes—twenty-two autosomes, plus x and sometimes y for those organisms currently called human—are the collective site out of or around which our bodies and their meanings swarm today, then the meanings of this text will be mobilized through the reader's hybridization with the twenty-three *chs* here. Just as genomics is that set of practices and theories that pursues not single genes or their products, but multiple genes, gene products, and interactions among multiple chromosomal loci, so too does this text ask for reading practices that span the *chs*, searching for new patterns and connections, forcing new articulations and crosses. Please, reader: let's be fruitful, and multiply.

Because we're going to need to—because nothing else will suffice for the geneXworld. The intensely experimental explosion of genomic demands multiple sets of affirmativeXcritical practices—literary, historical, ethical, political, and as many crosses as you can breed from them—that are just as experimental.

And just as *quick:* fast, and full of life.

DistanceXComplicity

January 1999. The Health Sector Database Act had passed. Michael Specter's profile of K.Co. appeared in *The New Yorker*, with more perfect timing than I could ever muster. I thought my project was over. Sure, I had my emissary's report to write, for some authority that remained to be identified. But the fat lady in full Viking regalia appeared to have sung her Wagnerian aria.

On the academic job market, I data-mined my material for professional talks, but a sense of closure was closing in. I was not particularly surprised by the passage of the legislation. I also didn't feel the combination of outrage and disappointment that Skúli and other Icelanders so clearly felt. Lack of appropriate affect, perhaps, but it seemed more a simple function of distance—and not merely geographic, but also disciplinary or professional. No matter how undersigned I actually was, I nevertheless habitually signed as "ethnographer" or "historian of the life sciences," a position that was supposed to be at some remove from my object of study. I had obligated myself to an ethic of distance—not because of some personal or professional virtue, but because this ethic was a productive force.

An ethic of distance keeps knowledge *becoming*. It's an ethic of alterity, of actively searching for or soliciting disruption and interruption. It's an ethic of refusing the oversignedness that can descend on one so easily, with the comfort of certainty and assuredness. (Indeed, Michel Foucault wrote of something similar in an essay titled "For an Ethic of Discomfort.")[1] An ethic of distance is an ethic of the fissure, an ethic of the *gjá* that opens any ground under your feet.

Which would include the ground of distance itself. And distance fissured becomes complicity.

XX

Questions of how one presents or represents an other—another culture, another set of practices and understandings, another nation or community, another individual, another set of silences—should be troubling. An ethnographer should feel and act on the basis of a sense of uncertainty, puzzlement, and other forms of active concern about the adequacy or propriety of one's strategies and methods for undertaking fieldwork and for undertaking the task of writing. Proven truths and methods are forever in need of the supplement of experiment. At least that's how I had learned to see it, although others disagreed.

In the introduction to his book of ethnographic essays on contemporary Iceland, anthropologist E. Paul Durrenberger inveighs against "the elitist escapism that parades under the banners of reflexivism and postmodernism." He elaborates:

Some of the postmodern folks speak of "experimental moments." I am not sure what that means. It seems to me that a lot of their language is intentionally indefinite to enhance the aura of word-magic. I kept my eyes open for experimental moments, as I did for ghosts among the Lisu when I was in Thailand, but since I am not certain what an experimental moment is, I am not sure I ever experienced one. Fieldwork is a lot like life itself, part of it. As Robin Fox says, you don't get a practice life; life is on-the-job training. So for fieldwork, and I don't really know what an experimental moment would be. Readers will find no experimental moments here.[2]

I found almost nothing but experimental moments when I was in Iceland, and the demand seemed only to intensify with time. The repeated reference here—the phrase "experimental moment" really seems to irritate—is to the subtitle of George Marcus and Michael Fischer's book, *Anthropology as Cultural Critique: An Experimental Moment in the Human Sciences,* a formative book in my professional education and an important book in the discipline of anthropology as a whole. The book describes multiple recent inventions by those human scientists called "anthropologists" as they attempt to do interpretive justice to the peoples, concepts, objects, rituals, exchange practices, and other events of the globalizing, shape-shifting contemporary world. And not just the ex-

otic "native people" that anthropologists were concerned with traditionally, but Taiwanese factory workers, Japanese and American high-
energy physicists, molecular biologists from Seattle to Berkeley, and
many other familiar strangers—or strange familiars, to accede to the operations of the chiasmus. Since the question of what should happen to
the methods, concepts, and texts of an anthropological tradition oriented
around distant, different "thems" when its practitioners turn to analyze
those previously thought of as "us" remains exactly that—a question—
Marcus and Fischer wrote that ethnography needed to become experimental: inventive, risky, searching, and at pains to probe a whole range
of fissures, including those that punctuate anthropology's own concepts,
methods, and texts.

Their book was, as Durrenberger suggests, only one in a "parade" of
texts that probed the limits of traditional methods and theories and the
ways in which their practitioners became entangled and enfolded in those
limits—a parade far too long and colorful to summarize here. That kind
of "reflexivity" was also a major theme in the fields of science studies that
I, in my education as historian of science, had gravitated toward. Marcus
and Fischer thus became a crossover point for me as I began behaving
more and more like an ethnographer, and as the phenomena that drew
my interest—genes, money, and other promises—displayed "postmod-
ernist" characteristics that demanded some sort of reflexive analysis.

This kind of analysis is troubling and disturbing on multiple levels—
indeed, you could say that reflexivity is nothing else but self-generated
acts of troubling and disturbing, much as one might say that "postmodernism" refers to those troubling and disturbing events and phenomena
within "modernism." One might also say that the postmodern is like the
eruption of the future within the modern.

Or it's like being contacted again by your long-distance advance man
when you weren't expecting to be disturbed again.

XX

In February 1999, an article by Jeffrey Kahn, of the University of Minnesota's Center for Bioethics, titled "Attention Shoppers: Special Today—
Iceland's DNA," ran on CNN's interactive Web site as part of its "Ethics
Matters" series.[3] In less than precise language, Kahn commented that "a
company called Decode negotiated the right to Iceland's genome for $200
million," which seemed, thought Kahn, "like a bargain basement price."

"Should a country sell its people's genetic information?" asked Kahn, via CNN. "Do we need to worry about protections in the kind of large population-based genetic research that Decode is undertaking?" After these questions, readers encountered the order words: "Post your opinion here."

Several Americans were among the first to obey, register,[4] and weigh in. Very American, in one case at least, as Dan wrote: "A man's body is his property by right if not by law, and his DNA also. That Iceland's government would so use its citizens speaks louder than any words how like chattel it considers them. The American way, individual consent for individual sale, is the right one and just. Free men would have no other."

"This HAS to be the last straw," typed Larry. "What else are corporations going to 'buy' from the world's patrimony? Countries already feel free to consign the plunder of their woodlands, wetlands, and rainforests to rapacious corporations. . . . In my head, I keep hearing the words 'endowed by the Creator with certain inalienable rights' . . . . . . Among these, surely, is the genetic information we are all born with. Is some corporation next going to 'negotiate' the purchase of certain of (all of) our freedoms so that we have to buy them back?"

Marie expressed similar sentiments: "Decode sounds like something from the *X-Files*. We can't give up our right to privacy to Big Governments or Big Drug Companies, or Genome projects without knowledge of what their goals are." She also wondered if the Trilateral Commission might have a hand in this and reminded readers that "last summer CNN had an article on a 1996 law passed in [the] USA that all citizens would be required soon to have all medical information from birth to grave on a micro-chip, in some form either implanted on our body, or perhaps a new 'smart medical card.' They say the reason is to have all one's medical history, allergies, etc., right there in case of emergency care and to have everyone in the 'system.'"

The next posting claimed to correct "gross misrepresentations of facts" present in Kahn's article. "The kind of exclusive rights to a nation's DNA you refer to is, as far as Iceland is concerned, pure fiction. . . . No one is being granted such an access in Iceland, nor will anyone be. Any Icelander who wishes to donate blood samples for genetic research can do so. . . . The samples are used only by active and informed consent of the donors, as required by law." Anyone desiring "accurate information" on these issues was directed to the Web site www.database.is. The posting was signed only "Dr. Árni Sigurjónsson, Iceland."

Marie was immediately swayed. "That makes more sense," she replied.

"I wonder if CNN is just trying to start something. They didn't give much for facts." But the next morning saw a posting from Eiríkur Steingrímsson, a mouse geneticist at the University of Iceland whom Kári Stefánsson described as "the most brilliant young scientist in Iceland" to *New Yorker* writer Michael Specter. (Eiríkur hardly returned the compliment: "Kári Stefánsson shoved this bill down our throats," he told Specter. "That is what we object to the most. If he had done this the correct way it would have been over with already. There would not have been any opposition.")[5] Eiríkur's posting was brief and flatly factual: "It may interest readers to learn that Dr. Árni Sigurjónsson is an employee of deCode Genetics and that the website he advertised is sponsored by the company. An alternative view is presented by the Association of Icelanders for Ethics in Science and Medicine [Mannvernd] at http://www.mannvernd.is."

Other Icelanders weighed in and supplied multiple straight facts; they also identified themselves and their affiliations. In addition to Skúli the advance man ("historian of science at the Max Planck Institute"), there was the population geneticist Einar Árnason (whose posting queried the purportedly "factual" genetic homogeneity of Icelanders, a topic to be taken up later), and the retired psychiatrist from the University of Iceland, Tómas Helgason. Bogi Andersen ("Assistant Professor of Medicine, University of California, San Diego") chimed in with a lengthy critique of the database legislation, which included an endorsement of the American value of "individual consent for individual sale" expressed by Dan: "We refuse to give Americans exclusive rights to that sentiment, especially since the database is a tool for American venture capitalists to take their company, deCODE, public." Bogi closed his remarks with a barb directed at Árni Sigurjónsson: "How telling for the ethics of deCODE that Dr. Sigurjónsson would enter this Ethics discussion without declaring his competing financial interest in this matter."

Dr. Sigurjónsson soon replied: "Being criticized for not revealing who I work for, I can inform the participants in this discussion that I did not mention this for two reasons: (1) The previous participants had not told us who they work for, so this kind of information didn't seem to be a part of the netiquette here. Furthermore, (2) I did not speak on behalf of the company but only for myself. My purpose was to get some key facts straight." He added that "the problem that some of the critics have with a private enterprise working on this project must sound very strange to American ears. Why should the federal government keep our healthcare data, rather than private companies such as deCODE genetics in Iceland, or, say, HCIA (Health Care Investment Analysts) in Baltimore?"

It was at this point that Skúli contacted me again. I had seen neither the original article nor the postings that followed. Skúli brought Kahn's article on the CNN Web site to my attention and encouraged me to enter the "discussion." Whatever my skewed views of bioethics—I still defer an entry into that fissure—a request from a friend hits me with more ethical force than some abstract principle. I registered with CNN, and experiment in complicity number 1 followed quickly:

As someone with "American ears," I can tell Dr. Sigurjónsson that it doesn't sound at all strange that citizens of Iceland are critical of deCODE. His question, "why should the federal government keep our healthcare data, rather than private companies?" has at least one obvious answer: democratic control and oversight, however difficult and imperfect that might be. There are plenty of people in the U.S. who share the concerns of many Icelanders about the increasing privatization of genetic and other medical information.

Personally, I'm not against buying and selling DNA or genetic information, per se. Two things do bother me, though: 1) when the majority of people get a bad deal, as I think has happened in the Iceland/deCODE case; and 2) when scientists like Dr. Sigurjónsson at genomic corporations like deCODE arrogantly dismiss anyone who disagrees with them as ill-informed or simply confused.

Like Skúli Sigurdsson, with whom I attended graduate school, I am a historian of science who is researching the science and business of genomics. I visited Iceland in September 1998, gave several lectures, and spoke with many scientists, doctors, and citizens there, including a number of deCODE employees. Since we are trying to stick to "facts" and not arguments, I'd like to put just a few things on record, based on what I've observed about the situation first-hand.

Dr. Sigurjónsson writes that the information in the central database will be "anonymous," and that it will be safer there than it would be "in other, similar databases around the world." These aren't facts, but arguments, and ones which have been cogently criticized by (among others) the medical database expert Ross Anderson. Dr. Anderson went to Iceland as a consultant to the Icelandic Medical Association, and has published his critique of the deCODE database on his web site (http://www.cl.cam.ac.uk/~rja14/iceland/iceland.html). The fact is that the security and anonymity of the deCODE database remains the subject of disagreement among experts.

It's also true that hundreds of media commentaries covered these events in Iceland; whether that constitutes a "thorough debate" is a matter of interpretation. But here's another fact: if deCODE had had its way, that public discussion would not have occurred at all. In the final days of the spring 1998 legislative session, the first version of this bill was introduced into the Icelandic Parliament, with the intention of getting it through in a hurry, with an absolute minimum of public debate. A few concerned scientists and doctors, utterly surprised by this bill which claimed to have their full cooperation, were able to slow things down and open up the necessary space for debate. So it hardly seems fair that deCODE employees now get to point proudly to the extensive public attention this issue has received, when deCODE would have preferred to have none of it.

Finally, an opinion. Dr. Sigurjónsson's rationale for not stating that he worked at deCODE in his initial posting is so feeble that it's laughable. His defense amounts to 1) no one else said where they worked, so why should I?; and 2) it doesn't matter where I work, since I'm my own man and only want to get "some key facts straight." It's astounding that Dr. Sigurjónsson could even imagine that the fact that he worked at deCODE didn't matter to this debate—that he was just like everyone else posting here! As we say for American ears: gimme a break! If an employee of Eli Lilly stood up in a town meeting without identifying himself or herself, and started telling people the "facts" about the latest Lilly drugs, the first two questions that every fisherman, farmer, and pharmacist knows to ask are: Where do you work? And why should I trust what you call "facts"?

DeCODE representatives need to understand that their social position entails a different, more demanding set of social protocols and responsibilities. Full disclosure is the bare minimum. It's also about time they stopped being so intent on setting everybody "straight" with their version of the truth, and started doing a better job of listening seriously to the people who differ with them. Because the future of corporate genetics and medicine in diverse societies is anything but straight: it's twisting and complex, and fraught with uncertainties, risks, and interpretations as much as promises and facts. And it's because we're going to encounter a lot of unexpected curves in the fast lanes of this genetic highway that we're going to need social and political mechanisms that respect and encourage differences, and even conflict. I'd feel a lot more optimistic about what's going down in genomics in Iceland—and in the U.S. and everywhere else—if just once someone like Kári Stefánsson stood up and said: we've got business interests that we're trying to establish and protect, but we also acknowledge that on the social level, this is hard and complicated and we don't have all the answers—so let's find a way to talk.

> Dr. Michael Fortun is a historian of science, specializing in the
> ongoing history of genomics, and a founder of the Institute
> for Science and Interdisciplinary Studies in Amherst, Massachusetts

XX

These statements, like almost everything else I undertook or underwent in and around Iceland, were an experiment, a probe into a set of relations: with a friend, Skúli; with a new genomic NGO, Mannvernd; with a corporation, deCODE; with a disciplinary field, ethnography; and with a public, Marie and Larry and Dan and Jeffrey and other CNN habitués. The experiment responded to the question: what could the undersigned promise to each of those entities? Which, since the promise is the performative speech act par excellence, is another way of asking: what could my words do?

While no one else may have put the question in this form, I was hardly in a unique situation. The eruption of deCODE and the Health Sector Database scandal had done for the biocommentary industry (allow me this shorthand for now) what the Blue Lagoon hot baths were doing for Iceland's tourism industry: providing a steamy zone of volatility in which visitors of all sorts could immerse themselves. There were all the journalists, from *Nature Biotechnology* to *The New Yorker* and a host of newspapers in between. There came undergraduates like Laura Bingham doing a senior project in the Barnard College anthropology department and law school students like David Winickoff. There were television crews from Finland and filmmakers from France and Canada. There came the diverse academics who often get clumped under the heading of bioethics, but ranged from the feminist-Marxist analyst of science Hilary Rose to legal scholar Henry Greely.[6] There came the bona fide bioethicists like Jon Merz, Glenn McGee, and Pamela Sankar.[7] And there came senior anthropologist and noted Foucault purveyor Paul Rabinow, no stranger to the "banners of reflexivism and postmodernism."

I have foregrounded the strangeness of my own ethnographic encounters to emphasize the need for some form of experimentalism as ethnography assays new subjects in new situations, but it seems clear that others have arrived at a similar point regarding Iceland, deCODE, and the HSD. Noted anthropologist Marilyn Strathern did not travel to Iceland, but did write prefatory comments to Hilary Rose's study, published by Britain's Wellcome Trust, the sponsor of Rose's engagement. "The interest of [Rose's] report," Strathern writes, "lies in the question it raises for anyone interested in the consultative process, where consultation is not just a matter of finding out what people think or dealing with public opinion but is itself an organ of government."[8] Reflexivity is not a choice, but an effect of these kinds of doubled situations and crossed identities. The ethnographer is enmeshed or folded within the phenomena being studied, consulting people about the process of consultation.

Rose was particularly successful at something no other ethnographer, including myself, had achieved or even attempted: analyzing the differences gender made in the events surrounding deCODE, the HSD, and lived relations of care and concern. Having noted that specific achievement, Strathern lauds Rose more generally for detailing "the specificities of the Icelandic case": "how a particular biotechnology firm sought to validate its procedures, how public debate did or did not get off the ground, and how it was that a purely market approach to genomics entailed national legislation." The result, says Strathern, was "a real life story of how political will was mobilized" (3).

Ethnography, experimental or otherwise, demands that kind of specificity. Paul Rabinow demonstrates this in his two studies of biotechnology carried out before his deCODE work: his account of the invention of a major biotechnical process, *Making PCR,* and *French DNA,* an account of another genomic project with a nationalist edge written from the advantageous perspective of the invited, if not included, insider. But the demand for specificity is most acute when one of the things at stake is that most volatile of substances, democracy, and here Rabinow does not meet the demand.

Rabinow ended up in Iceland a few weeks after I first visited in September 1998, but by a different trajectory and to a different location. He was invited by the Icelandic anthropologist Gísli Pálsson, whose previous work detailed the culture of Icelandic fishermen, particularly the fleet captains who became tremendously wealthy with the introduction in 1983 to 1990 of a quota system, which gave them a guaranteed percentage of the annual national catch (see "IcelandXWorld").

Like my advance man Skúli, Gísli Pálsson booked Rabinow for a public talk, complete with photograph and write-up in *Morgunbladid*—surely no other daily newspaper has ever featured pictures of two ethnographers within a one-month time span! Rabinow had microphones jammed in his face too, seeking pronouncement on the then-pending legislation. Sigurdsson and Fortun (SF) would later appear on panels together and twin their writings in journals and Web venues; Pálsson and Rabinow (PR) went one better and faster, coauthoring one of the first academic articles on deCODE, "Iceland: The Case of a National Human Genome Project," which appeared in *Anthropology Today* in October 1999.

Were SF and PR twinned twins, then? We certainly shared a sense of complicity, to use a term that PR invoke at the end of their article, between writers and the written about:

George Marcus has recently argued (1998) that anthropologists are moving from a relationship of 'rapport' with their informants to one of 'complicity.' Complicity is an ethically and epistemologically much more complex term than rapport and one that no doubt many anthropologists will feel less immediately comfortable with. But the old tropes of rapport associated with earlier relations of ethnographic production are now too closely tied to a colonial context that often facilitated it but was too infrequently analysed, to a presumed psychological relationship in which only one member spoke and wrote, to a view of two cultures facing each other across a clear divide. Complicity blurs and complicates these niceties even if it does not entirely eliminate them.[9]

What PR say is true: complicity is a much more appropriate, but also a difficult, complicated, and uncomfortable trope for ethnographic engagements in contemporary biofields. Relations of complicity are not so much a product of choice as they are an effect of habits and similar sedimentations and folds in one's own geology of morals. Complicity is an extensive set of becomings that happen just on or over the edge of one's consciousness. Complicity is hard to read.

Given such a complex trope, it would be a mistake to simply state that SF were "complicit" with Mannvernd and the "opposition" to the HSD, while PR were "complicit" with deCODE and the "establishment." Nor should the fact that one could hyperlink to the PR article from the front page of the deCODE Web site, where it was featured for a while in 2000, be allowed to solidify a simplistic definition of complicity. If it's apparent anywhere, complicity will be nestled in the deepest folds *(pli)* of a text.

In the PR article, the figure of deCODE CEO Kári Stefánsson appears exactly once: "DeCode has been the focus of controversy from the start. On the international scene there has [been] extensive coverage, in the world press and on major TV channels, of the company, its charismatic director (Kári Stefánsson), the scientific project, and the database DeCode proposes to construct" (14). I have found it interesting and important to detail the particular manifestations of "charisma" displayed by this central figure, rather than glossing over the topic quickly. Where the PR article does not once mention Mannvernd, I think the emergence of a new kind of NGO of scientists, physicians, and others in a nation that has almost no history of such NGOs is an ethnographically interesting event— not to mention that Mannvernd initiated and ran the most comprehensive bilingual Web site on what was happening with the HSD controversy.

In an article ostensibly about ethics and ethnography, Mannvernd isn't mentioned and Kári gets off easy with the label "charismatic." The PR article makes only repeated reference to an ethnographically vague class of "opponents" and "critics"—nothing like "prominent scientists from the university and the hospitals," or "the Icelandic Medical Association," or "many Althingi members not part of the ruling coalition." It's in this realm, where "political will was mobilized," that the PR article fails most noticeably in delivering the specificities that ethnography, ethics, and their combinations most acutely demand.

PR note that deCODE "was funded by venture capital funds coordinated in the United States. Of course, in this moment of globalizing capitalism such monies have no nationality. There is, however, an insistent desire to give money a nationality, especially by spokespeople for 'ethics,' largely as a means of attributing 'responsibility' for its effects. Ethnographically, this discourse of ethics and responsibility, and a subject to whom they might be attributed, is a core component of what might be called contemporary genomics machinery" (14).

The abrupt contradiction between "venture capital funds coordinated in the United States" and "such monies have no nationality" may be unavoidable. But in a specific case such as the deCODE one, I think this contradiction or chiasmus demands to be explored and elaborated in ethnographic terms: in what circumstances does money appear to have no nationality, and in what circumstances does it appear attached to the initials U.S.? And as later chapters will detail, it's not just "spokespeople for 'ethics'" who exhibit the desire to "give money a nationality"—unless one considers an organization like the U.S. Securities and Exchange Commission to be a spokesperson for ethics. As a high-level abstraction, a "globalizing economy" can be understood only by diagramming the transactions and exchanges that occur across the financial and regulatory systems of (in this case) Iceland, the United States, and as we'll soon see, Luxembourg and Panama. Monies have nationalities.

Leaving aside for the moment the matters of the "contemporary genomics machinery" and its "spokespeople," the passage from the PR paper quoted above continues: "Although deCODE is legally a United States company (most biotech companies in the world are given a fictitious Delaware location for legal, tax, and patent advantages), it operates entirely in Iceland and has had a majority Icelandic ownership from its foundation" (14).

Here again, nationality appears both as a "fiction" and as fact, and the contradiction only ends inquiry rather than begins it. The "giver" of this fiction is left unstated, unlike the ethics spokesperson who "gives" nationality to money. But the "givers" of corporations are a swarm of lawyers, legislators, judges, and the national legal systems they work within, and if deCODE's Delaware identity is thus to be considered a "fiction," then one must at least admit that this is a very large, elaborate, and compelling fiction. The statement that deCODE "has had a majority Icelandic ownership from its foundation" is not deconstructible in this same manner; it is only wrong, as we'll see.

Let me stick with the deconstructible chiasmus rather than the simple error, and turn to the matter of "ethics" and it spokespeople. Under the subheading of "the politics and ethics of representation," PR advance a critique of a 1999 op-ed piece in the *New York Times* written by Harvard University population geneticist Richard Lewontin. This critique is undertaken by PR in order "to illustrate some basic pitfalls of skirting basic ethnographic work while rushing to draw global conclusions."

While not averse to the rush to global conclusions in other parts of their text, PR delve into specificities here. Indeed, some basic eth/ical/nographic work on their text would begin by noting that practically an entire page of dense two-column text, in a five-page article, is devoted to Lewontin and his op-ed. While Kári disappears behind the single adjective "charismatic," many more damning and florid phrases attach, directly and indirectly, to the name of Lewontin: "his incendiary piece," "aberrant," "technocratic authority or humanitarian universalism," and finally and most egregiously, a long paragraph that is supposed to provide "troubling examples of what we anthropologists have come to call 'Orientalism'":

Although [Edward] Said's use of the term has been criticized as being too categorical, it does provide conceptual help in highlighting certain representational practices. Thus, Lewontin heaps scorn on the corruption of Mexico and Indonesia; he expresses his shock that "a northern European" nation has been duped by a capitalist plot that he can see through "even from thousands of miles away" at Harvard. Three paragraphs later Lewontin proclaims Iceland "does begin to sound like Mexico." Actually it begins to sound like Cambridge, Massachusetts, and the ever-growing number of biotech companies and governmental reform missions, that Harvard and MIT professors are associated with. It also sounds exactly like Orientalism. Disdain for democracy and deploying contemptuous representations of other people is bad politics, bad ethics, and contributes to the corruption of truth. Unlikely as it may appear to them, even powerful Americans profiting from their positions at world centres of prestige and power might have something to learn from those "thousands of miles away." If people are not commodities, as Lewontin maintains, why treat them as if they were, assuming that they are mere pawns in the games of self-interested investors and (other) prestigious professors? Lewontin's piece is a small example of how moralism and ethnocentrism can blind. (17)

Lewontin is placed in a position of power, persuasion, and profitability of such a remarkable quality that it has to be described, analyzed, and denounced at length, while leaving utterly undetailed the numerous ways in which Kári and deCODE exerted extraordinary political and cultural power that could certainly qualify as "disdain for democracy." There is

no mention that deCODE continually broadcasted exoticizing if not ori-
entalizing tropes of Iceland's "isolation" and Icelanders' "unique homogeneity" and "cooperativeness," using them to establish deCODE's position of profitability in Iceland in a way that Kári could never have
achieved in Cambridge, Massachusetts. There is also no mention that Kári
repeatedly "heap[ed] scorn" and deployed "contemptuous representations" of *absolutely anyone*—"native" or "foreign" physicians, scientists,
journalists, database experts, or professional associations—who demonstrated the temerity to question or criticize any of Kári's or deCODE's
moves or desires.

To further our understanding of complicity, I would say that the PR
piece is complicit with what it purports to critique: it enacts its own bad
politics and bad ethics and makes its own contribution to the corruption
of truth. It is a small example of how moralism and ethnocentrism can
blind a text to its own representational practices even as it positions itself
to illuminate the representational practices of others.

XX

As mentioned, for those without access to the journal of the Royal Anthropological Institute, you could get to the PR piece for a few months
through the front page of the deCODE Web site. If you surfed there in
July 2000, perhaps looking for information on deCODE's upcoming initial public offering as required by U.S. financial regulations, you would
have found the link to the PR article in the bottom right-hand corner, just
under a photo of Kári escorting King Abdullah of Jordan and president
of Iceland Ólafur Ragnar Grímsson through the deCODE labs. (Not that
nations matter any longer in the "globalizing economy.")

The Web site had recently been redesigned and featured the new de-
CODE logo. When I first visited Iceland in September 1998, I had asked
for and received a couple of deCODE T-shirts; they had the old deCODE
logo on them and a slogan that translated as "deCODE Genetics . . . for
better health." The logo, which was splashed all over company documents
at the time as well as the T-shirts, shows an outlined Iceland with the lens
of a gargantuan, all-surveilling magnifying glass hovering over it. Visible
through the magnifying glass were the four letters ATCG, the smallest
possible metonym for the genes contained in the interior of the nation
(figure 7).

By 2000, the deCODE logo had changed to a far more benign image

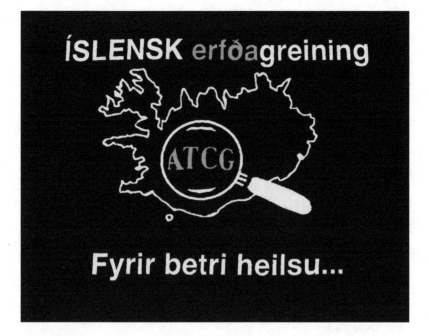

FIGURE 7. The old logo of deCODE Genetics

of two stylized figures, with the blank space of a helix fissuring them. Joining them. This was undoubtedly a necessary PR move.

XX

It's not my place to rate my own politics and ethics or to titrate the corruption levels of my truths. Nor am I prepared to develop a full analysis of my complicitous relations, which would proceed with the help of Kim Fortun's analysis of "advocacy" in international environmental politics.[10] Instead I will simply supply a few more signs of my becoming complicit, upon which future evaluations might be based.

While the PR piece was linked to deCODE's Web site, I turned two of my conference talks into an article for the Mannvernd Web site, "Experiments in Ethnography and Its Performance."[11] Why? First, because I was asked to write something by an organization whose members had given me generous gifts of time and words in my first visit to Iceland. Second, because I was planning a second trip to Iceland, I wanted people

there to see what I was saying about their situation and how I was saying it. Third, because I wanted to contribute to a Web site that had become a valuable source of information for the international scientific, medical, and other professional communities who were interested in these
events and who occasionally swarmed over their island.

When I went to Iceland for the second time, in March 2000, my time
and interviews were saturated by three themes. One was the registration statement that deCODE had just filed with the U.S. Securities and
Exchange Commission, announcing an imminent initial public offering
(IPO) of their stock on NASDAQ. This is discussed in detail over the
next few chapters. Second was the question of ownership of genetic information, which was being played out internationally through a statement by President Bill Clinton and Prime Minister Tony Blair (treated
in the "PublicXPrivate" chapter), and nationally through the emergence
of a new Icelandic organization, Fair Compensation. Fair Compensation
was encouraging Icelanders to opt out of the Health Sector Database
and join a collective that would demand some form of compensation for
the clearly valuable information that deCODE was seeking to extract
from their bodies.

I also want to briefly mention another thread, one that wove itself into
this unfolding pattern of complicity. Indeed, it was a story of multiple
complicities, all centered on the question of payments by deCODE to Icelandic political parties.

During my time in Iceland in March 2000, I was in frequent contact
with the media relations office at Rensselaer Polytechnic Institute, which
had sent out a press release about my research in Iceland. The world of
gene maps and sequences and genomic companies and their ego-inflated
CEOs has become grist for the daily news these days, and I can hardly
blame the institution of higher education that had by then employed me
for speculating on my (admittedly limited) cultural capital as ethnohis-
torian of genomics—I get some small percentage return on the transaction, after all.

I had told the office about one story I was hearing from multiple
sources: that the political parties in Iceland had received money from
deCODE. There had been two Icelandic newspaper articles about this.
One dated from December 1998, in the final days of parliamentary debate on the HSD. Stefán Jón Hafstein, a senior editor of *Dagur,* Iceland's
most liberal newspaper, had commented on the "very special treatment"
that deCODE was receiving from the government, including being al-

lowed at that very late date to rewrite the legislation (which deCODE had also helped draft). Hafstein posed a direct question to Prime Minister Davíd Oddsson and Minister of Foreign Affairs Halldór Ásgrímsson (of the Independence and Centrist parties respectively, forming the governing coalition): "HAVE THE INDEPENDENCE PARTY AND THE CENTRIST PARTY ACCEPTED MONEY—OR BEEN PROMISED FINANCIAL CONTRIBUTIONS—FROM THE ICELANDIC deCODE GENETICS OR PARTNERS ALLIED TO THE COMPANY?" "The question is not an accusation," Hafstein noted. "However, it is certainly based on suspicion," and was "not being asked without reason."[12]

About a year later, Valdimar Jóhannesson asked, "Are Icelandic politicians for sale?" in the more conservative pages of *Morgunbladid*. Jóhannesson had been a candidate for Parliament with the Liberal Party in the spring elections of 1999, but the party did not receive enough votes for him to be elected; in the spring of 2000, when I met him, he was the head of Fair Compensation. His November 1999 article rang with rhetoric not atypical of Icelandic speech:

Hereby we formally request an answer from the Independence Party and the Centrist Party regarding the truth of the claim that these parties have accepted a large sum of money, a contribution worth as much as half a million US dollars, from deCODE Genetics, the parent company of Íslensk erfdagreining, or from related parties.

It is alleged that the Independence Party accepted 20 million IS krónur and the Centrist Party 17.5 million to grease the company's momentum and especially to help the bill on the centralized health database clear the Althingi. At the passing of the bill into law, the stocks of deCODE rose to thirty times their original price making the company worth a total of 40 billion krónur.

Icelandic voters deserve to have full disclosure of such bribery, granted the rumor has basis in reality, so that the nation may rise from its slumber and realize what sort of government holds the reins of power in Iceland. The nation must guard against the predator's claw, it must cease to sleep on the watch, it must show will and stop accommodating liars and cheaters.[13]

Both Hafstein and Jóhannesson knew full well that campaign finance laws in Iceland provided total secrecy and that their demands were likely to go unanswered. Which they did.

But the stories continued to circulate in the spring of 2000, and through the efforts of the Rensselaer media office, Kristen Philipkoski, who covered the genomic beat for *Wired* magazine, decided she wanted to talk to me about the stories I had been hearing in my interviews. So now the consulter was being consulted, to use Marilyn Strathern's terms. I was experimenting with complicity—with Mannvernd and with the media—but a complicity that retained some measure of distance.

I have written about this episode at length in a previous article, so I will not rehash all the details here.[14] I had to make some quick judgments regarding the value of what can only be called rumors, albeit multiple and quasi-independent rumors that had circulated in the Icelandic newspapers and among the scientists and doctors tagged as "the opposition."[15] At one point, I was on the phone with an anonymous reliable source who "gave me his word"—and in the genomic economy, as we have seen, swearing, promising, and oath taking are often all you get—that 19 million krónur had been transferred into the bank account of the Independence Party, the conservative party that had led the database legislation to passage. I told Philipkoski what people had been telling me, told her about the newspaper articles, and gave her some names and numbers of people to call. Her story, "Genetics Scandal Inflames Iceland," was posted at 3:00 A.M. Pacific time on March 20, 2000.[16]

Did I regard these stories as true? Let me take my cue from Hjörleifur Guttormsson, the Icelandic member of Parliament who "filibustered" during the final days of the HSD debate, whom Philipkoski quoted: "'Nothing decisive can be said about the rumors,' said Hjörleifur Guttormsson, a former member of the Icelandic parliament for 21 years who voted against the database bill. 'Those are only speculations and you have to decide yourself if you believe it or not. The only thing that is certain is that deCODE made quite an effective lobby work, directed towards parliamentarians not to mention the media.'"[17]

I would depart only slightly from this and say that while nothing *certain* can be said about rumors, one can nevertheless speak decisively—indeed, in the case of rumors, speaking *is* deciding. And as far as their being "only speculations" go, I *decided* that they were far less speculative than the many stories I routinely read or hear about the imminent gene discoveries or the future business prospects of one genomic company or another. Or I could say, the stories of payoffs were more worth speculating about than many of the stories about biologies and economies that fuel genomic enterprises. So I too speculated in the media economy of genomics, filling my account with the accounts that I had heard over and over in my interviews, from multiple sources that I regarded as reliable, and with enough "supporting material" to underwrite their value in a complex economy.

And I could also say: The story is true. I promise.

XX

I don't know how many hours Skúli gave to journalists, other scholars, filmmakers, and everyone else who became interested in the deCODE-HSD business. Those hours must have accumulated on the scale of months. Skúli played advance man for legions of touring professionals who came to Iceland to consult and be consulted, and the journalistic, ethnographic, and historical record is much the richer for his work. Indeed, all the Mannvernders were exceedingly generous with their time, often at the expense of their own work and interests.

Back in the States, the complicity intensified as my name got around, and I too wound up becoming a source—mostly on background, but I was always aware of the need for a quotable phrase. Matt Crenson of the Associated Press, Kitta MacPherson of the *Newark Star-Ledger,* and James Meeks of the *Independent* in London are only a few of the reporters for whom I played the distance/complicity chiasmus, providing them with excess detail and tangled connections crossed with stabs at pithiness.[18]

In these cases, my complicity with the media sparked no pangs of regret or self-examination. Not simply because each of these articles was, in the end, quite critical of what was happening in Iceland, but also because it was evident in the outcomes as well as in our interactions that the reporters and the undersigned ethnographer had done their due diligence. We had questioned, pondered, detailed, self-critiqued, laughed, snorted, worried, and doggedly pursued to the best of our abilities in the limited time we had. An honest recognition of complexity and uncertainty accompanied—somehow, somewhere—each flat assertion. We crossed our complicities with distance.

If I overplayed my hand once, it was with a reporter for the Viennese newspaper *Der Standard.* At the Society for the Social Studies of Science annual meeting in Vienna in September 2000, Skúli and I spoke on a panel together, and on the margins of this professional economy Skúli had been contacted by a journalist. In his semiquixotic mission to keep critical perspectives on deCODE in print, Skúli asked me to join him. The fact that I failed to see how an article in a Vienna newspaper would make any difference to events in Iceland was incidental; my friend and advance man had asked me to do something he thought important, and I was happy to comply. Happy enough, anyway.

Jürgen Langenbach interviewed us in an old café. Skúli had directed him to my previous conference talks that I had made into the more or less coherent "Experiments in Ethnography" contribution to the Mannvernd Web site. In those talks I had begun working out the KeikoXK.Co. . . . *Spiel,* they might say in Vienna—act, game, gamble. Jürgen was taken by the analogy and asked me to elaborate: "'1998 sind unter enormen Medienspektakel gleich zwei Helden nach Island zurückgekehrt, Keiko, der Wal aus dem Film "Free Willy," und Kári, der Chef von deCODE,' erinnert sich Wissenschaftshistoriker Mike Fortun (Rensselaer Polytechnic Institute), 'ich war damals gerade in Island, und die Analogie der Inszenierungen war schon stark.'"[19]

Skúli got in one of his cultural critiques, too, inveighing against what he called the "sagamongering" of so many Viking-happy media accounts. "'Für mich ist das keine "Island-Saga,"' berichtet Skúli Sigurdsson (University of Iceland, Reykjavík), 'sondern eine Bürokratie, die wie bei Kafka mit den Bürgern umspringt.'"[20] Skúli's trope made for a good headline— "Island: Kafkaeskes Gen-Fischen"—while I was content that at least one journal of record somewhere in the world published photos of Keiko and Kári, "zwei Helden," side by side (figure 8).

As long I was going to have to cross ethnography with media work, I much preferred this oblique tack, which I hoped would spark a connection between the media spectacles surrounding two homecoming heroes. Maybe I just preferred being mistaken for a *Wissenschaftshistoriker* instead of an "ethicist," as I was in *Business Week*: "'This company presumed that everyone consented to be in this database unless they opted out,' says Michael Fortun, an ethicist at Rensselaer Polytechnic Institute in Troy, N.Y., who is advising the Icelandic foes of deCode's plan."[21]

Let me split a few hairs, since X also marks the spot of hairline differences that matter enormously: I was, in this period (and still am), becoming complicit with Mannvernd. I was not "advising" the "foes" of deCODE (who, for the record, I would have described as "critics of the HSD Act," even if the deCODE-HSD distinction was far from clear). Unlike some ethicists I know, I had little in the way of advice to give anyone. I don't necessarily share the bioethicist's faith in the principle of informed consent as some universal good or right. But in this specific case, in a nation of less than 300,000 people, in the high-flying late-1990s, with a database of health records licensed to a monopoly interest headed by a man whose multiple volatilities were becoming well documented, I can comfortably say: informed consent is necessary.

Nor do cash contributions and other forms of corporate influence in governmental affairs particularly shock my American ears. And I'm not so starry-eyed as to think that "informed democratic debate," especially on a matter like genomics, is easily achievable or even necessary or desir-

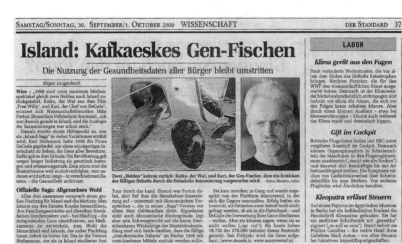

FIGURE 8. Keiko and Kári side by side, "zwei Helden" (two heroes) in *Der Standard* (Vienna), Sept. 30–Oct. 1, 2000. Reprinted with permission.

able; most people have enough to think about without adding the science and business of genomics to the list. And, finally, ethnographers or ethicists becoming complicit with genome corporations is not a phenomenon that offends my moral sensibility; any genome company ready to talk a six-figure salary for an in-house *Wissenschaftshistoriker* will find a receptive ear here.

But complicity should not blind an ethnographer to his or her own representational practices, obscuring one's own participation in what one critiques in others. Complicity should not be an excuse for ethnographers to resort to the shorthand of the philosopher or pundit and to write within a truncated discourse of "democracy," in which "some 700 newspaper articles in the press, 150 television programmes, a series of town meetings, and endless discussion and debate both within the Parliament and the shopping centers" is said to constitute "nine months of national debate."[22]

Or as Skúli has himself argued,

A draft bill had been faxed by deCODE to the Ministry of Health and Social Insurance at the beginning of September 1997. . . . Hence, it seems utterly misleading to describe what happened with concepts like democracy, or standards of reaching decisions. Yet, Paul Rabinow did so on Icelandic State Television in the middle of July 1999. He was asked what he thought about the HSD debate. In his answer, with the logo of deCODE in the background, he concluded by saying: "So, I think that what I am saying in two words is that the process has been democratic and passionate. I think it is time to move on to the next set of debates, both in Iceland and outside Iceland to make sure that this is done well so other countries can follow a model of what Iceland has done." The emphasis on how democratic events in 1998 had been in Iceland was repeated by Gísli Pálsson and Paul Rabinow, and they said concerning the passing of the HSD Bill: "This decision was clearly the product of informed democratic consent, whatever one may think of the substance of the bill." They then noted that some of the opponents had questioned democratic procedures. "Such a critique of democracy would, of course, necessitate accepting a subject position of technocratic authority or humanitarian universalism that are themselves the topics of lively critique."[23]

In a similar vein Paul Billings, a responsible geneticist by the usual metrics of responsibility, reassured readers of the *American Scientist* that "after a broad-based public debate, employing democratic institutions including a free press and independent legislature, the country imposed limits on this new biomedical effort. . . . The construction of science and its associated enterprises by the people of Iceland is paradigmatic; it represents an example of the assertion of national principles and sovereignty over international science and biotechnology. The outcome of gene hunting in Iceland may be better in the end than in North America or Europe."[24]

I would hazard further speculation and say that in no nation in the world can the process of democratic governance be summed up in terms of deliberation and "discussion" of information. Ethnography entails opening up, through one's own careful speculations and those of others, the near certainty that the Health Sector Database Act passed in Iceland less through a process of "discussion" and more through the mechanisms of greased palms, backroom deals, quid pro quos, "gentlemen's" agreements, back scratchings, blackmails, and other colorful expressions given to the actual workings of actual democracies around a globalizing globe where nations still matter.

Distance more than complicity demands that an ethnography of genomics and democracy in Iceland account for the fact that the prime minister passed the pen between the representatives of deCODE and Roche, inking the $200 million promise of February 1998 that truly launched deCODE as a company and altered the political economy of Iceland. Distance more than complicity makes it necessary to recall that former president of Iceland Vigdís Finnbogadóttir was on deCODE's board of directors, lending enormous credibility to the project, until she mysteriously and abruptly resigned just days before the HSD bill was passed. Distance more than complicity makes it necessary to remember that deCODE wrote the first draft of the government's legislation for the HSD and that both deCODE and the Icelandic government tried their best to push that legislation through late in the spring 1998 parliamentary session—tried their best to avoid not only public "democratic" discussion, but *any* discussion at all within the scientific and medical professional communities.

And distance more than complicity makes it necessary to state that in the summer of 1999 the "democratic" government of Iceland abruptly dissolved its National Bioethics Committee—whose members had been nominated by the major Icelandic biomedical institutions and professional associations and that was advocating widely accepted practices of informed consent that deCODE believed too restrictive—and replaced the committee with a government-appointed set of members who proved more amenable to deCODE's interests.[25] That Kafkaesque story is detailed in the following chapter.

NonXGovernmental Organization

Under the sign of complicity, the undersigned and Mannvernd became more enfolded as 1998 folded into the twenty-first century: not more identified, not more united, not more harmonized, not more assimilated, but more enfolded—involved in a complicated manner. Surely this is what all those exhortations one hears these days in the academy to "get involved" means? To get hyperbiologically entangled, exceeding the comfortably understandable economies of "for" or "against"?

I spoke under Mannvernd's auspices each time I returned to Iceland. I participated in some of their meetings, at which there was always a table full of sweets and, as Halldór Laxness wrote regarding similar gatherings in more than one of his novels, "prodigious amounts of coffee." In the meeting hall or around the table I would almost always see Tómas Zoëga, the psychiatrist at the National University Hospital who was one of the signatories of the 1998 letter to *Nature Biotechnology* that helped bring the deCODE events to national and international attention. Tómas also helped bring about the demise of the ethical, social, and legal disaster that was the first draft of the Health Sector Database legislation, and his leadership role in the Icelandic Medical Association kept the IMA working hard to make deCODE comply with standards of data storage and transfer, protocols of informed consent, and other legal and ethical principles established by the relevant international bodies. Alfred Árnason, a retired and fiery human geneticist, was another familiar presence. Both Tómas and Alfred gave generously of their time in formal interviews and informal conversations, and I'm sorry that demands of narrative and space have squeezed them into an unjustifiably brief mention.

Also active in Mannvernd were numerous other physicians, retired and active, other health professionals like Anna Atladóttir, a medical records secretary at the National University Hospital, a philosopher or two, and others. Sigurbjörg Ármannsdóttir was an active participant; as a leading member of an advocacy group for people with multiple sclerosis, she donated DNA to Kári in the pre-deCODE era for his MS research. When she lost confidence in the man and the work, she tried for years to get her DNA sample returned or destroyed, to no avail.[1]

Mannvernd was mostly men, for those interested in advancing future speculations on the promises of gender analysis,[2] and aside from Eiríkur Steingrímsson the mouse geneticist, Skúli was one of the youngest members. I had fantasies of enlisting Björk for a benefit concert to fix that generational problem, leveraging her newfound fame as a movie star in *Dancer in the Dark* (in which she played the mother of a child who has inherited her blindness), but we were both always too busy or too lazy.

I can't do justice to all the people who made Mannvernd happen and instead must limit my account to the two people who, along with Skúli, became my closest interlocutors: the psychiatrist Pétur Hauksson and the population geneticist Einar Árnason. I'm reluctant to describe them, although reading too many *New Yorker* genomic profiles has impressed the efficacy of this style upon me. I'll let Kitta MacPherson—a reporter for the *Newark Star-Ledger* whom I spoke with extensively before and after her visit to Iceland in 2000, passing on the same gifts of time, information, and opinions that Skúli and other Mannvernders had given so many journalists— do the job for me. MacPherson included physical descriptions of these men in her careful, substantive, and critical newspaper articles about deCODE and the HSD. Pétur Hauksson was a "sad-faced, gentle-spoken psychiatrist who founded Mannvernd, a non-profit human rights group, in October 1998." Einar Árnason was "a respected population geneticist at the University of Iceland . . . whose eyes crinkle like Santa Claus when he is amused."[3]

So paired are these two in my imagination that the original title for this chapter was to be EinarXPétur. They grew up down the road from each other; both of their fathers worked at Reykjalundur, a famous social welfare organization founded in 1945 as a "working home" for tuberculosis patients, which still operates today as a private enterprise owned by the Icelandic Association of Tuberculosis and Thoracic Patients. It's in Mosfellsbaer, the district a short distance from Reykjavík where Pétur still lives, near the farm where Halldór Laxness was born. Each studied abroad, as so many of Iceland's scientists and physicians have: Pétur in Denmark, Einar in the United States. They both returned, as so many Icelanders have, with non-Icelandic spouses—a phenomenon that bears upon the "homogeneity" of Iceland to be discussed later.

And now they were both active in Mannvernd, tirelessly . . . OK, *continually* analyzing, responding, publishing, speaking, testifying, sound biting, and Web posting an interminably long chain of texts for Icelanders and for international readerships. This coalescing of physicians, scientists, health workers, historians, philosophers, and others into Mannvernd, in a nation with almost no history of such NGOs, was surely one of the brightest spots in the new Icelandic genomescape. Especially in complex, technoscientific territories like the lavaXland of genomics, governmental organizations are not up to the demands of governing. The state needs a supplement; governing increasingly demands nongovernmental organizations.

XX

One of the few exceptions to Iceland's historical lack of NGOs is another organization that Pétur helped found, Gedjhálp. That story, as Pétur told it to me in September 1998, illustrates some of the same political and social dynamics, double binds, trade-offs, and "schizophrenic" opposites that Mannvernd would also have to negotiate—messy complexities that Pétur admitted enjoying:

> *Pétur:* It's an advocacy group for mental health patients and others interested that has existed since 1979. . . . It started as a grassroots movement, and is now much more organized, and is running services like halfway houses and sheltered homes and effective support services for the most chronically ill patients. The hospitals ran some of these services, but there was a need for much more. There was a debate in the association. . . . Some people wanted to hang on to the grassroots movement, and other people—like me—wanted to do something about the problems we were complaining about. . . . We were stronger in this debate, and I'm sorry to say that some of the people have left the association gradually. . . . But this is the way most of these organizations have developed . . . grassroots movements have turned out to be great research and service institutions. Of course, they lose some of their possibilities as grassroots movements to have an effect, but I think we can still have a lot of effect on policy and decisions by being responsible. And that's what we are seeing today. At the same time that the minister of health is giving us [donating] a great big house, in a week or so, we

are seriously complaining about her work on the HSD and criticizing her to the European community. It's very, very serious. So it's a very divided job. Some would say schizophrenic. It's difficult, but I like it. I like these opposites . . .

Mike: So your life is going along normally, and you're involved in this work that you're justifiably proud of, and then—how did you first hear about deCODE?

Pétur: Oh, in the newspapers. I saw the pictures and read the articles and the interviews with Kári. But that was OK; they were just doing their work. And then very suddenly the database bill came along. And that I heard about from my colleagues who were involved, who had been called up and asked if they could come to the Ministry of Health in a couple of hours to say what they thought about this new bill that was going to Parliament in a couple of days. So they had this very short notice, and everything erupted. There was an unbelievable process in April, which ended up with everything being stopped. The health minister, who proposed the bill, withdrew it. And we're glad that she did that, and that was very courageous, because she was pressured by the prime minister enormously.

The public, when they heard about the bill, did not know how important this was. Even in my association, Gedjhálp, people there said OK, we are trying to understand this, and they were trying not to be negative or critical, because the hype was that this would be so beneficial to everyone. So nobody wanted to be negative. But when it was discussed, and they learned more about it, everyone was very strongly against it. Mostly because of the fact that the health information about the individual is that individual's private property. And therefore, informed consent should be obtained in every case. That was our main stand.

Originally, people were talking about payment for being involved. We figured that if one good drug would come out of it, then a reasonable price would be about one million Icelandic krónur for every consent. But people thought that was ridiculous, and that it could not be done practically. So people have stopped talking about the price of consent. It also hurts their pride: they felt they ought to *give* their consent. Which is the highest price. Skúli has perhaps told you about the Viking who came to Norway, and he had a polar bear, which was completely white. And the king of Norway asked him what the price was, and he was told it was not for sale. Then the king said he would pay this and this; "no, it's not for sale." Then the king doubled the price; "no, it's not for sale." Then the king said, but will you give it to me? And that the Viking could not refuse; it was the highest price. So the king's duty was to give him something also priceless.

That's what the Icelandic people want to do: they want to *give* this. Which is a much higher price than payment.

This conversation took place in early September 1998. The database legislation was still being debated, and Mannvernd had not yet formed. But a few weeks later, as the debate on the legislation went on, it began to look as though something more organized and longer term might need to evolve. When I interviewed Pétur again, on my next trip in March 2000, I asked him about that period and the decision to found Mannvernd:

Pétur: We discussed the pros and cons of organizing. I was one of those who was in favor of creating this organization, mostly because I thought we could be more efficient—it would be easier for us as individuals, and we could have more results. Also we could be more powerful than we could as individuals in many respects—collecting money, for example, for spreading information. And we could be more powerful legally.

Then again, the cons were that it would dampen the individual's energy—which has happened. Maybe that would have happened anyway. But that's what we debated.

Mike: This was while the database legislation was still being debated. What was the mood of people—optimistic, pessimistic?

Pétur: A bit of both. People were still sort of in a state of shock, and we were just hoping for the best. We debated whether we should just continue to point out the various drawbacks and problems that the legislation had. If we did that, and our criticisms were listened to, then we would be partly responsible for it. That was one of the things we debated very early on, and I think we made the morally right decision, to try to prevent a greater disaster. So some of the things we pointed out were listened to—we demanded that the Ministry of Health include some form of opt-out clause, for example. Formal opinions were addressed to the parliamentary committee in charge of the legislation. I went before the committee twice, once as chairman of the mental-health alliance, Gedjhálp, and once for Mannvernd. But by the third debate, the committee didn't want to hear any more opinions.

But the minority opposition called us, and they had a meeting of their part of the committee without the majority—this was very strange—but called in several individuals and organizations who wanted to present their opinions. Which is a democratic right, and a tradition—either you are asked formally for your opinion, which makes your opinion stronger, or you can just request to give it. But that very sacred tradition was violated, and that made the opposition extremely angry.

Mannvernd was actually a very young organization then—only a few weeks when we got our first job, presenting these opinions. And presenting alternatives. We were often asked, "what would you like instead?" So we worked out elaborate alternatives—for example, how distributed databases could be used, instead of a centralized one. And how the existing databases, like the cancer registry, could be developed and strengthened. And we explained why the research results from those databases would be more exact and not as biased as the results from a big, monster database. And also how this could be financed, without a monopoly. We made very elaborate proposals on that. And of course, how this could all be done with informed consent. We did all this when the organization was very young.

Then we tried to inform the public. We tried to collect money to pay for advertisements, and that was a very difficult job. We collected money mostly from companies—we had a treasurer who was very active in that context. But one full page ad was very expensive, and the next five days it would be followed by a full page ad from deCODE. And where we had to wait several weeks to get our ad in, deCODE had it in right away. Also we tried to collect money to send an information brochure to every home in the country, but we weren't able to raise the money.

But we made various demands to the director general of public health [Sigurdur Gudmundsson], who was responsible for informing the public, to improve the brochure that was sent to all the people. We criticized the wording of that pamphlet and were actively involved in trying to rewrite that. It turned out to be extremely neutral. It was like something a lawyer had written—nobody read it. It was dull colors, even. And small print. No one remembers getting this thing in their mail, but it went to everyone.

Mike: What could Mannvernd do that the professional societies, like the Icelandic Medical Association, couldn't?

Pétur: We could do a lot of things, like the ad campaigns. Or like stating our opinions to the media, especially after the organization had become known. Like now, reporters take the initiative themselves and call me and ask my opinion. But it's difficult, in that we often don't have time to organize a formal opinion about all the things the government or deCODE do now. But we can use the kind of "surprise element," the immediate reaction—we can move quicker, since it's a group of people with relatively shared opinions. It's a very grassroots style or quality.

The board meetings are usually rather open—other people are invited to come—we call it the Big Board. I think it's only a couple of times that the board has met alone, when we have to take certain decisions. There's no voting; we make decisions by consensus. We discuss it, and if there's somebody opposed—like the pamphlet we were planning: that caused a lot of debate. I liked to tease the scientists who were there: it has to be so perfect, and they are so careful, so it takes a lot of time.

We haven't done many large meetings. We had one with a couple of hundred people—when Simon Mawer came, author of the novel *Mendel's Dwarf.* And we had a large crowd when Paul Rees came—a Danish doctor, elderly, who sits on the Council of Europe Bioethics Board. He said that this idea of a population database would last five minutes in Denmark and would never be discussed again.

Mike: What was it that he thought would make it last only five minutes in Denmark, as opposed to Iceland?

Pétur: He said that he has done studies on informed consent, about how much people understand when they are signing. And he has asked people in Denmark how long they take to understand this and make an informed opinion, and he says the minimum is one day. That's the minimum time there that people take to understand what they are signing. And also they understand, if you ask afterwards what they have signed means, they understand. Even the depressed people. So it's mostly this aspect of informed consent.

Mike: Did Mannvernd get involved in any way in encouraging people to opt out?

Pétur: Yes, it was like a ground rule: whenever you said anything in public, you should always end with, "Remember to opt out. And remember to opt-out your children, too." We don't say anything without it, and try to get it in whenever we can. And that's one of the things that we agree on: to recommend that people opt out. But that was only after we tried to reach an agreement—we tried to offer alternatives. And our chairman at that time had two meetings with the prime minister, just the two of them. And before the law was passed, the prime minister assured him that he didn't have to worry, because it's very easy to change the law, he said. So after a couple of months had passed, after the legislation had passed, our chairman went to him and said, now you can change the law. And he said: it's too early. Of course, the prime minister is a great supporter of the database and he was not going to change the law. But it was only after that that we could say we had tried to reach an agreement, we had offered alternatives, we had many proposals—our last and final demand was some sort of consent, and when that was not accepted, we began to recommend that people opt out.

Mike: What's the worst-case scenario for you, of the database not being anonymous?

Pétur: I think the worst-case scenario is not a single dramatic event, but the more general effect of people not being able to trust their doctors. That's the worst thing. This can happen even without any disclosures or law breaking. And that's happening already. People are being more careful. People are asking, will this go into the database? What will happen to my specimens? Why are you writing this down?

Mike: I also know from experience that having an organization like this is a real challenge—I think you're right, that the threat here is not any one specific incident as much as it is this general change in cultural practices involved in going to the doctor. And that's a very hard thing to educate about, and organize around, and make direct arguments about. The public hears great things, and its immediate, and the idea of long-term, slow degradation of a culture of trust is a very hard thing to get your head around.

Pétur: Yes, it's very hard to explain. But we don't like to publicize horror stories—that's another of the things we've agreed on: not trying to scare people. We haven't gone public and said that some information will leak out, or that someone will break into the database—some computer experts have done that. But we haven't done much of that. We have said that information that comes out of the research will be misused to discriminate against patient groups. And also that if it's true that the whole thing is worth $200 million, then theft is a real danger: someone just walks away with it on a disk in their pocket.

Also, we agreed that we should not criticize single persons. We have not criticized the CEO of deCODE personally. A lot of people are spreading stories, but we do not participate in that. We're asked questions about him personally, but we don't answer that. And I'm very glad of that.

And we agree that Mannvernd is not opposed to deCODE; deCODE is not our opponent. We are opposed to the database law. DeCODE is the main spokesman for that law, so to speak, so we have to address that. But we have not criticized the company. They might be doing a good job in their genetic research; that's not our concern.

Early on, one of the things that people didn't agree on concerned information abroad—whether we should speak to foreign journalists. Some people said that this was like criticizing Iceland and that we would be seen as traitors. That is a very sensitive issue. But the end result is that we do this a lot, and there is no argument about this anymore. But still there are people who say we have to watch out and not look like we are criticizing deCODE, because that's often the first impression people get abroad.

XX

The Health Sector Database, and the campaign to opt out of it, remained central to the work of Mannvernd. As a result, the issue of consent—informed, open, broad, or "presumed"—remained central as well.

"Presumed consent" as it was eventually enacted in the HSD legislation warped time, as we've seen: the entire population instantaneously found itself, on December 17, 1998, in a new present that came from a new past in which they were all—including the dead among them—presumed to have given their consent to have their medical records included in the database, and they now had the right to opt out in the future. Unless you were dead, in which case you had simply consented. (A lawsuit in Iceland's Supreme Court would eventually challenge this provision as unconstitutional.) And the associated principle of "broad consent," which deCODE was seeking to use in its genetic research, as we'll see below, effectively opted one out of having any say in future decisions, since a blood sample donated for research on a particular disease could be used broadly for any research purpose that might be invented in the still-to-come.

Let's first look quickly at the record of opt-outs maintained by Mannvernd on their Web site. It's safe to say that the curve in figure 9 is not a smooth or regular one. From January 1999 through June 1999, the opt-out rate was exponential; if the right-hand portion of Mannvernd's graph were not visible, as it would not have been in June 1999, there would have been no reason to expect a different future, no reason to think that the exponential withdrawal would not have continued.

However, among the Icelandic population that deCODE, multiple journalists, and even other ethnographers have characterized as a remarkably well-informed citizenry avidly digesting hundreds of media stories in their careful democratic deliberation, there seems to have been a misunderstanding that opting out would not be allowed after June 17, six months after the legislation was passed and, somewhat coincidentally and ironically, Iceland's independence day. A clause in the original legislation suggested that data entry would begin six months after the legislation had passed, and no one had clarified what this might mean. Once information was entered into the HSD, Icelanders were told, it could not be withdrawn, even if one subsequently opted out; it seems that people thought they had missed a window of opportunity if they had not acted by June 1999. Figure 9 shows that the opt-out rate decreased dramatically, and the curve marks how a poorly understood future shapes a present, now past. It also marks the question whose answer can only be speculated on: what other futures were unhinged in this swerve?

Opt-outs continued at a slower pace until January 2000 when, after many delays, the Icelandic government formally granted the database license to deCODE. The opt-out rate again climbed dramatically, as Icelanders thought again about future readings of their medical records. Finally, the curve reaches a limit of patience, attention, or care around twenty thousand Icelanders, a not insignificant 7 percent of the population. Only

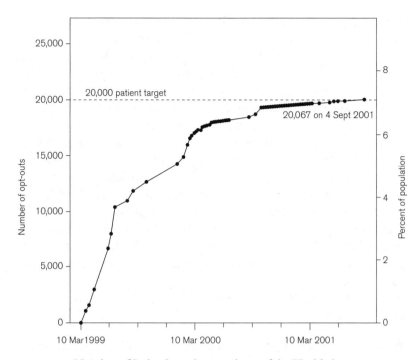

FIGURE 9. Number of Icelanders who opted out of the Health Sector Database. Adapted with permission from Mannvernd, www.mannvernd .is/english/optout.html.

a fool would read twenty thousand as a natural limit, though—a future somehow programmed into Icelandic culture. This unnatural curve in time should be read instead as a swarm intelligence's reading of an ever-opening future, where new events promise new swerves.

What did Icelanders think they were opting out *of*? There was and still is a great deal of confusion about deCODE's database, or more exactly, databases: what would be in them, how they could be accessed, the conditions under which they were to be constructed, the security and encryption measures taken, and other issues. DeCODE did not help matters much, referring at various times and in different documents to the GGPR, the DCDP, the HSD, the IHD, or simply "the database."

In the "Non-Confidential Corporate Summary" that was making the rounds in the summer and fall of 1998, deCODE told potential investors that it was "constructing a large database—called the GGPR database— that will contain the Genotypes, Genealogy, health history/Phenotype of a large proportion of the Icelandic nation, and Resource use in the Icelandic healthcare system."[4] What deCODE wanted to construct, then, or at least what deCODE told its potential investors it wanted to construct, was a *single* database containing these different kinds of information: DNA sequence and mapping information, genealogical information, health care records, and systemic data about the national health system's resource use.

By June 1999, in a new document for investors, there was no reference to a GGPR database; the entity was now called the Icelandic Health-Care Database, or IHD: "deCODE Genetics is currently negotiating with the Icelandic government to compile a database that will contain phenotypes of a majority of Icelanders. The law authorizing the creation of this health-care database further allows the linking up of the healthcare data with information about genotypes of consenting Icelanders and the genealogy of all Icelanders."[5] The desire for unification was still there, but it was now to be achieved through the linkage of three different databases.

Yet another object exists in later documents filed with the U.S. Securities and Exchange Commission—the deCODE Combined Data Processing system, or DCDP:

We are presently devoting substantial resources to the development of the deCODE Combined Data Processing system and its components. We plan to continue to devote substantial resources to this development for the foreseeable future. We cannot be sure that the deCODE Combined Data Processing system will result in marketable products or services. Our intended method for cross-referencing genealogical, genotypic and healthcare data is central to the development of the deCODE Combined Data Processing system and is unproven. The success of our database services is contingent upon:

- the development of the Icelandic Health Sector Database and collection of genotypic data;
- compliance with governmental requirements regarding the Icelandic Health Sector Database;
- the security and reliability of encryption technology;
- the cooperation of the Icelandic healthcare system;
- the ability to obtain blood samples from consenting Icelanders and consents to the use of their genotypic data by cross-referencing through the deCODE Combined Data Processing system[6]

In addition to making for a shifting target, this interconnection of multiple databases created multiple problems. Mannvernd's Einar Árnason described some of them when I interviewed him:

Einar: This cannot work, because the database will be biased. That's been my major criticism. In one of their published articles, deCODE says when you strip the personal identifiers and anonymize the data, you can nevertheless include certain information about the individual. But as the number of bits of data increases, you nullify the anonymization. So you cannot have lots of bits of information. But that's what is happening here. You're going to build this database with a lot of bits of information, because you're going to collate everything together, and that means you will get very heavy demands for privacy. And in order to meet those demands, you do away with the possibility of correcting data. The demands for privacy may get such that you cannot correct any errors. Errors will creep in, and because the system is supposed to be so safe, you cannot correct any errors. And that's a consequence of protecting the data: you get errors.

The second reason the database will be biased is because of the opt-out clause. . . . Because the perception is that it's dangerous, by at least some, and they opt out. And they tend to be politically active people, who read, and so on, and not the lesser educated people. And we know disease goes by class. So it's not just noise; it's systematic bias. Also people who don't mind being in the database, but they will sometimes go to their doctor and say to their doctor: I don't want *this* to be entered into the database. So for example, a gynecologist: if a woman comes to me, and she has chlamydia, it probably means she has had an affair, so I will enter into the records something else: the flu. I will know what it means, but nobody else will.

So for certain things, especially venereal disease, there will be different kinds of records. Another doctor has said, "I will never accept that my health records will be used as scientific data; yesterday I saw fifty people, and I wrote nothing down." This kind of database cannot be built if you have 50 to 60 percent of the doctors against it. It cannot be done.

World-renowned medical database security expert Ross Anderson, brought in as a consultant by the Icelandic Medical Association to evaluate the HSD, stressed additional problems. "For example, deCODE proposed in 1998 that personal identifiers be protected by one-way encryption or by public key encryption. But with a population of well under a million, an opponent with access to the encryption key can simply encrypt the names of the entire population and look for a match. To provide privacy protection, the system would have to use random padding—but this would render the encrypted identifiers useless for their intended purpose."[7]

In other words, despite all claims to the contrary, the HSD was not and could not be based on anonymized data. As a dynamic database—new medical records as they came in had to be assigned to the right person, new medical data on opt-outs had to be deleted—it could not be anonymous, but had to be encrypted, and someone would have to have the key. This led Anderson to make an additional criticism, even more far-reaching than the first, in another analysis a year later:

The security target document appears to ignore two fundamental problems:

- that the parties against whom the privacy of patients must be protected are the operating license holder, the end users, the system developer, and the sponsor for evaluation;
- that these are for all practical purposes the same organisation ("deCODE").

This is as far as I am aware a unique situation in the history of secure systems evaluation. There have been other applications in which all the parties are mutually mistrustful; these range from nuclear arms control treaty verification to prepayment electricity meters. However in no application in my experience, or described in the literature, have the threats to one of the stakeholders been so concentrated.

As in systems like treaty verification and metering, third party threats—from outside hackers, disgruntled employees—are almost insignificant compared with the threat of abuse by authorised insiders.[8]

I expect that you might find all this confusing. I know I do, and I've been reading about it, talking to Icelanders about it, pondering it, and writing about it for years. Ambiguity, cross-statements, technical nuances, lies. Let me try to cut through at least some of that confusion with what might seem a counterintuitive tactic: adding an additional layer of confusion and ambiguity. In other words, I will open up yet another fissure, one that we've encountered before and one that we'll encounter again, the volatile entwining of the present with the future.

In an article that often bends over backward to give deCODE and the HSD every benefit of the doubt regarding compliance with Icelandic and European Union laws, regulations, and codified ethical principles, the three Icelandic authors (two of whom were then professors at the University of Iceland's law school) reserve an interesting criticism of the HSD legislation for the end of their discussion. They praise the drafters of the legislation for being "careful in making every effort to ensure that data on the database are rendered and remain anonymous" (although the authors have just devoted pages and pages to discussing the ambiguities of anonymity—and, as we just saw, anonymity in this case is impossible). But the authors then immediately qualify this statement in light of the interconnections between databases that exist in the deCODE case:

An exemption from the careful drafting of the Act, however, is the hastily drafted provision on the interconnections of data from the database with data from databases of genealogical and genetic data. On the safeguards related to such interconnections, only skeletal provisions are to be found in the Act and much trust is put on the Data Protection Committee and other public bodies responsible for monitoring and imposing specific conditions in practice. Quite clearly it is not possible to present any final assessment of the prospective health sector database at this point in time, as the details of the implementation of the Act are yet to be decided.[9]

To reiterate this crucial argument: the most important, most novel, most potentially lucrative, most possibly invasive, and hence the aspect of the situation most demanding of democratic deliberation—the *interconnection* of the medical, genetic, and genealogical databases—this was the aspect that was dealt with "hastily," never fleshed out but given only "skeletal" attention. On the most crucial matter, the Althingi gets the worst marks from the three legal experts who have gone to great lengths to give the Icelandic Parliament credit and to legitimate the legal basis of the HSD Act. On the most demanding question, according to the most generous analysts, the Althingi failed.

And in a twisted sense, they *had* to fail on this question. The law can't guarantee justice; justice is always deferred, always an open question "yet to be decided."[10] This "radical" point is clear even in this very nonradical legal analysis. The above analysis is entirely dedicated to assessing the legalities of the act in such a way as to resolve any lingering doubts or dissents. The analysis takes great care to consider all the Icelandic and European laws and regulations, all the possible interpretations and loopholes, all the relevant legal principles, so that it can in the end endorse the legislation and legitimate its codifications of privacy, security, and monopoly. *And yet,* this article, so dedicated to exposing the foundations of the law in general and the HSD Act in particular, and so dedicated to pronouncing those foundations sound and stable, also says, "quite clearly," that "it is not possible to present any final assessment of the prospective health sector database at this point in time, as the details of the implementation of the Act are yet to be decided." This article erases its own writing. It assesses the finality of its own assessments—quite clearly and quite rightly—as impossible and ends by marking them as "yet to be decided."

And yet, the Althingi, like these legal experts, had to decide what could really be decided only in the future. Which is why the Althingi's deferral to the Data Protection Committee and other bodies was both a failure and a success, or failureXsuccess. The Althingi *had* to entrust attention to the details of practice to these future bodies. The HSD Act could be enacted *only* in the future by other state bodies like the Data Protection Committee and the National Bioethics Committee. An unsatisfactory solution to an impossible situation, *and* exactly the right thing to do.

In theory. In practice, however, the Icelandic state would do exactly the wrong thing in that future that underwrote their legislation. Instead of deferring to the National Bioethics Committee, they dissolved it and assimilated it.

XX

John McPhee wrote one of his more famous geo-essays on the January 1973 volcanic eruption in the Vestmannaeyjar—the Westman Islands off the south coast of Iceland, which would enter the world media again when Keiko came "home" to the islands in 1998. "Cooling the Lava" recounts the eruption of the interlayered natural and personal events there, events McPhee channeled into a landscape of jagged black words across ice-white pages. The main flow of the essay details how a small pack of Icelanders struggled to cool the lava by dousing it with water—to save homes, but primarily to preserve the invaluable harbor that was home to one of Iceland's most productive fishing fleets. Around this main text flow, McPhee releases a long series of sinuous narrative side channels: about the lava bombs ejected from the crater to explode near people and houses; about mainlanders' sustained skepticism about the lava-cooling effort; about Pompeii and the Plinys; about the underground economy of beer and the above-board economy of liquor; about a fisherman who swims five hours in the frigid sea after his ship goes down; and about other taciturn, stalwart Icelanders who make our folkloric counterparts in Vermont or Maine seem like emotive babies.

"Cooling the Lava" is a tale of men and women trying to control a vast, volatile flow of magma that has burst through this fissure in their island off the coast of an island. McPhee explicates the work of "human intervention" in these geological forces, centered around the pouring of millions and millions of gallons of seawater onto the lava flow for over a hundred days. The Americans sent "invasion pumps," "developed to move gasoline from offshore ships to Omaha Beach" in World War II, that could shoot water five hundred feet in the air, with an output of thirteen thousand gallons per minute. People scrambled over the recently cooled crusts under which molten magma still flowed, placing sprinklers and hoses. Through this never-before-attempted technological-human kludge job, the lava flow was cooled, stopped, and the harbor saved. Maybe—causality in such complex events is hard to ascribe.

The entire episode was one of "effects that affected other effects and were ultimately so imponderable that no one could assign to people or to nature an unchallengeable ratio of triumph to defeat." For that particular event in that particular lava×land, McPhee suggests that "the true extent of the victory will never be known—the role of luck being unassessable, the effects of intervention being ultimately incalculable, and the assertion that people can stop a volcano being hubris enough to provoke a new eruption."[11]

This is how I think of Mannvernd's work on the HSD eruption—both of which still continue. Some safe harbor—a phrase we will encounter in financial contexts as well—has been preserved, somehow, in the midst of numerous defeats and not a little destruction, and the members of Mannvernd deserve great credit. Whatever one might think about the HSD legislation that was enacted in December 1998, the bill and subsequent events were vastly improved by the interventions of Mannvernd to "cool the lava," more so than had the matter been left to the Icelandic government and deCODE. And Mannvernd continued to provide programs and information that helped build a culture of critical scientific literacy on the issues of genomics and biomedical research. This is hard, thankless work, work whose effectiveness is in some sense incalculable, and certainly not easy to sustain, as anyone who has ever worked in an NGO will tell you. Finances and attention span are only two of the scarcities to be managed.

But if there is such a thing as the democratic nation-state, it is always in need of this kind of supplement, especially in the volatile territories of genomics. Because governing occurs in many nongovernmental contexts. And because democracy's arrival is always only ever promised, "yet to be decided."

XX

The happiest I ever saw Einar Árnason, when that unmistakable edge of sheer scientific glee cracked through his sturdy exterior, was when he was describing his research on kleptoparasitism among Icelandic birds. He probably spoke just as intensely about his more recent work on the population genetics of cod, but it's the kleptoparasitism work that sticks with me—in part because it's simply such a great word, totally strange but with vaguely familiar overtones; we know what a parasite is, and we've read funny newspaper stories about kleptomaniacs. But *kleptoparasitism?* Exhibited by *birds?*

This work of Einar's, carried out in the early 1970s, was coauthored with Peter Grant, one of the great evolutionary biologists of the twentieth century. Grant's work—which is also the work of his wife Rosemary, and the work of a flock of graduate students and postdocs—on the finches of the Galápagos Islands and the *observable rapidity* with which they evolve, is the subject of the Pulitzer Prize–winning book by Jonathan Weiner, *The Beak of the Finch.* A quick look at one of the scientific papers by Einar Árnason and Grant also gives a sense of how some of the methodologies of field biology apply to the worlds of NASDAQ and international finance—and how kleptoparasitism might be exhibited by animals other than birds.

Einar spent most of the spring and summer of 1973 on the cliffs near Vík, on Iceland's southern coast. He divided the days into two-hour periods. In the first hour, Einar recorded the number of skuas (these are the kleptoparasites) patrolling the cliffs in a 300x300x200 cubic meter volume of air, the number of puffins that arrived (a cute bird to us, a tasty meal for Icelanders), and the number of great black-backed gulls and other birds. In the second hour, Einar recorded the details of skua-puffin interactions, which went something like this:

At the sight of an incoming puffin, the skua approached rapidly in order to see if it had fish; upon locating a fish-carrier it started a chase. The chase was initiated from behind and above. During the chase skuas either flew below a puffin and attempted to grasp the fish dangling from its beak, or flew above a puffin and kicked at its back with the feet. The chase ended with the puffin escaping or dropping some or all of its fish. The skuas tried to catch the dropped fish in the air either by intercepting it or by diving after it. . . . When chases occurred close to the cliff and approximately parallel to it, the skuas invariably stayed on the cliff side of a puffin, thereby preventing it from landing. . . . Most chases started at a height of 100m or more, but the majority ended below 100m, often within a few metres of the ground. . . . Once a fish had been dropped, the skua tried to catch it in the air. Catching success was directly related to the height at which the fish was released by the puffin.[12]

You don't have to buy my kleptoparasitic allegory to appreciate the careful empirical and analytic methods displayed here. The same observational doggedness and fine-grained analysis also characterized Einar's multiple works for Mannvernd: his burrowing through reams of U.S. Securities and Exchange Commission filings, his reanalysis of genetic sequence data to argue that Icelanders are among the *least* homogeneous of European populations, his construction and maintenance of the Mannvernd Web site that kept an international community informed of every event in Iceland and everything written about the HSD in newspapers and journals in the United States and Europe. My treatment of these topics in later chapters owes much to Einar's different lines of work—basic, necessary work, and so often behind-the-scenes and unappreciated work.

I want to go behind a different scene than the cliffs at Vík, or SEC filings and mitochondrial sequence databases, to document another story of the truly thankless labor that Einar was involved in: the design of informed consent procedures and forms undertaken by the National Bioethics Committee (NBC), of which Einar was a member.

> *Einar:* After the passage of the [HSD] bill, the problem was that we [the NBC] had never done our basic work. The same sort of things kept coming back up again: was this informed consent? So we were working on the informed consent form of deCODE Genetics, and others as well, like the Icelandic Cancer Society. But the committee had no chairman, from September 1998 until the end of January 1999, because the minister of health did not appoint one. The vice chairman was reluctant to get into the informed consent forms and protocols, because he said he was only the vice chairman, and this was a job for the chairman, and what if a new one was appointed that wouldn't recognize the previous work, and so on. One of us went to the Ministry [of Health] to suggest that one of our members be appointed chairman, and we were just simply told that this was none of our business. And then the ministry appointed Gudmundur Thorgeirsson in January 1999. He was a doctor at the Heart Association, and he is on the advisory board of deCODE Genetics. One member of Parliament had made a formal request to the government, asking whether this was not a conflict of interest, since there were so many matters related to deCODE before the committee. And Gudmundur Thorgeirsson announced that he would step aside on all matters related to deCODE. So that made it difficult for the committee, since we had been running it ourselves, had just gotten a new chairman, and then he hands over the meetings to the vice chairman, who had previously not wanted to make these sort of guidelines. So the making of the guidelines was delayed again, because the chairman was only really functioning at half capacity.
>
> So eventually I was asked to make these "Draft Guidelines for Genetic Research." I could have done that in different ways. I could have said to the committee, OK, we have to do this from scratch. And that means we have to sit down and discuss every item of these kinds of guidelines. Or, I said, we can take something from somebody else that

has done this work, and simply translate it, adapt it to Iceland. We discussed that, and that's the route that I went. I started hunting around on the Internet and elsewhere, and eventually I found what I thought were five good guidelines. The best, I thought, were from Washington University in St. Louis—a very large school with a lot of genetic research. It's obvious that they have really thought about everything for their guidelines.

So I took those guidelines, translated them into Icelandic, and then I adapted them to Iceland. I also took some material from the American Society of Human Genetics, like their recommendations for consent in genetics research and on this issue of linked and unlinked data, anonymization, and so on. I discussed these kinds of terms and the four principles of informed consent: it has to be voluntary and competent, that's the first two things; it has to be informed; and finally it has to be comprehended. You have to have these four elements of informed consent, otherwise it's not informed consent. The first two are really to do with the individual, and the second two have more to do with the researcher: he has to inform, and he has to make sure—to his satisfaction, at least—you've understood what you've been told.

This is all in the draft guidelines that I wrote, some twelve pages. This also dealt with the issue of data, in the following sense. In the Washington University guidelines, they thought about it this way: data generated in scientific research is not really clinically validated data. So it may not be of clinical value, but it may be. So you as a participant, if the researcher says "this may be relevant to your health," then the participant has to sign the form saying you would like to know or not like to know. And then even if the person has said he does not want to know, the researcher may find something that he would like to transfer nevertheless. The Washington University guidelines say that all transfer of information must get referred back to the patient—if the researcher wants to do that, he will have to submit to a subcommittee a proposal on how the people would be approached again. That then is rereviewed, the mechanism of giving the information back. They clearly had thought about this extremely well, and I thought this was the best that I could find.

So I presented this to the committee at a meeting in June 1999. At a meeting in May, we had stopped several protocols from deCODE because we had to make these decisions. I presented to the full committee in June: the chairman and vice chairman were there, and some of the advisors as well, because this was a major "thinking" meeting. I had also given all the references I had used in the English versions: the Washington University guidelines, the American Society of Human Genetics, the relevant sections of the U.S. Code of Federal Regulations, and so on. They all thanked me for this and said it was a fine piece of work, and said it was a lot of material and we would have to study it as well. So the committee got a copy and everyone was going to study it.

But then they asked, have we reached enough of an agreement now about where we are heading, so that we can pass the applications from deCODE now? These are applications for research on particular diseases, the kind of research they're doing in collaboration with Roche and cooperating physicians. So these are basically applications from the collaborating physicians, and deCODE is a part of that. So they all have the same wording, and they're just sent by deCODE, but they're applications for specific disease research.

In these cases a patient was informed about that disease, and he or she agreed to participate in the research and give . . . blood. The reason why we stopped it is because there was this thing that they wanted to use the DNA for other diseases. We had been making changes to the informed consent form that they had been using, and until that time they had this thing that they could use [a blood sample] for "related diseases" without asking, but if they were unrelated diseases, they were going to ask the Data Protection Committee. So that was the problem we had stopped them on.

And then we decided at this meeting that we could nevertheless give them the go-ahead for this research, based on the understanding of the committee at that time, which was to stop that practice when you only have consent for the particular disease that you have informed them about. That's what informed consent is; you cannot have it "open." We told them that they would have to change the informed consent form they had presented along with their proposal, that they could go ahead with their research, but it was for that specific disease.

I think this meeting was on the 22nd or 24th of June. Then July is vacation. I was going up into the mountains on a twelve-day horse ride. While I'm away, a letter comes from a deCODE lawyer . . .

The letter from deCODE—technically, from the company Íslensk erfðagreining—came to the chair of the NBC, Gudmundur Thorgeirsson, a physician on the advisory board of deCODE. It had three numbered points, and number one got right down to business:

1. Demand

a) Íslensk erfðagreining ehf. (ÍE) hereby demands that the National Bioethics Committee rule that Einar Árnason, member of the National Bioethics Committee, nominated by the Institute of Biology University of Iceland, step aside in all matters that are now before the committee and are connected to ÍE in any way.

b) It is demanded that all unfinished matters according to item a) will be reevaluated if Einar Árnason has taken part in preparation and decision making of said matter.

c) Further, it is demanded that Einar Árnason step aside permanently in all matters related to ÍE and that may be placed before the committee later.

d) We request that the National Bioethics Committee reply to this demand in writing after it has reached a decision.[13]

It's a curious thing, this "demand" addressed to an agent of the government. It's not a request for a review, it's not a suit filed in a court of law (although pertinent laws would be cited in point 3): it's a demand.

Points 2 and 3 discussed how, in the long public debate "both within Iceland and abroad," many "strong statements" had been made, but that few had "exaggerated to the extent that that Einar Árnason has. . . . Einar Árnason has taken great pains to defame the company both in speech, and as can be seen clearly, in his writings." As evidence of Einar's imputed inability to provide the "fair and objective treatment" that was the "important legally protected right" of deCODE, the demand included two letters as an attachment—letters written by Einar and sent to the *Times* of London and to the *New York Times,* neither of which had actually been published by the papers. Einar had posted them on the Mannvernd Web site, and the deCODE lawyer had downloaded them from there.

> *Einar:* So then the committee met on July 16 or something like that. They said he's [Einar] not here, so we can't discuss this while he's away. So they postponed the discussion and set a meeting for August 4th.
>
> The first Monday in August is a banking holiday, so the weekend before is a major travel holiday in Iceland. I had come back from my horse trip, seen this letter and just laughed at it, thinking it was crazy. My advisor who had been at the meeting on the 16th, he had just laughed at it too. So we didn't think anything more about it. So I came back from the horses on Monday, and then on Thursday we went to the east on another vacation. And then on the news on Friday, the day before this weekend, we heard that the Minister of Health had fired this committee.
>
> *Mike:* You heard it on the news?
>
> *Einar:* Yeah. Yeah. And when I came back, on August 3 I think, there was another letter for me.

Einar posted deCODE's letter and related documents on the Mannvernd Web site, for all those interested in understanding how "democracy" actually goes down:

Ministry of Health and Social Security, Reykjavík, 29 July 1999

(To members of the National Bioethics Committee)

The Minister of Health and Social Security today signed the enclosed regulation on biomedical research. On its enactment the old regulation nr. 449/1997 concerned with the same matter is void.

Due to changes in the appointment of the National Bioethics Committee appointments according to the old regulation are void at the enactment of the new regulation. Nominations to the National Bioethics Committee according to the new regulation have been solicited and it is expected that a new committee will be appointed soon.

You are hereby given best thanks for your work on the National Bioethics Committee.

On behalf of the Minister,

Ragnheidur Haraldsdóttir (sign)[14]

Einar has never been one to mince words about deCODE. In those unpublished letters to the London and New York newspapers, he had written things like, "deCODE genetics has evoked the myth of the homogenous Aryan Icelanders to entice foreign investors. And in Iceland the company has rallied support for its plans by inventing genetic nationalism, declaring that the Icelandic DNA is superior to all other DNA."[15] But I asked him if this episode had nevertheless marked a change in his attitude toward deCODE, or if it was more like one more domino had fallen.

Einar: It was a very serious message that I got there. I realized that the government is completely in the hands of Kári Stefánsson. He just phones the government and tells them to fire the committee, and they do it. It can't be any other way. There's no coincidence, that they send a letter trying to remove me, the troublemaker on the committee, and they are then told that can't be done, there is nothing wrong with stating your opinion in public—that's what they must have told them. So then what is the recourse? Throw out the committee. That means the government is in the hands of Kári Stefánsson. He just decides. Just the same way that we learned that he had faxed the government the draft HSD bill. And that is absolutely incredible. Of course, we knew that there was a cozy relationship. But that it was this way, that he could really basically tell the government to throw away the regulatory structure . . . I thought he might infiltrate, like he had infiltrated with Thorgeirsson, our committee chair who was on the advisory board of deCODE. But this isn't infiltration, this is just *whhhhhhsshhht,* you throw it out! I mean, you see infiltration of regulatory bodies everywhere. But this kind of a method I've never seen. So to be honest, this really hardened my attitude quite a lot.

The *Icelandic Medical Journal,* and a lot of people also found this really disturbing. I got phone calls from people who said, how do I get out of this thing—the database? And then the *Icelandic Medical Journal* had an editorial, and this made a splash in Parliament and in the papers and so forth.

Mike: Has the minister ever had to defend this move?

Einar: The defense is basically, the director general of public health [Sigurdur Gudmundsson] had recommended this. And then the director general of public health said "yes, I said something like that, but the decision is the minister's." The *Icelandic Medical Journal* interviewed him, and you should really read his statements, because they give you a sense of the nonsense of it. Let me give you one example. He said that there was a need to have a lay person on the committee, and the previous committee had been all academics. And there was a need for the education minister to appoint someone.

But then who did he appoint? He appointed a nurse. He also says that the method of nomination is not important, but who is nominated. That's what he says.[16] If that is true, if it is only important who is nominated, and not who nominates—we had a nurse on our committee, nominated by the Association of Nurses, so he is saying that his nomination is better than the one nominated by the nurses themselves.

That's what government officials get away with in Iceland . . .

This is not all that different from what government officials anywhere get away with. One U.S. journalist with whom I spoke at some length compared Iceland to Rhode Island—both small states controlled by some kind of mafia, he said. So just where is the boundary to mark the differences between Iceland and the rest of the world?

IcelandXWorld

> The conflict of the ocean currents with the submarine ridges, and vice-versa, causes a mixing in the sea: upwelling at the continental slopes and anti-clockwise currents with deep, vertical mixing in the seas around Iceland. Together with winter cooling, this process of mixing serves to facilitate the dispersal of oxygen through deep waters and the movement of nutrients upwards to the surface layers. These conditions, coupled with others such as a fairly extensive continental shelf and the rays of the sun, form an ideal environment for the recruitment and growth of marine life, the basis for the existence of fishing grounds around Iceland and all human life within the country.
>
> Nordal and Kristinsson, *Iceland: The Republic,* 49

Conflicts, mixings, upwellings. A geological and oceanographic viewpoint is useful for reimagining this place that is constantly described as "isolated." Jóhannes Nordal and Valdimar Kristinsson's handbook on Iceland, published by the country's Central Bank, describes the fecund effects of submarine ridges outside national borders, beyond any land where you could plant a flag. At a silent depth that's difficult to plumb, formed by forgotten ancient processes, the submarine ridges work on temperature gradients, rechanneling them into new collisions and collusions. Opposites — no, *differences* meet and swirl turbulently. The subsurface redirects the surface flows. Fish love it. Fishermen love the fish. The nation loves the fishermen. National prosperity, with its new gradients of wealth, emerges on shore. As do other conflicts, mixings, upwellings.

Like Nietzsche, the Central Bank of Iceland recognizes that any force is always "coupled with other" forces. Isolation is impossible; there's always an *and:* ridge *and* gradient *and* currents *and* oxygen *and* nutrients *and* fish *and* "all human life within the country."[1] It's possible to speak of Iceland's "unique geographical position," as Althingi member Hjörleifur Guttormsson did back in "TrustXGullibility," but that's not a statement about isolation; that's a statement about Iceland and the United States and Europe and the flowing substances — water, words, wealth — that connect them. Let's continue diagramming some of these flows.

XX

One answer to the question "Where is the limit of Iceland?" would be "three miles offshore," but only if you were a fishing boat and only if it was 1901. That was the territorial fishing limit declared by Iceland at the time, although Denmark was in the business of declaring such things for Iceland in 1901. Non-Icelanders had been fishing that close to Iceland since at least the fifteenth century, and this historical fact, as we'll see in "SameXDifference," raises some questions about the other kind of "isolation" that Iceland has been said to enjoy, genetic isolation. But as far as fish and fishing boats were concerned, Iceland might have been far away, but it was certainly not isolated — it was aswarm. So in 1901, other nations in effect had promised not to fish in Denmark's Iceland for fifty years, a promise that carried through past Icelandic independence in 1944. But when the time limit on the international promise to the Danes had passed, the newly sovereign Iceland+3 expanded the fishing limit to 4 miles in 1952. All nations again promised to recognize the new line where Iceland stopped and the rest of the world began — except for the British.

The British began a boycott of Icelandic fish, but this blow to Iceland's chief industry was absorbed by new markets at both poles of the new Cold War, the United States and the Soviet Union. As nations the world over began debating the merits of a transnationally recognized 12-mile fishing limit at a 1958 United Nations conference provoked by concerns about endangered fish stocks, Iceland cut to the chase and declared it. All foreign fishing vessels left the Iceland+12 territory on September 1, 1958 — except for the British ones.

Thus began the first Cod War, that gradient within the Cold War.

Britain sent in the Royal Navy to protect its trawlers, preventing the Icelandic coast guard from arresting their crews. A deal was struck in 1961, when Britain promised to recognize Iceland+12 in most places, in exchange for three years of fishing in other choice places somewhere between Iceland+12 and Iceland+6. Also in the treaty was what historian Jón Hjálmarsson calls "a questionable clause," although this characterization might itself be questionable; the clause held that isolated Iceland would recognize international binds and would seek approval from the International Court before extending the limit again.[2]

Iceland extended the limit again in 1972. A coalition of the Progressive Party, the People's Alliance, and the Union of Leftists and Liberals in the newly elected Parliament of 1971 decided it would be Iceland+50. Britain and West Germany protested, arguing that the International Court had not been consulted. Iceland asserted its isolation again, saying it need not have consulted the International Court. After an appeal by Britain and West Germany, the International Court ruled that their ships had the right to fish in places within Iceland+50. Iceland lodged a protest with the court and went ahead and declared the 50-mile limit anyway.

Cod Wars, the sequel. The British and West Germans brought in reinforced tugboats and continued to fish. The Icelanders had a "secret weapon," as all war stories require: clippers pulled by the Icelandic coast guard vessels craftily sailed among the protective tugs, getting between the trawlers and their nets, cutting the lines. By the summer of 1973, the British sent in frigging frigates, counterharassing the Icelandic coast guard vessels and even ramming them on occasion. Not grasping the different demands posed by swarms of fish and swarms of U-boats, the British required their trawlers to behave like a wartime convoy, staying in small groups. Easy to protect, lousy for fishing. One fishing boat captain broke ranks; finding him fishing off on his own, the Icelandic coast guard fired a couple of "shots across his bow," one of which happened to go *into* the bow. The hapless fisherman was about to surrender when the frigates arrived to prevent his arrest.

After a threat by Iceland to withdraw their ambassador to Britain if the warships didn't leave, a deal was struck once again: Britain would respect the new Iceland+50 after two years of fishing in certain areas—but with no big technology-enhanced factory trawlers. The West Germans were not so quick to negotiate, but as the Cod War with them went on, larger events took over. The International Court denied Iceland's appeal and pronounced the 50-mile limit illegal. "Iceland remained undeterred," writes Hjálmarsson, although "in violation of international law" would

be another way of putting it. By 1974 and a new United Nations conference on the law of the sea, many countries were talking about 200-mile
limits. A new governing coalition was elected in 1974, and the Progressive Party and the Independence Party took this opportunity to be in
the political vanguard: starting in 1975, they declared, it would be Ice-
land+200.

The reinforced tugboats and British frigates returned. Cod War III.
More rammings and clippings. This time, Iceland actually did withdraw
its ambassador from Britain. But as Belgium, West Germany, and other
countries agreed to the new limits, and as international opinion began to
support the 200-mile limit, and as NATO put pressure on its two cod-
warring members who were supposed to be unified within the Cold War,
Britain saw the writing on the wall. When the European Community itself, of which Britain was also a member, announced it would extend its
territorial fishing limits to 200 miles, the game was up. Cod War III officially ended on June 1, 1976.

XX

Members of the Icelandic coast guard were revered as national heroes.
The fishermen themselves, given their importance to the national economy, had held that kind of symbolic status for a longer time, in a much
more deeply layered way. The various fish imprinted on the reverse of Iceland's coins are a constant reminder, jingling daily in your pocket, that
this particular kind of biomass is literally (albeit with the ghostly strangeness that accompanies all processes of valuation and commoditization)
convertible to cash.

The anthropologist Gísli Pálsson, whose parallel interests in the de-
CODE events were discussed in "DistanceXComplicity," has analyzed the
political, economic, and cultural crosscurrents of the Icelandic fishing
world as it developed over the last century. What Pálsson calls "the con-
tested character of a nation" got hashed out over the better part of this
century vis-à-vis fish.

Fish first gave rise to the competing discourses of the nation's "common property" and of the right to efficient exploitation of that common
property, discourses that were again debated in the deCODE events. "The
fishing territories are the common property of all Icelanders," wrote an
Icelandic politician in 1926, "to be jointly exploited by them without interference, according to the laws and regulations in force at each moment

in time."[3] A county-level official wrote more effusively in 1930, when the fishing limit was a mere Iceland+4 and the Icelanders were still governed by Denmark. The official argued to expel foreign vessels from Iceland's waters: "When this has been accomplished, *then, at last, we Icelanders will have reclaimed for ourselves Iceland as a sovereign state,* and then, both on land and sea, we can begin to sing in a free and mighty voice 'Rejoice Iceland's millennium!'" (Pálsson, 63).

In a nation dedicated to at least the rhetoric of equality, it surprised some observers when, in 1983, in response to dwindling fish stocks produced by a technology-enhanced and growing fishing fleet, a system of quotas was installed. In the new fish regime, each boat was allocated a certain percentage of the reduced total permissible catch, based on that boat's average catch over the previous three years. This in effect legislated and locked in inequality among the 667 active fishing vessels and their skippers.

The quotas were supposed to be a temporary measure, mandated by the ecological goal of "sustainable exploitation of the fishing stocks." Somebody in the government figured out that this phrasing could be improved upon, and "efficient production" was born, and by 1990 the quota system was made more or less permanent. Quotas also could be bought and sold, like any other commodity.

It wasn't long before quotas became "less transient and more akin to permanent property rights," writes Pálsson. Like a hidden submarine ridge, this ambiguous relationship between a fishing quota and a permanent property right created conflicts, mixings, upwellings. Ninety-one percent of Icelanders polled in 1991 said they were opposed to changing the "common property" basis of the fisheries. Politicians and fisheries officials denied that any such change had taken place, since the legislation still said that fish were the common property of the nation, and the quotas were merely temporary use rights that, despite the extension of the "temporary" into the indefinite future, should not be confused with private property.

Other government agencies, and their endless supply of printed forms, are less tolerant of such ambiguities. Quotas have to be reported as property by fishermen on their tax forms, and if they sell the quotas this counts as income that also has to be reported. And the Supreme Court has ruled that holding permanent fishing quotas indeed represents private property subject to taxation. The end result is that fishing quotas, according to Pálsson, have "the transitional and somewhat anomalous status of being the public property of the nation, in name, but in effect the private property of boat owners" (66). The whole process, in the rhetoric of the political campaigns of the early 1990s, amounted to the "biggest theft in Icelandic history."

Time marches on, and new candidates for biggest this and most heinous that emerge. There are bigger fish to fry now, if not steal. Trawling for cod seems so quaintly historical. Trawling a nation's genealogical history and collective bodily fluids in a search for valuable information and, maybe, actual useful substances—now *there's* an industry for the future. And as we'll see in "GenomicsXSlot Machines," a lot of the capital netted through the fishing quotas got dumped into deCODE at the height—depth?—of the speculative wave of 1998–2000.

XX

Like all industries of the future, genomics is replete with the phrases and concepts of the industries of the past. Mining is a popular trope—data mining, genome mining—but another term also became popular: "gene fishing." This description of what scientists and technicians engaged in genomics were doing was usually used in a derogatory sense, and usually by scientists themselves. "Genomics and gene expression experiments are sometimes derided as 'fishing expeditions,'" David Lockhart and Elizabeth Winzeler of Novartis's Genomics Institute observed in 2000. They had a simple response: "Our view is that there is nothing wrong with a fishing expedition if what you are after is "fish," such as new genes involved in a pathway, potential drug targets or expression markers that can be used in a predictive or diagnostic fashion."[4]

Or, as John Weinstein, senior scientist at the National Cancer Institute and a pioneer of multiple gene expression analysis, complained in a 1999 letter titled "Fishing Expeditions" to *Science* magazine, "Some referees, editors, site visitors, and study sections have tended to disparage other -omic studies as 'fishing expeditions'—often because the hypothesis that drives the generation of a molecular database relates to the nature of information and its utility, rather than to biological specifics." What this part of the life sciences establishment didn't seem to get, Weinstein was arguing, was that, "beyond semantics, -omic research appears to require a different mind-set from the more traditional study of one gene, gene product, or process at a time. Often, one generates a database of molecular information with only limited ability to predict what about it will prove most useful." It's not what huge genomic databases can do, it's what they promise. With genomics, in other words, you *had* to be out ahead of yourself, where the only future was a featureless, oceanic, promising one: *it's out there somewhere, I'm sure of it* . . .

The moral for Weinstein was a simple, almost folksy one: "If one is going to fish, it is best to do so in teeming waters with the finest equipment and flawless technique."[5]

A fishing license, some fishing limits to keep other people out, and perhaps a government-sanctioned fishing quota system would be of use as well, although these kinds of basics tend to get overlooked in the glare of fine equipment and flawless technique that we associate with doing science. DeCODE got some version of all of these from the Icelandic nation in the first such arrangement of its kind, but certainly not the only one. Estonia quickly followed suit, as did the Sweden, Tonga, and the United Kingdom. Latvia, Newfoundland, and the Marshfield Clinic in the U.S. state of Wisconsin also got in on the act. All were trying to leverage the genetic characteristics of a particular population, along with their medical records, into a scientific and commercial resource for developing "personalized medicine." "Population Databases Boom," ran the title of a 2002 *Science* article, which pointed out that "4 years after deCODE sparked international debate on population databases, ethical questions still loom large." *Science* suggested that it was "not clear" that these population-based databases "will deliver on their most ambitious promises," quoting prominent geneticist David Altshuler that "there are many, many opinions and not a lot of hard facts about this field."[6] But (or as a result), the boom kept booming.

The licenses, limits, and other terms of these national gene fishing expeditions were different in each case, often in important ways.[7] But they all shared the difficulty of needing to articulate a limit to the genome space in question, a limit that coincided in some ways with national borders, but in other ways did not—*could* not.

Early in the deCODE history, in 1998 with the Althingi vote still in the future, Kári Stefánsson commented in an interview: "Should biological materials be collected for genetic studies of indigenous populations? Such groups sometimes justifiably object to the process. Scientists from the outside can arrive unannounced, extract blood from members of the population with vague promises of benefits, and then disappear, never to be seen again by donors. DeCode Genetics, Inc., the first Icelandic biotech company and one founded by Icelanders for Icelanders, does not operate in this manner."[8]

Not exactly "Rejoice, Iceland's millennium!," but you get the drift. The statement "the first Icelandic biotech company . . . founded by Icelanders for Icelanders" overlooks the Delaware incorporation, the board of U.S. venture capitalists and their $12 million in start-up money, the fact that Hoffmann-LaRoche was the single largest shareholder in the company, and an even wider, more tangled web of nonlocal relationships, especially financial ones, that we'll encounter later. So since we have to call it something, let's call deCODE an "Icelandic+n biotech company." Yes, there is something undeniably "Icelandic" about deCODE. And yes, there is something "globalized" about it. But this unstable equilibrium, Iceland-Xworld, has been happening for quite some time.

XX

In an article on the electrification of Iceland, my advance man Skúli quotes a 1945 letter penned by "a future member of the engineering elite," who described how capital flows were already changing "isolated" Iceland decades before globalization became the buzzword of the bio- and info-technology economies of the 1990s:

The prime mover in all these changes has, of course, been the tremendous capital flow of the war years, which has come like manna from heaven into this capital deprived country. Now for the first time in history there is sufficient domestic capital to start several enterprises, which in normal times would only have been conceivable had foreign venture capitalists thought it likely that they could make some money from it. Now the plan is to use some of these extensive funds to renew and build from scratch the fishing industry, on which the whole financial state of the country depends.[9]

This letter's author, Sigurdur Jóhannsson, would eventually become the civil engineer in charge of Iceland's road system and father of Skúli, another analyst of Iceland's political economy. He died long before I met Skúli, although I once met his mother, Stefanía Gudnadóttir, before she died in 1997. As spirits, both Sigurdur and Stefanía were presumed to have consented to have their medical records become data sets in the Health Sector Database, and Skúli could do nothing to change that bizarre fact created by the 1998 law.

Skúli's article on the electrification of Iceland discusses the expanding presence of the U.S. military in Iceland and its cultural effects. Twice during World War II, the British asked that they be allowed to establish military bases in Iceland. Twice Iceland refused. In what seems a rather genteel set of events, the British invaded neutral Iceland, and a diplomatic delegation brought a letter of explanation from King George to the Icelandic prime minister, who is said to have welcomed them politely, "since after all they were here."[10] Iceland's prime minister did tell them that they should nevertheless expect a formal protest from the Icelandic government. That night, after the protest had been filed, the prime minister addressed the nation over the radio, assuring Icelanders that the British were there only to keep Germany out, would not interfere in Icelandic politics, and would be gone when the war was over.

They actually ended up leaving just a year later, but the U.S. military kindly agreed to replace them, even though the United States had not yet entered the war. "They required an official request from the Icelandic government. Under pressure from the British, during the summer, when the parliament was out of session, the Icelandic government agreed to make this request without the knowledge of the public or parliamentary consent. This was unconstitutional. After the American troops had left for Iceland, an emergency session of the parliament ratified the request, since it was believed that Iceland could not be without military protection."[11]

The Americans brought in the first heavy construction equipment that Iceland had seen, building the airfield at Keflavík, which every visitor to Iceland still flies into, and the surrounding base. Trade with the United States rose. Iceland, cut off from Denmark by the war, began taking the political steps to dissolve the treaty that bound the two countries together, becoming politically independent on June 17, 1944. During the war, the United States was unsuccessful in its negotiations for a long-term lease of land for the Keflavík base, with the result that all forces left Iceland by 1947.

When the Soviet Union blockaded Berlin in 1948, and Norway and Denmark announced they would join the new alliance the United States had formed, the North Atlantic Treaty Organization (NATO), the Cold War heated up everywhere, Iceland included. An Icelandic government delegation traveled to the United States in 1948 and returned to argue that Iceland should join NATO, with the provision that no U.S. troops would be stationed at Keflavík during peacetime. As the proposal was being debated in the Althingi, a huge crowd gathered in the main square outside the Parliament building. The Socialist Party and its supporters demanded a national referendum on the issue of NATO membership. The conservative Independence Party brought out its own citizens' force, many armed with clubs. And, of course, the police came. A volatile situation. Not surprisingly, violence broke out. Eggs and rocks were thrown, clubs swung, teargas fired. It was Iceland's biggest riot, and it "left scars on daily life in Iceland that took a long time to heal."[12] The treaty was passed that same day, and Iceland became a member of NATO on March 30, 1949.

When the United States involved itself in the police action known as the Korean War in 1950, it argued that peacetime was over and that troops would be on the way. It was summertime in Iceland, and we have seen a number of examples of how democracy tends to function in the Icelandic summer. The governing coalition of the Independence Party and the Progressive Party called in its members for discussion and also invited the members of the Social Democratic Party; members of the Socialist Party (which would become Hjörleifur Guttormsson's People's Alliance) were not consulted. Within two days of signing a new defense treaty on May 5, 1951, U.S. forces began arriving in Iceland. They would remain there for more than fifty years.

XX

In his article on electrification, Skúli touches on one particularly transformative but not readily apparent effect that the combination of electricity and the U.S. military had on Icelandic society and history: the radio station at the U.S. base in Keflavík began broadcasting rockXroll, which members of Skúli's generation listened to on their sets in Reykjavík. As a veteran musician of Reykjavík's late-1970s punk scene recalled,

If I need to find one word to sum up living in Reykjavík in 1978, I think perhaps that it would be "isolation." Also, "boredom" and "frustration" come to mind. At the time, there was only one state run radio station which aired stuff like Icelandic news, educational programmes, talk shows, plays, classical music, German military bands, James Last, Icelandic folk singers and very little international pop music. . . . Other than that, most people who were into music tried to listen to US Army radio as reception conditions from Europe were not good, although occasionally the BBC or Radio Luxembourg got through. This meant that a lot of the pop music we heard was heavily inspired by the USA.[13]

Skúli played an old vinyl record of his for me, "Rock in Reykjavík," from 1982; Frídrik Thor Frídriksson, who went on to become one of Iceland's most famous filmmakers, made a documentary film of the same name in 1982. Both feature a band, Tappi Tíkarass, fronted by a sixteen-year-old Björk Gudmundsdóttir, who would go on to become a star with the Sugarcubes and then on to an even more successful solo career. She became an icon of Icelandic music, even if she was living mostly in the United Kingdom.

But is there really an "Icelandic music" for which one then becomes an icon? In that U.S. Armed Forces–driven punk scene of the early 1980s, Björk was screaming—literally and figuratively. And she has screamed in the same ways since, although, like many aging pop stars, increasingly more in the figurative sense. This fits with how Halldór Laxness characterized Icelandic music in *The Atom Station* as "on the other side of usual form":

The organist and the self-conscious policeman were sitting at the battered old harmonium with some barely legible scrawled notation in front of them. . . . For a long time they struggled their way through some sort of tunelessness, full of weird sounds that recalled the light over the countryside early in the morning before anyone is afoot. In the end, however, I seemed to perceive a melody emerging, but it came from such a distant place, in addition to which its wonders revealed themselves to me in so sudden a flash, that perception struck rather than touched me. And just as I was beginning to get palpitations over a new world, a fantastic and undiscovered world, on the other side of usual form, the two had stopped.[14]

The Icelandic landscape and lightscape would seem to have suffused its music. A half century later, music critic Neil Strauss, writing for the *New York Times*, speculated that a similar effect could be detected in the contemporary music scene in Reykjavík as it erupted, along with genomics, onto the global market:

Iceland is known for its surreal lunar landscape. . . . Its expanse of glaciers, lava fields and mountains are alluring yet harsh and inhospitable. The music aspires to the same sort of friction between the lush and the abrasive, whether it's in the skittering show tunes of Björk's soundtrack to "Dancer in the Dark;" the desultory dance-music of the nine-artist collective Gus Gus; . . . the experimental soundscapes of Sigur Rós; the whispering feedback-laced pop of Slowblow; the dense rock and light electrofusion of Ensimi and AmPop; or the ambient and natural sound bricolages of Múm. Even the country's more straight-ahead mainstream pop and rock acts . . . have something that is a little off in their music.[15]

I bought at least one CD by every one of these Icelandic bands, as well as many by more experimental groups like stillupsteypa. I was delighted when Sigur Rós started making it big as an opening band for Radiohead; any group that sings in its own made-up language deserves success. And with every Icelandic CD I bought, I also bought into this particular exoticization of Iceland even as I resisted others.

But I've become more judicious in my purchases over the years, better able to straddle the fissure rending Iceland's "uniqueness" without losing contact with it. Strauss, Laxness, and Miss E. J. Oswald, who likened the Icelandic landscape to the "difficult to follow" "music of the moderns" back in chapter 1, were all clearly responding to something shared between Iceland's landscape and its music, as were my own cultured ears. But I can make a long list of other music that I find to be "a little off," even while restricting the geographic locale to Akron, Ohio. And if glaciers and *gjá* have powered Icelandic music and a force like Björk, it should be clear that the U.S. Armed Forces have done so as well.

To put it another way, Icelandic music is also very much on *this* side of at least one usual form: capital. Weird sells. Icelandic soundscapes, like the landscape on which they may depend, can be marketed in an increasingly global economy. In 1999, the year after my initial visit, the first Iceland Airwaves music festival (backed by Icelandair) was held in an abandoned airport hangar. It showcased three Icelandic bands. The festival in 2004 featured 130 acts from Iceland, the United States, Germany, Finland, the United Kingdom and elsewhere, spread through clubs and other venues all over downtown Reykjavík. Swelling crowds flowed through streets that, over the same years that I was researching (1998–2001), continually sprouted new restaurants, new clothing boutiques, new coffeehouses, new clubs and bars. In a city where you couldn't buy beer in public until 1989, change was accelerating and invigorating.[16]

The new crowds drinking their Egil's beer as they celebrated Iceland's new millennium through the 3:00 A.M. Reykjavík streets on their way to the next happening place were not just the new techies who loaded the DNA samples into the automated genomic machine at deCODE but, increasingly, were foreign tourists. The Icelandic tourist industry was one of the fastest-growing sectors in the 1990s, second only to the fishing industry in the percentage of foreign currency hauled into the nation (tourism drew roughly 13 percent of foreign earnings). As genome stocks and dissonant music bubbled in the late 1990s, so too did the number of tourists, whose main reason for coming to Iceland was for the "Nature." In 1996, 58,800 tourists from Nordic countries came to Iceland; by 1998 that number was 68,900 and had ballooned to 91,600 in 2000. The 40,000 or so U.S. tourists who went to Iceland in 1998 had increased to more than 53,000 by 2000. And, most dramatically, U.K. tourists went from 27,800 in 1998 to over 45,000 in 2000. By 2002, these numbers had again dropped: to 73,000 (Nordic), 45,800 (U.S.), and 44,800 (U.K.). The upwelling had reversed.

XX

In "TrustXGullibilty," we saw Ugla the "mountain-owl" of Laxness's *The Atom Station* reflecting on the Althingi members' many sworn oaths to never sell the nation so the Americans could have their atom station. It was when the ministers "swore it on their honor" that Ugla "knew that now it had been done." But, she added, "there was one further thing that gave me an indication: they had started the bones rigmarole again."[17]

The "bones rigmarole" was drummed up by Two Hundred Thousand Pliers, the key figure in the fabled joint American-Icelandic company F.F.F. (Federation of Fulminating Fish/Figures Faking Federation) and owner of the Cadillac that the Atom Poet had (sort of) stolen. The bones in question are those of someone referred to in the novel only as "the Nation's Darling." "The Nation's Darling wants Pliers to dig up his bones," Ugla's minister and employer tells her, "so that we Icelanders of today can become the well-merited laughing-stock of history" (59). Laxness had no question about Icelanders' ability to make fools of themselves through one resurrection scheme or another.

"The Nation's Darling" is, in reality, Jónas Hallgrímsson (1807–45), "a naturalist and outstanding poet in the Romantic vein, who made a major contribution towards reinvigorating the lyrical tradition and purifying the language," in the words of an Icelandic historian.[18] He was one of a group of young Icelandic students in Copenhagen who in 1835 started a journal, *Fjölnir*, whose unwritten motto was a triple promise: "We will all be Icelanders, we will protect our language and our nationality, we will have the Althingi at Thingvellir." In an early milestone in Iceland's road toward full independence, the king of Denmark did restore the Althingi, with limited powers, to Reykjavík in 1845—the same year that Jónas Hallgrímsson, the Nation's Darling, died. In Copenhagen. Thorsteinn Gíslason commented in 1903 that Jónas had died like Moses, "leaving the band of his contemporaries on the edge of a mountain overlooking the Promised Land, the land of the future which they longed to inhabit: Iceland as they imagined it ought to be—and *might* be."[19]

Two Hundred Thousand Pliers enlists the help of a medium and holds a séance in the minister's house, with the minister's wife in attendance. "My friend the Darling," Pliers announces to the minister at the end of the spiritualist session, "has confirmed in your wife's hearing . . . what he has so often told me previously during seances: Iceland must have her bones. The Icelandic nation needs spiritual maturity and light. . . . The papers shall have it, the radio shall have it, the people shall have it. And if you defeat it in Parliament I shall go to Denmark myself and have him dug up at my own expense; I shall moreover buy the bones and keep them myself. Nothing shall come between my bones and his."[20]

Ugla soon forgets all about Pliers and his determined plan for national renewal via the embrace—monopolized, if necessary—of those remains that were most enduring in a pregenomic era. She has other things to be concerned about—like the fact that she is pregnant.

Ugla had been at the organist's house again, along with two other students of music, both policemen; they are named only as "the unself-conscious policeman" and "the self-conscious policeman." It's the self-conscious policeman who walks her home, having pilfered her key to the minister's house where she works and lives. Unable to get in and unwilling to wake anyone, Ugla goes home with the self-conscious policeman, a fellow northerner likewise migrated to the city. "I am not going to say how it happened or what it was," Ugla tells us. "I can only tell you the external causes." She models the taciturn contempt for interiority that she learned from her father: "My father was never angrier than when he heard talk of the soul; his doctrine was that we should live as if the soul did not exist" (Laxness, 77). (We will have occasion to learn more of Ugla's ethical sense in "EthicsXExpediency.") Beyond willingness or unwillingness, having more questions than answers about love in general and about this man in particular, Ugla beds with the self-conscious policeman.

She becomes pregnant, and her pregnancy furthers her radicalization. Ugla shocks the minister's wife when she tells her that she has been attending the meetings of a Communist "cell." The minister's wife asks what was discussed:

"The day-nursery," I said.
"What day-nursery?"
"We need a day-nursery," I said.
"Who needs a day-nursery?" she asked.
"I do."
"And who is to build it?" she asked.
"The public," I replied.
"The public!" she said. "And what manner of creature is that, pray?" (83)

Madam, the minister's wife, fires Ugla, but the minister tells her she can stay. Ugla's relationship with the minister intensifies; he is "the man who was to me the most unknown of all, the most incomprehensible and the most distant, even though he was closest to me of all in that mysterious disintegrating way which I shall never admit" (110). The minister, on the other hand, thinks he knows Ugla, thinks he comprehends her, and is clearly in love with her.

Ugla tries to convince the minister to press Parliament to build the day nursery. "Our wives want to have legitimate children," he tells her, "at least on paper; and preferably no competition. It is an attack on the wives' class to have day nurseries" Ugla reveals that she is pregnant. The minister changes his tune: "Do not be anxious, you can get from me all the money you want, a house, a nursery, everything. . . . I promise you that in this matter I shall behave as if I were inspired by a woman." "A pregnant housemaid," Ugla corrects him, seeming to know that abstractions like "a woman" should be shunned. She refuses to accept the minister's promise and returns to her home in the north to have her baby (139–41).

Months later, Ugla is surprised to find on her distant northern doorstep Brilliantine and the Atom Poet, those acquaintances of the organist and associates of Two Hundred Thousand Pliers. "The whole world—one station," the Atom Poet says in response to Ugla's shock. They've come, not in Pliers's Cadillac, but in a truck carrying two crates. One of them is supposed to contain the bones of the Nation's Darling, which they have come to bury. "We examined the crates and found addresses printed on them: 'Prime Minister of Iceland' on the one, and 'Snorredda Wholesale Company' on the other—two names for the same enterprise" (165, 168).

Ugla pries open the lid of one of the crates: "I recognized the merchandise quickly enough from my pantry work in the south: Portuguese Sardines imported from America, that fish which the papers said was the only fish that could scale the highest tariff walls in the world and yet be sold when ten years old at a thousand percent profit in the greatest fish country in the world, where even the dogs walk out and vomit at the mere mention of salmon" (168–69).

The other crate is duly opened; it contains exactly what it says stamped on its side: *Dansk ler,* Danish clay. "It was just as I had expected—in that crate too there was not much that was likely to enhance the nation's prestige. But yet, if one believes that man is dust and dirt, as the Christians believe, then this was a man the same as any other; but not an Icelandic man, for this was not Icelandic dirt; it was not the gravel nor earth, sand nor clay, which we know from our own country, but a dry, greyish calcareous devil like nothing else so much as old dog's dirt" (169).

That night, "Government messengers arrived in police cars to fetch the Portuguese Sardines and D.L." (173). Nothing more would be heard of the episode.

XX

Laxness was a member of the Red Pens, a group of writers in the 1930s and 1940s whose views on literature and politics are not difficult to speculate upon. Saying that his fictional prime minister and fictional Snorredda Company (with its American subsidiary F.F.F. making sure that the value of goods "increased at sea") are "two names for the same enterprise" is thus understandable, though a bit heavy handed. Sameness, as we'll see, is more troublesome than that. Nevertheless, what holds for sardines holds for genomics. They are the joint product of a government and corporate relationship simultaneously tight and antagonistic, deserving of a new stamp to mark its devilish contents: PublicXPrivate.

PublicXPrivate

The undersigned went to Iceland for the second time in March 2000. I was expecting a routine research trip now that the "debate" was "over." But somewhere in that electronic accessless time, when I was rounding up last-minute items, packing bags, getting to the Albany airport, getting through that airport and the next, getting frustrated with my inability to sleep in a cramped airplane seat over the Atlantic Ocean, getting my body to not think that it was three in the morning but seven and that it needed to ignore the ice pellets that were assaulting it horizontally as the wind whipped through the Keflavík airport parking lot where the Átak rental car was waiting, and then eventually getting to the Hótel Leifur Eiríksson— sometime in these body-intensive operations, a more virtual event had taken place: deCODE had filed its registration statement, immediately electronically accessible, with the U.S. Securities and Exchange Commission. DeCODE was planning to go public sometime in May, offering its stock for sale on the techcentric NASDAQ exchange.

Before I went to bed that night I had deCODE's S-1 registration statement. Einar Árnason had downloaded it from the SEC's Web site and dropped it off at the hotel for me, along with his preliminary comments and analysis; the man had not wasted any time in tearing into the hundred-plus pages of dense infotext.

So began a new phase of my research on promising genomics in a lavaX-land that now included that most volatile of territories in that most volatile of times, the U.S. stock market on the millennium's cusp.

XX

In early March 2000, the promising biotech economy was in full surge. DeCODE was probably hoping that the wave hadn't crested and that they could ride it to a quick and gloriously lucrative initial public offering. Things didn't turn out that way, although they may not have turned out all that different in the end. But the devil is in the details, they say, and the devils between March and July, when deCODE issued its IPO and raised a virtual bucketful of virtual capital ($180 million was a figure often mentioned, as if that was an indicator of actual value), were devils of volatility.

At that time, most commentary offered an answer like "reality" to the question, "What's behind the biotech boom?" Evaluations would be different in a few months, but in early 2000, conventional wisdom would have probably lined up behind Incyte Pharmaceuticals' (later Incyte Genomics) CEO Roy Whitfield: "I think it's really coming home to investors that genomics is really going to affect their lives in the future in a big way. The amount of information that people are getting about the sector is far greater than it ever was."[1] High stock values only reflected this underlying reality of a promising future, transmitted by secure information.

That explanation, as we'll see in a later *ch*, is the standard view of stock valuation: current price reflects future value. But even some commentators at the time recognized reality to be more complicated. According to Steve Flaks, an investment manager of a hedge fund specializing in biotech stocks, biotech executives at the end of 1999 and the beginning of 2000 were "in shock about how much money they can raise so easily. . . . All the rules are out the window right now."[2] Some analysts thought that the money "sloshing around" in biotech was coming from investors afflicted with "dot-com angst" who had pulled out of that sector and reinvested in biotech.[3]

Others were more sanguine. Ed Owens, manager of the $11.2 billion Vanguard Health Care fund, characterized biotech stocks in late February 2000 as "ridiculously overpriced" and forecasted a bust on the way. History and experience may have been some help to him; having managed the Vanguard fund since 1984, Owens had seen previous "boomlets" in the biotech sector in 1984, 1987, 1991, and 1995 each end disappointingly.[4]

In addition to these market forces, we also have to consider the amplified effect of bionews stories on the biowires. In mid-February 2000, the major genomic company Human Genome Sciences Inc. was awarded a patent on a gene involved in HIV transmission; values rose across the biotech board, and the major biotech stock indexes went up 20 percent in two days. HGSI was up over $29; Millennium was up $54; Incyte, up $59. The mechanism seemed obvious and rational, even if somewhat sloshy: patents are good for genomics, news about patents is good, investors reward good news with more investment, more investment means more value.

But other actors in this world of biofinance resisted such easy explanations. One story reported that while some "analysts said that . . . the [biotech] group continues to make good progress, there has been no fundamental change that would account for the rally. Instead it appears to be a combination of momentum players and major mutual funds returning to biotechnology."[5] Another voice tempered the description of investor "enthusiasm" provoked by the HGSI announcement and noted that "nonetheless, the validity of gene patents is uncertain." The story went on to quote HGSI CEO William Haseltine to the effect that that President Clinton was "dead right" to oppose "broad" gene patents, and that HGSI's patent program was "consistent" with the government view.[6]

The "government view" in question concerned a long-standing question about what kind of genetic information or material could actually be patented. The question had taken on renewed visibility as the "race" between the more-or-less private Celera Genomics and the more-or-less public Human Genome Project had heated up, as had tempers on both sides. Understanding this question of patents in the context of early 2000 requires that we backtrack to 1991 and tell the story of that other genomic man that everybody loved to hate, Craig Venter.

When we last encountered Venter in Ch 5, his new genomic company Celera had announced it would sequence "the human genome" on its own and beat the more public Human Genome Project in a race to completion. As sequencing rates on both sides shot up, civility went downhill. Relations between Celera and its scientists and the HGP's international consortium of scientists (many of whom were involved in corporate endeavors too) became acrimonious; terms like "slimy," "egomaniac," "dumb," "schoolyard brawl," and "grudge match" were employed by all parties and provided embellishment to the comparatively lackluster term "race."

The fundamental differences were over data access and ownership. At a 1996 meeting in Bermuda, the members of the international consortium had elaborated a set of principles concerning human genome sequencing: all data should be "freely available and in the public domain to encourage research and development"; "sequence assemblies should be released as soon as possible," preferably daily; and "finished annotated sequence should be submitted immediately to public databases."[7] It was often difficult to discern exactly how Celera proposed to handle the information it was producing, but there were clearly differences: some Celera data might be "freely available," but not "immediately," and Celera would also sell licenses and different kinds of access to the database and software tools it was creating. And by November 1999 Celera announced that it had filed sixty-five hundred "provisional patent applications," placeholders for future patents built on and around DNA sequence information.

A new round of talks began between Celera and representatives of the international consortium, attempting to come to some agreement about data access and ownership. Like many diplomatic negotiations in wartime, these talks started, stalled, broke off, and restarted. In early March 2000 the U.K.'s Wellcome Trust effected a different kind of sortie across the public-private front line when it publicly released a confidential letter sent to Craig Venter from Francis Collins, titular head of the public HGP, in which Collins laid out (relatively nonnegotiable) terms and set a (relatively unreasonable) deadline for response; "open warfare" broke out.[8]

This was the backdrop to the anxiety about gene patents that permeated the otherwise ebullient genomic world in early 2000. So one can understand why issuing a patent to HGSI was a newsworthy event. And despite Haseltine's expressed consensus with his government's patent policy, the facts of the case complicate matters. Britain's *New Scientist* reported that HGSI had in fact filed the patent on this particular fragment years before, before knowing its function, before knowing that it was involved in HIV transmission.[9] Haseltine, HGSI, and the CCR5 patent were exactly what President Clinton and Prime Minister Blair had in mind when, on March 14, 2000, they addressed the media about this issue of gene patents.

On that date, forty-five minutes before the anticipated media op with Clinton and Blair, a financial analyst for TheStreet.com issued an Internet bulletin titled "Listen Up, Genomics Day Traders!" TheStreet.com predicted an upsurge in the genomic market once Clinton and Blair reaffirmed, as was expected, that there would be no change in their governments' policies on access to and patenting of genetic information.[10] Clinton and Blair did make exactly such a statement and simply reaffirmed the status quo regarding patenting of DNA. Listening genomic day traders stood poised to profit on the new upsurge that should have followed this reassuring news.

Instead, the NASDAQ biotech index began to crash. The major genomic companies lost between 14 and 27 percent of their value overnight. Despite numerous reading cues, a swarm of investors failed to read the announcement as expected. Press releases from Celera, Millennium Pharmaceuticals, Incyte Genomics, and the Biotechnology Industry Organization welcomed the Clinton-Blair announcement as the affirmation of gene patenting, which in truth it was, but this did nothing to stop the bleeding. "Tony Blair and I crashed the markets for a day or two, and I didn't mean to," Clinton tried to explain a few weeks later.[11] The biotech index lost 37 percent of its value by the end of March, and the crashing continued.

Post-hoc analyses started immediately, and they were understandably conflicting. The highly regarded and highly successful Dresdner RCM Biotech Fund had been up 100 percent for the year at the end of February 2000, "benefiting from several months of excitement surrounding the impending completion of the human genome project," as reported by the *San Francisco Chronicle*. The fund then lost half its value from mid-March until mid-April. The *Chronicle* reported that fund manager Faraz Naqvi believed that "the trigger for the biotech sell-off was doubts about the possibility of extracting profits from the human genome sequencing project in the wake of comments from President Clinton and Prime Minister Blair's suggesting giving free access to data and research from the project," even though that's not what Clinton and Blair said, or even "suggested." At the same time, Naqvi tried to provide a more rational explanation, or at least a better rationalization, by suggesting that the biotech market "was already overheated, and that valuations were out of alignment with short-term expectations." (The Dresdner Fund performed better than many biotech funds. "It limped along until mid-May," the *Chronicle* continued, "when biotech stocks got another jolt of hype from the human genome project," so that by July the fund was back up 73.7 percent for the year.)[12] Another analyst for the firm Robertson Stephens argued that the crash started when "some of the investors who had bought in at higher prices during the financings dumped the stocks when they were battered," which was "partially the result of having a lot of new and inexperienced investors in the biotech sector."[13]

Two days after the announcement, Don Luskin, former CEO of Barclays Global Mutual Funds and vice chairman of Barclays Global Investors before moving on to cofound a company called Metamarkets, tried to read the events. His seemingly willful misreadings are instructive: "There will probably be recovery, but investors realize that the world has changed.

Yesterday's announcement reminded investors that biotech companies operate in a highly regulated environment, which is subject to sudden and capricious policy changes. It will be a while before investors forget this lesson."[14] But the world hadn't changed at all, aside from some ephemeral value becoming so ephemeral as to become nonexistent. What was truly remarkable was a swarm of investors thinking that the world nevertheless had actually changed. There had been no "sudden and capricious" change of policy; the political world had stayed the same and people panicked nonetheless. Of course the market is a "highly regulated environment"— which is also what makes it resistant to sudden and capricious change, and which is why Clinton would eventually go to such pains to clarify that he and Blair had not meant to change anything. Even the *perception* that U.S. patent policy was changing was enough to cause market madness; why would a head of state be fool enough to announce that he was actually going to do it?

Luskin also commented that "this whole sorry matter is an example of what happens when government policy and corporate innovation collide." This statement conveniently forgets that it was U.S. government policy in the second half of the 1980s that created the Human Genome Project, in part, to spur corporate innovation in the biosciences because the major pharmaceutical companies couldn't be bothered. And how, exactly, does something "collide" with what was just previously named its "environment"? The entire episode is an example of how genomic corporate innovation doesn't collide with government policy, but is heavily dependent on the environment called the state—its promulgation and enforcement of intellectual property laws, its encouragement of technoscientific developments that have no immediate market value, but plenty of promise.

The scientific press was actually relieved, in a stiff-upper-lipped, adversity-is-good-for-you kind of way. A *Nature Biotechnology* editorial thanked "Bill and Tony" for their statement and its effects, even if "they had little inkling of the result." It burst the bubble and put everyone "firmly back in reality." "Reality" was, as usual, undefined, but left only as the opposite of that previous state in which there was "all this money sloshing around" that might have led to a situation in which "biotechnology companies could have become too used to free-flowing funds," working "largely on the basis of feelings and fingers in the air." Metaphors of irrationality and irreality abounded in the editorial: money was being used "indiscriminately," "dot.com fever" had mutated into a "genomic infection [that] spread to other quoted biotechnology companies," and non-genomic companies "happily surfed on the froth of the genomics wave." Instead, thanks to the Bill-and-Tony "accident," everyone supposedly learned a few moral lessons, which *Nature Biotechnology* phrased in terms of habits: biotech companies had "learnt the good habit of exerting stringent control on R&D spending," and "research and clinical directors can resume their habits of applying stringent criteria to development programs."[15]

While other commentators may have agreed with the return-to-reality principle, they nevertheless questioned the reality of the Bill-and-Tony effect. "This was a red herring for an overdue correction," Mike King, a senior biotechnology analyst for Robertson Stephens in New York, told a writer for BioSpace.com. "The group had gotten ahead of itself, and when a situation like this crops up, the outcome of a 30 to 40 percent correction is almost predictable."[16] King's reasoning is not exactly transparent: How exactly does a sector of the economy "get ahead of itself"? How far ahead of itself does it have to get before there's a problem? What is it about economies, or value, that makes it possible for a group to get ahead of itself, to disconnect from reality—and then to "correct" itself, and for that correction to come not when it is *due,* as would be only proper in a restricted economy, but only when it is *overdue,* long past the proper term of debt and repayment?

XX

The biomarket crash—or dip, or "necessary correction"—happened in the middle of my March 2000 visit to Iceland, and it sparked some optimism among those opposed to an Icelandic genomic future centralized in deCODE and the Health Sector Database. Anything that might forestall, complicate, or even foil deCODE's ability to leverage a large amount of capital was a welcome development. Like most biotech and genomic companies at this stage of the game, deCODE was burning through a few million dollars a month and needed a heavy infusion of cash. But unlike other genomic companies, deCODE did not have multiple alliances or agreements with pharmaceutical companies; the company had only the $200 million promise from Roche, with pay-outs contingent on deCODE accomplishing several research milestones. Filing its registration statement with the U.S. Securities and Exchange Commission on March 8, deCODE was surely hoping to catch the huge biotech wave of the winter of 1999–2000; six days later, that wave had crashed, and deCODE would have to wait until the summer months for the next biotech stock market surge.

This story of the biotech crash is an index of the importance of stories in today's genomic economy—perhaps better described as tomorrow's genomic economy, since the "source" of value is located in the future. Biotech and genomic stocks are some of the best exemplars of what are called "story stocks" on Wall Street: stocks whose value, even more so than "regular" stocks, is contingent upon the kind of narrative that can be spun around them.[17] And as any literary theorist can tell you, a narrative is an extremely productive yet volatile medium, one peculiarly open to what is called, in many stories about stories, the future. As one media analyst said of the Clinton-Blair announcement that crashed NASDAQ: "Tuesday's sell-off of shares in biotech companies demonstrated that the same buzzwords that draw investors can also turn them away." Words buzz with a strange and powerful volatility.

Certainly, this dependence on language and the expectations it creates, the multiple and even contradictory anticipations language is capable of setting into sociological motion, seem *always* to be a feature of the economy and valuation—and not only in times of "irrational exuberance," to use Robert Shiller's phrase later deployed by U.S. Federal Reserve chairman Alan Greenspan. Shiller has described how speculative bubbles since the tulip mania of the seventeenth century have been blown up by narrative-dependent anticipations and how this process has always required the media for its production. In Shiller's analysis, one of the most important features of the great speculative bubble of the 1990s (if, indeed, it was a bubble) has been the intensification of this media effect in the economy, volatilizing value through multiple feedback loops that become increasingly self-referential.[18]

This was most evident with Internet stocks, Shiller argues, but is also an important feature in the genomic economy. The late 1990s through 2000 were becoming a time of daily and even hourly obsessive attention to genomic stock values through online news and stock services and a multiplicity of narrative forecasts, projections, and other anticipatory stories channeled through television, newspapers, and magazines. But what kind of thing is language, and what kind of a thing is an economy, such that the former can have such an effect—such contradictory effects—on the latter? What is it about economies that makes them subject not only to government regulation, but also to language?

Open FutureXSafe Harbor

> Forward-looking information occupies a vital role in the
> United States' securities markets.
>
> U.S. Securities and Exchange Commission, "Concept
> Release and Notice of Hearing: Safe Harbor
> for Forward-Looking Statements"

Maybe it's not simply *information* that animates markets in today's "information society." The U.S. Securities and Exchange Commission, that regulatory body most concerned with enforcing the disclosure of corporate information, here names the "vital" force as *forward-looking information*. Just what kind of force is in play here, when forward-looking information plays its role? Or: what is the place in the network, in the so-called information economy, that forward-looking information *occupies?* What kinds of reading practices does forward-looking information demand, and from whom? In a territory of forward-looking information, how does one decide between fact, speculation, puffery, hype, straight dope, and bald-faced lies? Most succinctly: how are promises to be made and taken?

I have developed an abiding interest in the workings of the U.S. Securities and Exchange Commission, based on ethnographic work with Kim Fortun on how the SEC understands and works on important abstractions—information, disclosure, truth telling, transparency, due diligence—in the pragmatic context of globalizing capital markets.[1] The SEC is an imperfect but important and interesting site for studying capital and its corporate entities. It provides a wealth of information on genomic companies and other corporations and is the place where the "self-regulating" securities industry that undergirds the U.S. capital markets is, in fact, regulated.

An important part of those securities regulations changed, however, with the passage of the Private Securities Litigation Reform Act of 1995 (the PSLRA). The change concerned how "forward-looking information" would be read by the courts, and how it should be read by someone sometimes called "the sophisticated investor" and other times called the more modest "reasonable investor." This is the regulatory framework that shaped the genomic companies. Companies like deCODE Genetics, Celera Genomics, Millennium Pharmaceuticals, and Human Genome Sciences Inc. have existed almost entirely in a historically specific regulatory framework of corporate disclosure—a framework that sanctions and encourages the promissory quality of the "forward-looking information" that has proven vital to these life-science corporations.

XX

In late 1994, the SEC issued a "concept release" calling for comments on proposed changes to the "safe harbor" provisions of federal securities law. The SEC asked "whether the safe harbor provisions for forward-looking statements . . . are effective in encouraging disclosure of voluntary forward-looking information and protecting investors." What is forward-looking information? The 1994 concept release made this distinction: "Required disclosure is based on currently known trends, events, and uncertainties that are reasonably expected to have material effects, such as: a reduction in the registrant's product prices; erosion in the registrant's market share; changes in insurance coverage; or the likely non-renewal of a material contract. In contrast, optional forward-looking disclosure involves anticipating a future trend or event or anticipating a less predictable impact of a known event, trend or uncertainty."[2]

Since its establishment in 1933 as part of the New Deal, the SEC had prohibited disclosure of forward-looking statements. With the 1929 crash fresh in its institutional memory, the SEC regarded such forward-looking statements as "inherently unreliable," the kind of speculative activity that had bubbled and burst the economy; in its role as protector of investors and preserver of trust in capital and its markets, the SEC worried that "unsophisticated investors would place undue emphasis on the information in making investment decisions." This philosophy prevailed for thirty years.

But in the mid-1960s the SEC formed the Wheat Commission to re-consider these matters and to speculate once again on the question of spec-ulative statements. Despite the fact that, according to the SEC's 1994 con-cept release, the Wheat Commission's 1969 report found that "most investment decisions are based essentially on estimates of future earnings"—that is, "based on" something that was, at least in part, spectral or speculative—the commission did not recommend changing disclosure re-quirements, apparently because that was how things had been done for thirty years: "[The] commission stated that its decision not to mandate disclosure of forward-looking statements was based on its desire not to deviate too far from its historical position of prohibiting such disclosure."

In 1972 the SEC announced its "intention" to promulgate rules that would still not require the disclosure of forward-looking information, but that would encourage voluntary disclosure, and the SEC promised cor-porations some limited protections from antifraud litigation. The SEC never issued those rules, citing "opposition from commenters," but de-ferred to the future, hoping that the issue would be taken up again by its newly formed Advisory Committee on Corporate Disclosure.

The courts, in the meantime, had begun to rule on similar questions revolving around "facts," "intentionality," and "prediction." In the case with the almost allegorical title, *Marx v. Computer Sciences Corporation,* the ninth U.S. Circuit Court of Appeals addressed the question of whether "predictions or statements of opinion could ever be considered to be 'facts' which could be said to be false or misleading for purposes of liability un-der the securities laws."[3] The court found that "while predictions could properly be characterized as facts, the failure of a prediction to prove true was not in itself actionable. Instead, the court looked at the factual rep-resentations which it found were impliedly made in connection with the prediction; namely that, at the time the prediction was made, it was be-lieved by its proponent and it had a valid basis."[4]

In its 1994 concept release, the SEC noted new trends in capitalism that suggested the need for change in disclosure requirements; the net-works were being rearticulated. There was "increasing interest" both by corporations and among analysts and investors in "enhanced disclosure of information that may affect corporate performance but is not readily susceptible [to] measurement in traditional, quantitative terms."

Among such qualitative informational items are workforce training and devel-opment, product and process quality and customer satisfaction. A large registrant considers one such item—product quality—to be so important to its profitability that it has chosen to make it a key determinant of executive compensation. Other companies are beginning to experiment with voluntary disclosure of the utilization of an intangible asset termed "intellectual capital," or employee knowledge. In this connection, another federal agency has urged more corporate disclosure of the use of measures of "high performance work practices and other nontraditional measures" of corporate performance.[5]

At the same time, some corporations expressed concerns about the increased risk of securities antifraud class-action suits that such disclosures might encourage. "Recent surveys," the SEC wrote, "suggest that this threat of mass shareholder litigation, whether real or perceived, has had a chilling effect on disclosure of forward-looking information." (The fine-print footnote to this statement discloses the source of the surveys: the National Venture Capital Association, the National Investors Relations Institute, and the American Stock Exchange CEO Survey. This list of names suggests a certain slant, whether real or perceived, to the survey.)

The SEC also included in its concept release suggestions from legal scholars about how the speculative status of forward-looking statements might be recodified. Law professor John Coffee offered a "bespeaks caution" doctrine under which "a forward-looking statement would be protected so long as it were properly qualified and accompanied by 'clear and specific' cautionary language that explains in detail sufficient to inform a reasonable person of both the approximate level of risk associated with that statement and the basis therefor." (The "reasonable" if not "sophisticated" investor returns as ideal assessor here, precisely when the sheer increase in the number of investors into the U.S. securities market might have called for some reconsideration of the security of these characterizations.) In addition, "the suggested safe harbor would not require that the forward-looking statement have a 'reasonable basis' . . . because, according to Professor Coffee, this requirement often raises factual issues that cannot easily be resolved at the pre-trial stage."[6] These suggestions—in which the volatile and hence litigation-inviting concepts of "fact," "reason," and "basis" are devolatilized by a second cautionary statement that simply names them as volatile—would become part of the new disclosure landscape.

The concepts released in 1994 by the SEC were soon gathered and picked up. What would become the Private Securities Litigation Reform Act of 1995 was introduced into the U.S. Congress early that year, as part of the Newt Gingrich–led Republican Party Contract with America package of legislation. The reform act was supposed to have multiple effects, the two most vital being a reduction in the number of "frivolous lawsuits" brought against corporations by their shareholders and the expansion of the safe harbor for forward-looking statements. The high-tech, infocentric corporations of Silicon Valley were a main force behind the act's passage. As an editorial in the *Washington Post* reported on the day of the final congressional vote (that would override President Clinton's previous veto of the bill): "When the price of a company's stock drops sharply, the present law invites suits on the questionable grounds that the company's past expressions of hope for its future misled innocent stockholders. This kind of suit has turned out to be a special danger to new companies, particularly high-technology ventures with volatile stock prices. . . . The bill would protect companies' forecasts as long as they did not omit significant facts."[7] *Money* magazine spoke in the name of protecting "small investors like you," and was more critical of the proposed legislation, characterizing it as "a license to defraud shareholders" by "help[ing] executives get away with lying." "High-tech executives, particularly those in California's Silicon Valley, have lobbied relentlessly for this broad protection. As one congressional source told *Money's* Washington, DC, bureau chief Teresa Tritch: 'High-tech execs want immunity from liability when they lie.' Keep that point in mind the next time your broker calls pitching some high-tech stock based on the corporation's optimistic prediction."[8]

But with promises and other commissive speech acts, as we learned from J. L. Austin and others in "PromisesXPromises," all one ever has is the volatile speech act itself; "one's word is one's bond," as Austin says, because to try to gauge the promise by what the "high-tech exec" *intends*— making the difference between a lie and an optimistic prediction one of interior "profundity"—in fact only "paves the way for immorality" (see Ch X). An impossible situation, yet something had to be done.

The Private Securities and Litigation Reform Act of 1995 accomplished many things, but one of the most important was to adopt a strong form of John Coffee's "bespeaks caution" doctrine, which expanded the safe harbor for forward-looking statements and protected corporations from shareholder lawsuits.[9] The PSLRA also sanctioned both "oral forward-looking statements" (such as what is said during an IPO "road show" or an investors' teleconference) and "written forward-looking statements" (such as ebullient press releases), as long as they were marked as forward-looking statements and as long as potential investors—"sophisticated" or not—were also directed to other, more "cautionary" texts, such as SEC filings.

The full and final effects of the PSLRA remain unclear. Whether the legislation has reduced the number of lawsuits (and whether there were, as certain surveys "suggested," so many of them in the first place), whether it has given CEOs "a license to lie," and whether it has increased market volatility while parting the sophistication-challenged investor from his and her money—all this remains uncertain, unknowable, or at least open to debate.[10] But some signs of this uncertain future are still worth reading and pondering.

In their delectably named article "Enter Yossarian," Elliott Weiss and Janet Moser analyze the catch-22 set up by the PSLRA: plaintiffs in securities fraud cases need to show that a company knowingly misrepresented matters in forward-looking statements, but can do so only by being granted discovery, which they can't get since they can't file suit based on forward-looking information now protected by the expanded safe harbor.[11] This fissure is also plumbed by Douglas Branson, who describes the effect as one of substituting "mere" words or ink for "due diligence":

The PSLRA provision provides that if a statement is "accompanied by meaningful cautionary statements," plaintiffs are denied discovery and the court must dismiss allegations as to the false or misleading nature of the statement. . . .

The effect of the PSLRA provision, as with stronger forms of the judge-made bespeaks caution doctrine, is to substitute mere cautionary words for the due diligence traditionally associated with preparation of statements in disclosure documents. Rather than building a due diligence file that, through research, establishes more than plausible, and often alternative, bases for making the statements made in the documents, securities lawyers will plaster forward-looking statements with cautionary warnings. . . . No incentive now exists for hiring the traditional, classical securities lawyer who quarterbacked the research and other effort necessary to do the due diligence exercise. Instead, Congress has placed a premium on buying and using ink by the barrel.[12]

Richard Rosen, who is sympathetic to the PSLRA, has discussed the case of *Parnes v. Gateway 2000, Inc.,* and suggests that "forward-looking" and "cautionary" statements can't be considered on their own. Rather, they must be evaluated within the larger machine that enables them to function, a machine that includes the old reliable "reasonable investor":

The plaintiffs claimed that the computer company misrepresented its obligations to pay sales taxes to states other than South Dakota. But the court pointed out that the prospectus warned investors that taxing authorities in other states had sought information regarding the sufficiency of Gateway's contacts with the states, that the company had not established any reserves and that it might be required to pay income or franchise taxes in other states. The court found that "any reasonable investor would be on notice that Gateway faced potential state tax liability for states other than South Dakota."

Gateway also warned that because of volatility of the computer industry, the introduction of new products was a risky venture and there was no assurance of success. This more generalized risk disclosure was also found to be sufficient, even though it says little that is specific to a company or its products. Yet there is no question that some courts would have found the latter statement by Gateway to be too general to be "meaningful."[13]

In "Yahoo!✕Finance," we'll look more closely at how such reasoning about disclosure and the reading demands placed on "any reasonable investor" worked out in the world of genomics. The general pattern that is supposed to hold can be glimpsed here in the Gateway case, however: the reasonable investor does not watch TV news puff pieces, read press releases or the newspaper articles based on them, or surf a plethora of investment Web sites, but spends all his or her time wading through downloaded reams of SEC filings.

Let's close out Rosen and this discussion of forward-looking information and its burdens with one last quote:

> Of course, it would be wonderful to have a rule that allowed courts and litigators unfailingly to be able to discriminate among the cases and to allow discovery to proceed only in those in which there was some reason to believe that, notwithstanding adequate cautionary language, the company's management really did know that the predictions were not likely to come true. But because no such rule could ever be constructed, any rule will either allow a few dishonest issuers to win motions to dismiss or will impose enormous costs on honest companies and their shareholders. Congress has struck the balance in favor of protecting companies and their shareholders—a balance which strikes me as absolutely correct. (657–58)

One might agree with Rosen insofar as it is indeed impossible to construct "unfailingly" discriminatory rules for calculating fissures, volatilities, and chiasma such as these opened up by forward-looking information. But it would be prudent and even reasonable to question the "balance" that he hyperbolizes as "absolutely correct," since it in fact depends on a far-from-certain calculus of the fissure: how does one know that, in the chasm opened up by forward-looking information, there won't be an "enormous" number of dishonest issuers and only a "few" costs to honest companies? Rosen's unsubstantiated calculation is little more than a political endorsement of the balance that Congress indeed "struck": a forceful cut that transfers many of the financial risks and the burdens of proof, discovery, and due diligence from corporations to their presumably sophisticated shareholders.

The volatile conjunction of safe harbor (however expanded or restricted) and open future was certainly intensified by the PSLRA of 1995. But the chiasmus of safety and risk, secured closure and speculative future, has always been a feature of economies—a fissure that economists have diagrammed and mapped, but never paved over.

ManiaXFundamentals

In 2000, the year of deCODE's initial public offering, there were an estimated sixty-seven biotech IPOs and secondary offerings, which raised a total of $39 billion—$30 billion more than was raised in the previous three years combined.[1] Was the great genomic run-up of 1999–2000 an instance of "financial euphoria," a "speculative bubble" or a "mania," in the tradition of the Dutch tulip mania of the early seventeenth century, the Mississippi gold (Banque Royale) or the South Seas bubbles of the early eighteenth century, or the speculative periods that preceded the stock market crashes of 1929 and 1987? Is the emerging genomic economy, after the precipitous decline that began in March 2000, still an example of "irrational exuberance" in the market? And is there a methodological and/or theoretical approach—historical analysis and analogy, economics, social psychology—that could resolve these questions without speculating?

A first cut, highly condensed and abbreviated, would suggest that the economic experts may be found on either side of the maniaXfundamentals fissure. Robert Shiller's *Irrational Exuberance*, John Kenneth Galbraith's *A Short History of Financial Euphoria*, and Charles Kindleberger's *Manias, Panics, and Crashes* privilege the mania side in their critical analyses of these episodes; for them, these market events exemplify periods of a certain kind of insanity to which the market is always prone. To represent the other side of this fissure I've selected Peter Garber's *Famous First Bubbles*, which criticizes the conceptual vacuousness of the "bubble" explanation and constructs an argument for the rationality, based on market fundamentals, of these same events.

Let's begin with Peter Garber, who analyzes the rhetoric of bubbles, manias, "herding," and panics in both the economic literature and in the popular media. He references famous instances of bubbles, like the Dutch tulip mania, "as prime examples of the madness possible in *private* financial markets." Both the Mississippi bubble and the South Seas bubble, on the other hand, were "grandiose macroeconomic schemes launched or aided by high government officials and supported by the entire apparatus of the governments of England and France."[2] This is an excellent reminder that the craziness of an event as volatile and complex as a speculative bubble is unlikely to be traceable to the market alone.

Garber also criticizes the rhetoric of "herding," in which investors are described as irrational or at least nonrational cattle or sheep, blindly following the pack. Garber argues that it is not only possible, but is often the case that large flows of investors and money may actually be reasonable and based on sound analyses, and hence the size and rapidity of a financial movement alone does not qualify it as a speculative bubble. Garber also points to the selectivity with which herding behavior is ascribed. "Keynesianism was a convincing theory once, and governments *herded* on the basis of Keynesian policy prescriptions. These tended to fail in their more overblown forms, after which governments shied away from such policies and imposed (*herded* around) stringent anti-inflationist policies. No one says, though, that we observed herding behavior on the part of governments during the 1960s and 1970s when they bought into Keynesianism and during the 1980s and 1990s when they got out en masse" (6). Garber's counterargument is a good Nietzschean riposte: *everything* humans do is herd behavior.

As for "irrational exuberance," Garber contends that Federal Reserve chairman Alan Greenspan "removed all meaningful content from the concept" when, three years after his initial warning that the Dow might be wrongly indexing value, he backpedaled when asked by a congressional committee if "irrationality" was still evident: "That is something you can only know after the fact."[3] Like the premodern definition of "bubble" that Garber cites from the 1926 *Dictionary of Political Economy* — "any unsound undertaking accompanied by a high degree of speculation" — the difficulty here is a temporal one: "we cannot know if we have a bubble until after it bursts," and it's only "after we find out that a commercial undertaking did not work that we can conclude it was unsound and then call it a bubble" (7). Garber contends that the recounting of these episodes are "rhetorical weapon[s] to be used in influencing modern policy out-comes," and that the main such outcome is an argument for "government control and regulation" of the market (12, 6).

But John Kenneth Galbraith, despite his status as head steer in the Keynesian herd, argues that something different than government regulation is needed: "Regulation and more orthodox economic knowledge are not what protect the individual and the financial institution when euphoria returns, leading on as it does to wonder at the increase in values and wealth, to the rush to participate that drives up prices, and to the eventual crash and its sullen and painful aftermath. There is protection only in a clear perception of the characteristics common to these flights into what must conservatively be described as mass insanity. Only then is the investor warned and saved."[4] Protection for Galbraith amounts to an immunization that comes not from a government vaccine, but from a kind of empiricism, historical and contemporary, that would prevent mass irrationality from taking hold. But is this kind of nonspeculative clarity so easy to achieve and disseminate?

Charles Kindleberger is perhaps clearer in his perception of the fundamental double binds or aporias at work in speculative events, and if he opts for the trope of synthesis, his rhetoric at the same time keeps the volatilities of his own necessary speculation in view: "A study of manias, bubbles, crashes, panics, and the lender of last resort helps us to move from classical thesis through revisionist antithesis to a more balanced synthesis. Or so I claim."[5]

Part of Kindleberger's (speculative) claim is that the problem lies not with speculation per se, but with "speculative *excess*" (13, emphasis added). As suggested by his preference for synthesis, Kindleberger is always at pains in his analysis to avoid "extremes," which for him includes monetarist fundamentalists: "The monetarist school of Milton Friedman, for example, holds that there is virtually no destabilizing speculation, that markets are rational, that governments make mistake after mistake." Such theories, Kindleberger suggests, "although not necessarily wrong, are too emphatic and leave too little room for exceptions" (13). So, where Galbraith claims that "clear perception" might allow one to distinguish between the necessarily wrong and the necessarily right, Kindleberger embraces the questions of emphasis and the inexorable forces of deviation, dissemination, and exception.

And while Kindleberger may claim, in the end, that he is pursuing a synthesis with his economic theory—an economic theory he admits would be derogatively referred to as "literary economics" (7)—his language along the way opens up other possibilities. Kindleberger's synthesis is one with multiple remains, residues, and other loose ends; Kindleberger's own bottom line is not really synthesis, but a volatile chiasmus. His text continually returns to "fundamental ambiguity," contradictions, conceptual and empirical "difficulties," and "dilemmas" or double binds. Speculation and its excesses guarantee such unstable outcomes and the subsequent need for unstable, pragmatic responses. A rich and lengthy historical record of speculative episodes involving "commodity exports, commodity imports, agricultural land at home or abroad, urban building sites, new banks, discount houses, stocks, bonds (both foreign and domestic), glamour stocks, conglomerates, condominiums, shopping centers, [and] office buildings" indicates that neither extreme nor simple resolutions are workable (9). While "markets work well on the whole, and can normally be relied upon to decide the allocation of resources," they "occasionally . . . will be overwhelmed and need help" (6). But the help can't take the form of a synthesis, since it must negotiate or traverse a double bind or dilemma: "the dilemma, of course, is that if markets know in advance that help is forthcoming under generous dispensations, they break down more frequently and function less effectively" (6).

The historical record suggests that "official warnings," "moral suasion or jawboning" (6), and other clear and present responses are ineffectual, or may in fact precipitate the crisis they aim to fend off. To describe what governments or banks must do to respond well to speculative excess, Kindleberger has to shift to a language that has more in common with the excesses of magic than with reason—a "neat trick" has to be performed, a "sleight of hand" that, if not invisible, is at least the inexplicable effect of a smoke-and-mirrors machine reflecting contradictions back on themselves. Not unlike a gene or a god, the "lender of last resort"—who must exist, but whose "presence should be doubted"—must "always come to the rescue . . . but always leave it uncertain whether rescue will arrive in time or at all, so as to instill caution in other speculators, banks, cities, or countries. In Voltaire's *Candide,* the head of a general was cut off 'to encourage the others.' What I am urging is that some sleight of hand, some trick with mirrors be found to 'encourage' the others (without, of course, cutting off actual heads) because monetarist fundamentalism has such unhappy consequences for the economic system" (12).

Fundamentalism has to be replaced—or so I claim—by a foundation without foundation, a ground with its ground mined under.[6] We require some tricked-out mechanisms of doubledness, that traverse chiasma without synthesizing them, that can leverage a better future with no point of purchase.

The disclosure mechanisms of the U.S. Securities and Exchange Commission are one set of such mechanisms that I think are worth experimenting with and worth improving. These mechanisms have to negotiate, in a pragmatic, day-to-day way, these same fissures of an unavoidably speculative economy produced by the crosses of mania with fundamentals. And in addition to their salutary economic effects, the blandly named forms of the SEC—the S-1 or the 10-Q—also harbor ethnographic material that can be leveraged, as both Icelanders and I found out, into multiple insights and strategic actions.

PromiseXDisclosure

The many stories about genomics that increasingly appear on television, in newspapers and magazines, and on the Internet reinforce the standard story that this is an industry based on "genetic information." Genetic information, it is said, will provide a foundation for new drugs, new diagnostic kits, new forms of therapy. But to the extent that the genomic industry is "based" on anything, it would be more accurate to say that it is based on the *promise* of genetic information—based on what genetic information *may become* in an anticipated, contingent, open future. This begins to account for why the value of companies like Celera Genomics, Millennium Pharmaceuticals, Incyte Genomics, and deCODE Genetics are "story stocks," dependent not only on genetic technologies but on that other set of technologies for simultaneously producing and evaluating anticipated, contingent futures: literary technologies. A genomic company may have gigabytes of "genetic information" in its databases, but the value of that information is far more promised than present—a value built on promising "platform technologies," promising drug targets, patents on promising gene fragments, and the future work of a talented, promising scientific staff.

We have seen how genomic companies, like their dot-com cousins that also emerged in the speculative economy of the 1990s, operated in the discursive space of the Private Securities Litigation Reform Act of 1995. One effect of this revision of U.S. securities law was that companies were required to analyze the genre of the press release within the press release itself, calling attention to how, like every other genre that partakes of the promise, the press release narrates an open future with forward-looking words or phrases such as "believe," "expect," "intend," "anticipate," "should," "planned," "estimated," and "potential," among others. The company then had to detail the "risks and uncertainties" that "could cause actual results and experience to differ materially from anticipated results or other expectations." A genomic company, in other words, was legally required to anticipate a different set of anticipations, narrate a different array of future expectations, each of which was a dense amalgam of technological and sociological contingencies. With such "cautionary language" in place at the bottom of the forward-looking statements of the press release, a genomic company would be in a "safe harbor," protected from future shareholder litigation.

It would be too quick to dismiss these genomic stories of designer drugs, widespread and accurate genetic tests, predictive medicine, and all the other anticipated products of "life sciences corporations" as "hype."[1] As should be clear by now, evaluating a future is never straightforward. The lavaX-land of genomics is multiply fissured: no safe harbor unthreatened by an open future, no economic fundamental not subject to some mania, no history without myth, and no truth that is not complicit with fiction. Just as every operation of language is essentially promissory and thus "unfounded" in the classical sense, there can be no science without speculation, there can be no economy without hype, there can be no "now" without a contingent, promised, spectral and speculated future.[2] *Promising*—and thus the *possibility* of hype, mania, intoxication—is as ineradicable from the science and business of genomics as it is from any other supplemental writings on genomics—including this one, to bespeak the necessary caution.

None of which belies the need for philosophical, literary, political, and cultural critique and analysis of the various micropractices by which genomic futures, with all their ineradicable contingency, are produced, valued, judged, narrated, and written. We have seen that one particularly interesting site for such analysis is the U.S. Securities and Exchange Commission, the federal agency most directly responsible for regulating what a genomic corporation can and cannot, and, occasionally, what it *must* say about a future that must nevertheless remain, in some measure, anticipated, promised, or hyped—unsaid or unwritten. Promise what you like; the SEC also makes disclosure *necessary*. The logic of the chiasmus is a twisted one: you must promise, *and* you must disclose. The S-1, the 10-Q, and every other form required by the SEC are just as inescapable as speculation or mania. Chiasma are double—which may not be what you were dreaming of, but it's not nothing.

XX

March 2000. That same main lecture hall at the University of Iceland, a somewhat less undersigned undersigned. There was a panel presentation and discussion aimed at the Icelandic public, one means by which Mann-vernd was keeping its promise of fostering ongoing, informed discussion about deCODE, the Health Sector Database, and genomics more broadly. Skúli spoke first, followed by Oddur Benedíktsson, a computer scientist at the university who had become an outspoken critic of the HSD, while some former students and colleagues worked or consulted for deCODE. They spoke—I probably don't need to add "passionately" and "at some length"—in Icelandic, leaving me once again to read only gestures, pos-tures, and the crowd, which was large and included a number of deCODE employees in the back row and along the side wall. In the discussion that followed our presentations, one of them said (with what I thought was just the right hint of sarcasm) how much he had enjoyed my "imagina-tive" reconstruction of the Húsavík junket and my comparison of Keiko and Kári, which I had recently posted on the Mannvernd Web site.

In my presentation, I again took the strategy of trying to avoid speak-ing directly about deCODE and the Icelandic context and instead pro-vided information and analysis of genomics more generally. Since de-CODE had just filed its S-1 registration statement with the SEC, I had the perfect vehicle for grounding my remarks in the context of the U.S. system of corporate regulation.

Which is where, despite much rhetoric to the contrary, deCODE ex-isted. Yes, there was the Icelandic company Íslensk erfdagreining—even two of them, as Einar Árnason pointed out to me, one incorporated as an "ehf" company and the other as an "hf," a legal detail whose implica-tions are as yet unclear. But these were wholly owned subsidiaries of de-CODE Genetics, incorporated in Delaware in 1996. So it boggled my mind to see deCODE described over and over again as "an Icelandic company." *Time* magazine, for example, while noting that deCODE was "equipped with $12 million in U.S. venture capital" (from U.S. venture capital firms with close links to Harvard and the University of Chicago, where Kári Stefánsson spent his American years), could nevertheless conclude by stat-ing that the "company is entirely owned by Icelanders"—quoting Kári with a flourish: "we are doing this ourselves."[3]

But on March 8, 2000, a new wealth of information became available to Icelanders: over two hundred pages of deCODE's S-1 registration state-ment with the SEC, easily downloadable from the SEC Web site by the more critically inclined journalists, by the biomedical professionals of Mannvernd, and by the six thousand Icelanders who had bought shares in deCODE from the Icelandic state banks at inflated prices on the "gray market." More on that later.[4]

Among this additional material for further speculation—material that had not previously been available to Icelanders, material with (for lack of a better word) some *heft*—was the fact that the single largest shareholder was Roche Finance Limited, with 4,483,334 shares, or 13.4 percent of the company. After Roche came Kári himself, with 3,125,292 shares of common stock, 9.6 percent of the total. "Entities affiliated" with the U.S. venture capital firms of Alta California Partners, Atlas Venture, and Polaris Venture Partners held another 7.1 percent, 7.1 percent, and 5.7 percent of the stock respectively, while individual venture capitalists and deCODE board members—men with classy names like Andre Lamotte, Terry McGuire, Guy Nohra, and Jean-François Formela—followed close behind with a cumulative total of 22 percent. Icelanders could do the math for themselves, and two things became clear: at least one member of an entirely new, extraordinarily wealthy-on-paper class of individuals was now living in Iceland, and the phrase "we are doing this ourselves" was something of a hyperbole.

When commentators describe what had been taking place in Icelandic newspapers, television, and radio for the better part of two years as a "public debate," it's necessary to recall that most of the material coming from deCODE and filtered into both the Icelandic and international media was a series of promotional predictions about gene discovery in Iceland, with virtually no scientific publications to substantiate these claims. What proliferated were tendentious, exoticist, and most likely wrong statements about the "unique" "isolation" and "homogeneity" of the Icelandic population;[5] vague nostrums about improving health and promoting scientific progress; and other assorted pieties, half-truths, and blatant lies. But now that deCODE was about to become publicly traded on NASDAQ, every press release that promised a future had to be accompanied by the necessary "cautionary statement" to establish a harbor safe from future shareholder litigation:

Any statements contained in this presentation that relate to future plans, events or performance are forward-looking statements within the meaning of the Private Securities Litigation Reform Act of 1995. These forward-looking statements are subject to a number of risks and uncertainties that could cause actual results, and the timing of events, to differ materially from those described in the forward-looking statements. These risks and uncertainties include, among others, those relating to technology and product development, integration of acquired businesses, market acceptance, government regulation and regulatory approval processes, intellectual property rights and litigation, dependence on collaborative relationships, ability to obtain financing, competitive products, industry trends and other risks identified in deCODE's filings with the Securities and Exchange Commission. deCODE undertakes no obligation to update or alter these forward-looking statements as a result of new information, future events or otherwise.[6]

So as part of the social price of its anticipated initial public offering in the U.S. securities markets, deCODE was required for the first time to publicly articulate the "risk factors" to which it was exposed. In my portion of that panel at the University of Iceland, I simply presented some of risk narrations that were now to be part of the "public debate." For many Icelanders, who had been treated to the most optimistic media pronouncements for the previous two years, this was a real eye-opener: fifteen pages of deCODE's SEC filing were filled with a different kind of speculative statement, the kind that tries to anticipate what could go wrong. Without going into the paragraphs of fine print, just some of the subheads from the registration statement offer a window, in capital letters, into the scientific and political economy in which deCODE and other genomic companies operate. I put them on an overhead for all to see:

WE MAY NOT SUCCESSFULLY DEVELOP OR DERIVE REVENUES FROM ANY PRODUCTS OR SERVICES

OUR BUSINESS MODEL IS BASED ON UNPROVEN APPROACHES

IF WE CONTINUE TO INCUR OPERATING LOSSES FOR A PERIOD LONGER THAN ANTICIPATED, OR IN AN AMOUNT GREATER THAN ANTICIPATED, WE MAY BE UNABLE TO CONTINUE OUR OPERATIONS

IF WE DO NOT MAINTAIN THE GOODWILL AND RECEIVE THE COOPERATION OF THE ICELANDIC POPULATION, WE MAY BE UNABLE TO PURSUE OUR GENE IDENTIFICATION PROGRAMS, PHARMACOGENOMICS OR FUNCTIONAL GENOMICS EFFORTS, COLLECT GENOTYPE DATA OR DEVELOP THE IHD [integrated health database]

OUR RELIANCE ON THE ICELANDIC POPULATION IN OUR GENE DISCOVERY PROGRAMS AND DATABASE SERVICES MAY LIMIT THE APPLICABILITY OF OUR DISCOVERIES TO CERTAIN POPULATIONS

OUR DEPENDENCE ON COLLABORATIVE RELATIONSHIPS MAY LEAD TO DELAYS IN PRODUCT DEVELOPMENT AND DISPUTES OVER RIGHTS TO TECHNOLOGY

ETHICAL AND PRIVACY CONCERNS MAY LIMIT OUR ABILITY TO DEVELOP AND USE THE IHD AND MAY LEAD TO LITIGATION AGAINST US OR THE ICELANDIC GOVERNMENT

THERE IS INTENSE COMPETITION FOR THE DEVELOPMENT AND MARKETING OF PRODUCTS BASED UPON THE IDENTIFICATION OF DISEASE-CAUSING GENES

USE OF THERAPEUTIC OR DIAGNOSTIC PRODUCTS DEVELOPED AS A RESULT OF OUR PROGRAMS MAY RESULT IN LIABILITY CLAIMS[7]

Such statements are no more and no less speculative than the optimistic "forward-looking statements" of press releases announcing isolated genes and lucrative corporate alliances and promising biocompounds or drug targets. There's no more reason to allow oneself to be taken in by speculative genomic pessimism than by its cheerier sibling. But these statements stake out a far more complex and dense social, scientific, political, legal, and ethical terrain of genomics—a sociotechnical terrain that, like the geology of Iceland, is fissured, jagged, austere, expansive, and prone to slippage and eruption. Such a complex and harsh space requires extensive and detailed diagramming, querying, and analyzing—a practice that the SEC calls "due diligence." When navigating in the unknown territory of an anticipated genomic future already arrived, I suggested to the gathered Icelanders, the speculative pessimism strikes me as the more valuable tool.

That was about all I had time for on that March 2000 panel, and my remarks consisted of what I thought my main responsibility was: to inform people about the kinds of new information that would have to be disclosed as a supplement to the promises already trumpeted, where they could find it, and how to begin evaluating the uncertainties, risks, and infelicities that are a feature of all promises. And supplementarity, I stressed, was the order of the day: disclosure was not the same as closure.

In theory, the SEC requires "full disclosure" of a company's financial holdings and liabilities, properties, research and licensing agreements, and the economic and technological risks and uncertainties the company faces, all in the name of guaranteeing the "transparency" of the U.S. securities market. But in practice, disclosure is always a question of particular accounting requirements and methods, loopholes, intentional or inadvertent omissions, and the particular enforcement strategies of SEC staff, who work with less-than-perfect information and some degree of opacity.[8] (And consider an additional layer of opacity: how likely is it that most investors today, especially the day-trader variety, even read these registration statements or the other documents that the SEC demands and disseminates? See some of the "sophisticated investors" featured in "Yahoo!XFinance.")

For example, in the case of deCODE's one major alliance at the time, that with Hoffmann-LaRoche, it's impossible to understand how the $200 million promise that had catapulted deCODE to fame was actually structured. Maybe I'm just not one of the sophisticated investors, but I would have liked to see some of these blanks filled in:

(a) Major Research Programs. Subject to the terms and conditions of this Agreement, for each Major Research Program then in effect on the relevant due date, Roche shall pay to deCODE the following amounts, which shall be due and payable as follows:

< PAGE > 33
[CONFIDENTIAL TREATMENT REQUESTED]

< PAGE > 34
[CONFIDENTIAL TREATMENT REQUESTED]

< PAGE > 35
(b) Minor Research Programs. Subject to the terms and conditions of this Agreement, for each Minor Research Program then in effect on the relevant due date, Roche shall pay to deCODE the following amounts, which shall be due and payable as follows:
[CONFIDENTIAL TREATMENT REQUESTED]

< PAGE > 36
[CONFIDENTIAL TREATMENT REQUESTED]

< PAGE > 37

And if I were potential investor, or especially if I were an Icelander on my way to an appointment with an Icelandic physician who had struck a collaboration agreement with deCODE, I would have liked to see similar fissures filled in, such as:

COLLABORATION AGREEMENT
BETWEEN
THE ICELANDIC HEART ASSOCIATION, HJARTAVERND
AND ISLENSK ERFDAGREINING EHF.

If ÍE or its parent company, deCODE genetics Inc., succeeds in contracting for the sale of individual Research Projects or their conclusions or sells the results of a Research Project to a third party, HV will receive as its share [CONFIDENTIAL TREATMENT REQUESTED] of all payments to ÍE or to deCODE genetics Inc., . . .

If ÍE or deCODE genetics Inc. concludes a contract with a third party pursuant to Paragraph 2 above, ÍE will pay to HV [CONFIDENTIAL TREATMENT REQUESTED] on signature of such contract, and thereafter an annual amount of [CONFIDENTIAL TREATMENT REQUESTED] during the course of the Research Project in question, the total amount never to exceed [CONFIDENTIAL TREATMENT REQUESTED]. In the event that the Research Project is concluded in a shorter time than five years. . . . HV will receive on such conclusion the amount which remains unpaid of the [CONFIDENTIAL TREATMENT REQUESTED] for the Research Project in question. . . . This payment is in addition to and independent of the [CONFIDENTIAL TREATMENT REQUESTED] payment pursuant to Paragraph 2 of this Chapter III.

I would have especially appreciated such financial information once I had seen—as I could for the first time in the SEC disclosure of March 2000—the informed consent form I would be signing when I used the services of a physicians' group that had a deCODE agreement. I think item number nine would have given me pause:

9. I consent to the biological material and data collected on me being preserved in encoded form so that both may be used later for research on other disorders than those specified above, provided that such research is conducted for the purpose of discovering mechanisms which could lead to a cure or preventive measures.

Even if I wasn't aware, as most residents of Iceland and other lava lands were unlikely to be, that such an "open consent" clause was well outside the international norms for genetic research (people with, say, multiple sclerosis usually give a blood sample for genetic analysis toward MS therapies and must be approached again if a scientist wishes to use that blood sample for future research on other conditions), I think I would have nevertheless recognized that the clause establishes a particular relationship to the future—the one called "signing your future away."

But one of the most interesting bits of disclosure in deCODE's first statement to the SEC is a settlement agreement between deCODE and Beth Israel Deaconess Medical Center, where Kári worked just before founding deCODE. The disclosed document and its signatories settle a 1997 suit filed by Beth Israel (Civil Action No. 97–3046 in the Suffolk Superior Court of Massachusetts) and illuminate the more cutthroat aspects in today's economy of biomaterials and bioinformation. Let's simply read this bit of disclosure as is, in its sobering, formal legal language:

SETTLEMENT AGREEMENT BY AND BETWEEN
THE BETH ISRAEL DEACONESS MEDICAL CENTER
AND
DECODE GENETICS, INC.

This License Agreement (hereinafter, the "Agreement") is effective as of the 31st day of December 1997 (hereinafter, the "Effective Date") between Beth Israel Deaconess Medical Center (hereinafter "BIDMC"), a nonprofit corporation existing under the laws of the Commonwealth of Massachusetts and having its principal place of business at One Deaconess Road, Boston, MA 02215, and deCode Genetics, Inc., (hereinafter "deCode") a corporation existing under the laws of Delaware and having its principal place of business at Lynghals 1, 110 Reykjavík, Iceland.

WHEREAS, utilizing BIDMC facilities and resources Dr. Kári Stefánsson performed a study of multiple sclerosis and identified linkage to an approximately 200 kb segment of DNA;

WHEREAS, Dr. Stefánsson has identified at least two genes in the HLA region which are associated with myelin-forming cells and are candidate genes for multiple sclerosis;

WHEREAS, Dr. Stefánsson also began systematically sequencing the DNA from the 200 kb segment using facilities and resources of BIDMC;

WHEREAS, the parties have agreed that any Technology (as defined below) made by Dr. Stefánsson identified above, between November 1, 1993 and the Effective Date, shall be jointly owned by the parties.

NOW THEREFORE, in consideration of the premises and mutual covenants and conditions set forth below, BIDMC and deCode agree as follows:

There follows twenty pages of hard-core, bad-ass legal text that makes clear, in no uncertain terms, who either had the better lawyers or the better case. The settlement dictates that an *undisclosed* cash sum be paid to Beth Israel, that a "[confidential treatment requested]" number of shares of Series A preferred stock in deCODE be granted to Beth Israel (this turns out to be 130,000 shares), plus all manner of licensing, marketing, and ownership rights in any products or "know-how" that might be spun out of this molecular chunk of someone's body. Beth Israel risks absolutely nothing, gets a dollop of gravy, and receives an option on the future; deCODE paid up and agreed to pay still more if the future works out favorably—but most importantly, deCODE gets out of court.

So Kári and Beth Israel had "agreed"—which might be a contract to a lawyer, but is a promise to an ethnographer—to joint ownership of "Technology." Kári was less than duly diligent in keeping this promise. A tiny stretch of DNA yielded promising results in experiments and analysis— not definitive, but promising. Work was done toward the extraction of 200,000 bits of information coded by these molecules, information that linked up in promising ways with other information about the condition called multiple sclerosis. It still looks promising. The authorities learned of this work, somehow; there are stories about laboratory locks changed, computers impounded, grants frozen. Kári was moving on, returning to his natal country and to a company that will ask to be entrusted with the nation's databased medical records and biobanked tissue samples.

This is just one of the stories that can be told from this and other material disclosed by deCODE as part of its obligation to the capital markets in the United States and the world. What's its value?

What's the value of the sequence information for a certain 200 kb fragment of DNA extracted from a person ill with multiple sclerosis? Still promised.

XX

Even though I knew "full disclosure" and "transparency" were formally unachievable, informally I wanted to see if I could fill in some of those blanks. I filed a Freedom of Information Act request with the SEC asking for disclosure of this "confidential treatment requested" material. A month or so later I learned that my request had been denied; the rationale was that such disclosure would harm deCODE's competitive position. In an appeal, I explained that I was an ethnographer and a historian, not a corporate rival or even an investor, sophisticated or otherwise, and that I wanted the material only for a book I was writing. This, too, went nowhere.

But due diligence, I reassured myself, was all about exertion and effort, and actual future payoffs were only a bonus. When Mannvernd asked me to assist in writing a letter to the SEC, detailing what they thought were insufficiencies in deCODE's risk disclosures, I was happy to give my complicity one more twist, even if I was less than optimistic about the outcome. Given all Mannvernd had given me, I felt that sort of diligence was due them.

The project turned into a seventeen-page letter, plus a thick bundle of attachments, written mostly by various parties in Iceland but with contributions from Troy, Boston, San Diego, and [confidential treatment requested]. With the same kind of doggedness he displayed in his other scientific research, Einar Árnason took the lead in stacking up the facts, figures, and occasional rhetorical flourishes. I contacted a former SEC lawyer and got some advice on how best to proceed, as well as the office — the Health Care and Insurance Group of the Division of Corporate Finance — where the letter should be sent. The lawyer also suggested sending it to NASDAQ, which Mannvernd eventually did.

Mannvernd's letter foregrounded what they believed was the greatest threat to the future existence of the Health Sector Database, the fact that a large number of physicians in Iceland had stated explicitly that they would not cooperate in its construction:

A large fraction of the Icelandic medical community is opposed to handing over medical records to the database without their patients' prior signed statements permitting such transfer. A large number of doctors has made public announcements to this effect. A list of the names of 181 doctors refusing to hand over data from medical records without the written consent of the patients are included. . . . All the doctors at the Kópavogur health clinic . . . , in Iceland's second largest city, have stated that they will refuse to hand over data to the database. A large fraction of doctors in Hafnarfjördur and Akureyri, Iceland's third and fourth largest cities, will not send their patients' data without their patients' written consent. . . . These doctors may be ordered by their superiors to hand over records, but they have stated that they will refuse, because it would be a violation of their oath of confidentiality. Therefore they are preparing legal action, not disclosed in deCODE's S-1, which would constitute a risk factor.

The annual general meeting of the Icelandic Medical Association (IMA) declared "I. The Annual General Meeting of the Icelandic Medical Association (IMA), held at Hlídasmári 8, Kópavogur [Iceland], on 8 and 9 October 1999, is of the opinion that the National Data Base Act is deficient, as no provisions are made for the informed consent of patients and the Act may thus undermine the confidentiality that needs to be established between doctor and patient." . . . The World Medical Association stands solidly behind and supports the position taken by the IMA (published for example in the British Medical Journal 1999;318:1096 . . .). The Icelandic Psychiatric Association has adopted the following resolution: "The meeting of the Icelandic Psychiatric Association held 7 February 2000 demands that no medical data be handed over to the Health Sector Database without the consent of the patient."[9]

This kind of resistance, Mannvernd argued in an attempt to cast all this as a business risk, would at the very least keep the HSD from having "a quality label attached to it," and therefore it "cannot be marketed successfully. This, therefore, constitutes a risk factor for investors, not disclosed in deCODE's S-1."

The letter went on to argue for another related effect from this kind of social resistance, documenting the increasing opt-out figures from the database, which by then had reached over seventeen thousand, or 6.3 percent of the population. Mannvernd added that they also believed "that the government of Iceland has misinformed the public regarding opt out," citing the "common misunderstanding . . . that there was only a six month period for opt out because of a clause in the Act on HSD stating that the HSD could not be created until six months after the Act was passed." (See figure 9.) "Mannvernd considers the HSD to be unethical and unconstitutional," the section wound up, and just to make the business risk explicit, ended with "Mannvernd will use all legal means to increase opt outs in order to halt the creation of the database."

Situating itself in the discourse and codified agreements of international human rights, the letter charged a number of violations of international laws and standards, starting with the 1964 Helsinki Declaration of the World Medical Association. This was violated by clause 9 of deCODE's informed consent form, quoted above, and by the provision that data once entered into the HSD could not be removed, even if the patient subsequently opted out; the Helsinki Declaration does not provide for "open consent" and stipulates that participants in any research must be able to withdraw completely from the research at any time. Mannvernd also insisted that the data in the HSD would not be anonymous, but would be "personal data," and thus subject to European Community regulations requiring that informed (rather than the HSD Act's "presumed") consent be given. In sum, Mannvernd argued, "this breach of international ethical rules could mean that research done with these methods will be become highly suspicious and will not be considered valid in other countries. . . . This can affect approval of agencies such as the U.S. Food and Drug Administration and EC regulatory bodies. Therefore this constitutes a risk factor for investors that has not been disclosed in deCODE's S-1."

Mannvernd listed a variety of conflicts of interest that had also not been disclosed. There was a conflict between access to the HSD and its oversight:

According to Article 5 of the HSD Act The Ministry of Health and Social Security and the Director General of Public Health shall at all times have access to statistical data from the database. These are, however, also the government agencies directly responsible for the appointment of the National Bioethics Committee (NBC). The NBC is also given a role in overseeing use of the database including the use by the Ministry of Health and Social Security and the Director General of Public Health. This is a structural conflict of interest.

Mannvernd also insisted that there was a basic conflict between the database itself and the opt-out provision:

The Director General of Public Health clearly has a vested interest in the database according to Article 5 of the HSD Act. According to Article 8 of the HSD Act the Director General of Public Health shall ensure that a coded register of the persons who opt out be maintained and be made available to those who prepare data for transfer to the database. The Director General of Public Health shall also produce forms for giving opt-out notice, and shall ensure that these are available at health institutions and at the premises of self-employed health workers. Furthermore, the Director General of Public Health shall ensure that information on the HSD and on the rights of patients shall be accessible to the public. The greater the opt out the less valuable will be the database to the Director General of Public Health. There is, therefore, a structural conflict of interest between the vested interest of the Director General of Public Health and his role as a guardian of opt-out rights.

The constant effort to translate what Mannvernd considered to be serious social, political, legal, and ethical transgressions into the category of "business risk factors" may seem forced or stretched. But this strategy was required, since material business risks were the only things that concerned the SEC. So the Mannvernders opted to play on the only terms allowed it, and the group squeezed every issue they wanted to address publicly into this procrustean category of business risk. I admired the seriousness and sincerity with which Mannvernd played this game of forcing information disclosure as required by law, although it might appear quixotic to some. But these were people who, when I accompanied them to a presentation they gave at the Harvard Law School on the deCODE-HSD case, asked me to take them on a side trip to Lexington and Concord to see the bridge memorialized as the start of the revolution that made the United States a more rather than less democratic nation. If they had so clearly heard that famous shot as far around the world as Iceland, I was not about to second-guess the trust they placed in democratic ideals like "corporations should tell the truth as required by the laws and regulations of U.S. governing institutions." Quixotic, yes—and just.

Moreover, deCODE had already disclosed, as mentioned above, that the necessity of "maintain[ing] the good will and receiv[ing] the cooperation of the Icelandic people" constituted a business risk. By its own terms, then, anything deCODE did that might result in losing the much-ballyhooed "cooperativeness" of Icelanders would be subject to the SEC's disclosure requirement. So Mannvernd included every fact, event, and issue that could possibly bear on this matter.

One such issue was a set of financial folds whose implications were far from clear, making the need for further disclosure especially significant. It seemed that five million shares of deCODE stock had somehow gone from the company in Iceland to an "anonymous" holding company in Luxemburg and then back to Iceland through the state banks. The path of these five million shares is further traced in "GenomicsXSlot Machines," in which we also find out that, in addition to the well-known pair of "black markets" and "markets" ("white," as usual, is simply assumed), there exists the volatile space that is neither black nor white, nor is it black *and* white, but is referred to as the "gray market." Several thousand Icelanders would find out just how volatile that space is.

Yahoo!XFinance

DeCODE's imminent initial public offering, announced in March 2000, was placed on hold as NASDAQ tumbled through the spring, possibly in response to the loose-lipped comments of BillXTony on gene patenting. Many genomic-companies-to-be did the same, anxiously biding their time for a more propitious moment. Eventually, the market made enough of a recovery that deCODE's underwriters, Morgan Stanley, decided to go ahead, first offering the stock on July 17, 2000. Some eleven million shares were sold, grossing $198,720,000. Morgan Stanley took nearly $17 million of this as commission and expenses.[1] The IPO was clearly a financial success, for both deCODE and its underwriters. We'll take a more detailed look at the services provided by Morgan Stanley to earn their $17 million, but for now we'll focus on a less elite set of investors.

U.S. Securities and Exchange Commission regulations, as we have seen, often refer to a "sophisticated investor" as their ideal subject: the person who makes rational decisions about his or her money, about other people's money, and about the corporations in which these monies might be invested. This population of sophisticated investors swelled in the 1990s, and online securities trading sites multiplied, all in the expanded "safe harbor" for forward-looking statements dredged out by the Private Securities Litigation Reform Act of 1995. In this chapter we'll look at how deCODE was discussed in the period immediately before and after its IPO in July 2000 on these online investing sites: Raging Bull and—the most appropriately named site for the genomic and dot-com economy of the late 1990s—Yahoo!Finance.

I don't claim that the people presented here and their ways of speaking are "representative" of anything: the online investor, the day trader, or even just the genomic enthusiast. For one thing, they make up a limited sample. As of May 2001, when I began writing, there had been 22 postings about deCODE to the Silicon Investor site; 399 postings to the Yahoo!Finance board; and 617 postings to the Raging Bull site. To make matters even murkier, some people would often post on one of these publicly accessible bulletin boards, only to exchange e-mails directly with each other, invisible to public technologies. And then, as we'll see, trying to sort out who people are and how their comments about stock values are themselves supposed to be valued—how seriously are you willing to take someone pseudonamed "Casinomom"?—becomes a tricky affair. If the question, "how do you tell a counterfeit genomic company from a genuine one?" is a volatile one, the question "how do you tell counterfeit remarks concerning the counterfeit/genuine status of a genomic company from genuine remarks about the counterfeit/genuine status of a genomic company?" is, obviously, multiply volatile. So the excerpts and commentary here should be thought of in the empirical sense: less as *representative of* something, and more as a simple *presentation of* people and the things they wrote about deCODE, genomics, and the stock market of the late twentieth century.

Two general points, statements for which only my generally trustworthy character is security: most of these people were not just investing in deCODE, and not just in genomics. They were speculating across the bubbly tech spectrum, from genomics, biotech, and the health industries more broadly, to software, Internet companies, and assorted electronica. Some people were in it for the short term, others for the long, but a whole lot more were trying to day-trade the volatile margins emerging and dissolving every hour. And while we have seen "sober" advice about reading SEC filings rather than the "forward-looking statements" purveyed by corporations and the media, many of the postings and the discussion therein centered on news stories and what they portended for stock values. Despite occasional references to "DD"—due diligence—there was a noticeable lack of numbers and specificity. Instead, the discourse more closely resembled the keikophony of Keikomania and relied extensively on the exoticizations of Iceland, deCODE, and especially Kári, which popular coverage of these events promulgated.

Icelanders themselves were some of the most avid purveyors:

Ya I'm Icelandic alright, and proud of it tooooooo.
We do love this company here in Iceland. The whole nation went upside down

when Kári came to Iceland after years at Harvard as a professor with the script of his idea.

We have a biotech company with this uniqe database of medical reccords counting back a 100 years or more, all available for DeCode to exploit, not to mention our Sagas that we can read back for many centuries, mentioning all kind of illnesses. By the way our language and writings has not changed significantly over centuries. Also the genetic pool of Icelandic people are relatively pure caused by the isolation of the country through the centuries.

Kári Stefánsson, CEO is a strong leader and after having experienced his skills, both as a scientist and CEO, I have no worries about DeCode for years to come. The man is simply brilliant in every way, and we do not see his kind to often. Further more he has build up a fantastic team of top professionals that makes this company first among equals.

I bought in at 26 and I'm going to hold this one for ever.

In my oppinion the financial world is going to put DCGN in the front row, realizing its potentials, great management team, powerful allianzes like Hoffman Laroch, among the best equiped labratory's in the world, and lastly but not last DATABASE OVER A WHOLE NATION.[2]

Casinomom (with four dollar signs after her name, Raging Bull's rating system to help people value comments) provided another example of forward-looking, media-infused analysis: "I read somewhere that this company has one of the most ultra sophiticated labs in the world. . . . I gotta go find that article. will post when I do."[3] She too felt the "Harvard guy" was not only "brilliant," but "ethical" to boot:

You know siggi- I tell you, I am not hyping nor being dramatic. I did a lot of dd on this one before I bought and I really deep in my heart thought we could become a cra [Celera] as well. The Harvard guy who is the CEO seems brilliant to me (and ethical as well which is extremely important with genetic research) The conditions of the research are so unique . . . and from what I have read the results can be had faster than in other companies. This company has already targeted a couple mutated genes having to do with premature labor and osteoarthritis. what is they find something huge in terms of disease???? Then we hit the home run![4]

Later, in response to CNBC's interview with Kári after the IPO, Casinomom enthused, "Wasn't he impressive? So knowledagble, so forthright . . . really, most of the CEO's that come on cnbc are just embarassing . . . more concerned about the camera than the company's business. I liked this CEO's focus on the ethics of the use of the genomic info they are learning."[5]

When analysis did become more sophisticated, it also seemed to become subject to more questions:

Someone just sold a BIG BLOCK . . . worth $263,000 . . . makes you wonder why?

Today's money flow . . . in +3.9M and out -$2.6M which is a positive sign . . . BUT! again if we break down who is buying and who is selling, we see four big ticks selling -$1.2M and only one buying tick total $0.7. . . . so the buying was done mainly again with very small blocks . . . 166 bought and 89 sold . . . usually if there is something behind the corner the smart money can smell it first, right? So my question is why are they selling and not buying?[6]

Careful analysis and skeptical questions about a promissory genomic market, surely the sign of honest inquiry and due diligence — or a despicable ulterior motive:

Why are you so interested in DCGN if you think this one is a looser? My guess: YOU WANT TO BUY IT CHEAP!!! Good Luck, it was a Nice Try but it's not working :) Use a better approach the next time![7]

In this speculative economy, "sophisticated" analysis is indistinguishable from clever deception. Do you trust a fellow online trader who shows some financial savvy and investment acumen — or is that person all the more suspect? The more "sophisticated" the investor — the very quality extolled as fundamental by the SEC — the more capable of deception he or she would be. But this undecidable knot doesn't prevent these people from slinging their savings around cyberspace.

No one seemed as absolutely gung-ho as someone called Decodege — a name which, intended or not, I could only read to rhyme with "protégé." (His exuberance led some to suspect he was a deCODE employee, but this too was an undecidable; investors had to decide for themselves.) In August 2000, after a month of post-IPO sluggishness and inactivity, some on the Yahoo!Finance deCODE discussion board began to get impatient. Decodege posted a few badly spelled messages:

I thing you Decode lovers will be verry happy when the news are coming out next week? Decode set to fly.[8]

If you think Kari. dosent hawe any news after 6 month of saying nothing you defenantly dont know the man.

He is sonthing else.

cant say any more now sorry[9]

DECODE IS GOING TO AT LEST 80 BEFORE YEARS END I HAWE 10.000 SHERS NO-1 IN MY PORTFOLIO. DECODE WILL TAKE OFF I KNOW. MARK MY WORDS. LONG DCGN. . . . [10]

In the immediate post-IPO period, this brand of enthusiasm, combined with exhortations for patience, ran high across the Yahoo!Finance board: "just stay cool and relax. DCGN will GO UP for SURE . . . HANG ON, the fun is almost here !"[11] "DCGN to 40 . . . you must be joking. I cannot recommend this stock highly enough . . . hitting 55 is accurate by Sept 7–14. This company has news . . . wow."[12]

Nervous questioning punctuated the effusiveness, but never really punctured it. When Flunked_biology101 asked if "the lack of news since the end of the quiet period is the reason why we have tumbled in the last 2–3 days?"[13] he/she/it was reassured by Ribozyme (self-identified as "female" and as being from "Earth") in remarks that situated deCODE in the broader economy:

I don't think the lack of announcements has a lot to do with the drop in the stock price. Its more to do with a huge choice of new IPO stocks available and a withdrawl of money from companies like AFFX, DCGN etc. and investing in new IPOs. Nasdaq movements in recent days upwards, typically involve share value increases in the IT, internet, telecommunications stocks which further decreases interest in biotechs. So hold onto your biology books. This company has not yet begun to fight. This stock is about to throttle up.[14]

On August 18, messages like the following began appearing on the Yahoo!Finance board and on the other online investing sites:

News today will put DCGN on the map and screens of the fund traders.[15]

DCGN will close at 35 today here is why:
1. The news is huge
2. DCGN is very undervalued
3. Genomics is a hot sector[16]

Sure enough, deCODE and Roche issued a press release describing what was supposed to be their most recent achievement:

Kári Stefánsson, CEO of deCODE genetics noted that, "We have made significant progress towards finding a novel gene that, depending on the presence of certain molecular variations, contributes to the common form of Alzheimer's disease. This work underscores the feasibility and power of studying common complex diseases using Iceland's unique resources." Jonathan Knowles, Head of Global Research at Roche added, "We are very impressed by the rapid progress made by deCODE genetics towards identifying genes that play important roles in the molecular pathology of common diseases." Roche plans to initiate discovery and development programs for new diagnostics and therapeutics building on this genetic information. deCODE genetics has received an undisclosed milestone payment from Roche for this accomplishment.[17]

No forthcoming publication in any kind of scientific journal was mentioned, nor would any be forthcoming over the next few days, weeks, or months. Any investor sophisticated enough to actually try to find out anything more specific—what is "significant progress"? is this a gene, or a merely a locus or region that contains a possible gene somewhere on it? what is this gene supposed to do, or in what soberingly complex biochemical pathway does it exert its action, on the way to the massively and sadly intricate disease event called Alzheimer's?—would be unable to find anything in the published literature.

But only an aging crank who had grown up with some pre-1970s Mertonian or Popperian view about how science works would be so churlish and traditional to inquire about scientific publications as a guarantor of the Real in this day and age. A promise alone—"we have made significant progress"—is sufficient to trigger a previously promised milestone payment from Roche and to create an event in the larger economy. Datamining the NASDAQ Web site shows the trading trend that occurred around this heavily mediated event:

Date	Closing Price	Shares Traded
08/16/2000	24.000	789,700
08/17/2000	24.563	453,100
08/18/2000	27.000	2,441,100
08/21/2000	27.438	660,600
08/22/2000	27.250	428,500
08/23/2000	25.125	339,900[18]

The volume of shares exchanged on August 18 multiplied dramatically and the price bubbled briefly, both from nothing other than the announcement of a promise, before returning once again to the previous trade volume and a lower share price.

All of which exactly fit the expectations of the people in the game:

Just looking at volumes . . . DCGN IPO'd one month ago today. The first 5 days' volumes: 13.4M, 3.8M, 1.5M, 0.73M, and 1.36M. Since then it hasn't traded more than 0.8M shrs.

Until today, that is, where we have 2.3M shares traded with one hour to go. So this news obviously has gotten the co. some attention.

As has been pointed out, the CEO is on CNBC sometime between 4 and 6 ET.

Notice one good pop and we've already got someone on the board talking short squeeze. It never fails.[19]

All it took was Joe on CNBC to mention that DCGN has successfully located a gene associated with Alzheimers and the stock goes up 2 points immediately. Here's to more news.

THAT WAS EASY . . . MADE OUT GOOD ON DCGN . . . THX FOR THE AD-VICE . . . WORD IS MCDE HAS NEXT BIG NEWS . . . HOPE IT DOESN'T GAP UP ON MONDAY SO I CAN GET IN . . . GOO LUCK[20]

XX

Some of the more sophisticated—and hence suspect—postings came from Jabbiz, who seems to have done some homework and actual analysis. As the summer of 2000 expired, Jabbiz speculated about deCODE's future through a comparison with the experience of another company, Orapharma:

Here is what will happen to DCGN . . .
Orapharma planned to raise $64 million in an IPO around March 7. . . . Orapharma's key product had already passed all three stages of clinical trials and had a good chance of making it to market in 2001.
Overall, however, I couldn't give Orapharma very high marks. I accused the company of using deceptive marketing on its Web site. I also talked to CEOs at rivals and analysts who noted that Orapharma is one of about five companies competing in a market with a potential of only a few hundred million dollars. And even that market isn't expected to materialize for a few years.
The company had a great IPO, netting $77 million at $18 a share. At least Orapharma turned out to be a steal for institutional investors who flipped the stock. It began trading at $30.25 but never went much higher. It's currently trading around $9—a much more realistic price.
DCGN will drop like a rock after 1/18/01 [the expiration of the lockup date; see below] if not before it. IMO can not have $1B market cap at today's market without revenue and positive earnings.[21]

As autumn settled in, the speculators began anticipating January 2001's expiration of the lockup period, when insiders would have the opportunity to sell their deCODE shares for the first time. Usually, this event causes a dip in a stock's value; this was especially true for the high-tech stocks that had their IPOs in the late 1990s, and even more true of the biotech stocks at this precise moment in time: many lockup periods were expiring more or less simultaneously, and there was marked concern about a flood of shares drowning interest, enthusiasm, and value.

Days, and even weeks passed—it must have seemed an eternity in this speculative microcosm—with no news from deCODE and no movement other than the random downward walk of NASDAQ across the board. One poster tried to be reassuring, but ended up sounding like one more patriotic Icelander pushing vague boosterism:

DCGN will move up when it's time. This is the best recent BT stock that I know of. There is only 1 Iceland on earth.[22]

[One month later:]

As far as I know this is one of the best biotech company, and there is only one Iceland on earth. I believe institutions have been accumulating this stock heavily. Just wait and see . . . a ticking time bomb. This is not a daytraders' stock.[23]

On October 11, 2000, deCODE stock dropped dramatically, and one message board participant asked frantically:

News today? I haven't found anything. What's happening? Something must be up to make it drop $3.25 !! Anyone else know anything???[24]

Reyjo2, an Icelander, could only suggest the possibility of a negative news story:

Here in Iceland we hear of a "story" in Der Spiegel in Germany portraying Mr. Stefánsson very negatively. Now, if that's the reason for todays drop (and not simply the free-fall of everything else on Nasdaq etc.), then I wouldn't worry. The story is from the sparsely populated group "Mannvernd" in Iceland whose sole purpose is to harm DCGN as much as possible. Why? Who knows? News-hungry reporters "buy" such "stories" every once in a while. Anyone familiar with deCodes' gestational period 2–4 years back? "Stories" like this one were in the news here in Iceland every day, often quoted from "respectabel" sources from abroad!
Now, as I said, IF that IS the reason, I'm not worried, but, as I haven't had the time to surf the Net . . . , I would not know.
I have no connection to deCode other than my few thousand shares.[25]

One might say that a $40,000 connection (my conservative estimate: two thousand shares at $20 per at the time) is a connection worth taking into account as one evaluates Reyjo2's evaluations. "Stories," "respectabel," and even "buy" receive the destabilizing, skeptical scare quotes when this noun, adjective, and verb are associated with "Mannvernd," as if this entire exercise that Reyjo2 is smack in the middle of—writing and reading messages on an Internet investing bulletin board, which might be said to exist entirely "abroad"—isn't one of buying or selling stories whose respectability and source is always a dice roll. It's also indicative that whatever the reason for the drop, Reyjo2 thinks that finding it is a matter of surfing the Internet.

Those who gave no credence to Mannvernd's "stories" or what "respectable" foreign sources were saying remained optimistic:

Believe it or not, deCODE will go abaove $100 by the end of this year or early next year. What deCODE genetics is doing is a pioneering work in human genetics and pharmacogenomics. There will be no internet type bubbles in this stock until the maturation of biotech industry. Soon big news will come out from this and other BT companies that will match the annoucememt of first draft of human genome sequence.[26]

A new discussant named Partyspoiler (some speculated that this was Jabbiz posting under another name) seemed to sense uncertainty and anxiety on the board, and weighed in at some length in a tone that accorded well with his name:

Believe and suffer!
Not only insiders are waiting for the lockup period to end. Lots of suckers followed the hype in the small but influential media in Iceland and acted up on it and bought shares in this company. The lockup covers all owners of shares before the IPI date.
I'm told by Icelandic friend that even a local community of 300 person also invested in this, also lots of people took loans and bought shares with the same attitude as buying lottery tickets. These people are victims of lousy local media and reporters who do not any DD and just echo the crab they are spoonfed by.
This company will loose huge amount of money this year and the next few years.
They will feed you on a regular basis on postive news, quite remarkable news from medical point of view, but avoid any income issues.
Your only comfort is that the company got so much money in the IPO that 10% interest on that capital will probably go a long way to cover their losses if they do not spend to much on the lavish facilties in Reykjavik city center.
You will unfortunately see 18 soon and then lower price.
Good luck to you here, you are going to need it.[27]

(Around this time I, too, began wondering what might happen around the expiration of the lockup period in January 2001. I decided to make one more trip to Iceland so that I could be there to see what, if anything, would occur. That event—which also tells us more about the people to whom Partyspoiler refers, the ones who took out loans to buy deCODE stock—is treated in "GenomicsXSlot Machines.")

By October 19, when these messages had been posted, deCODE had fallen off more than $7.50 in a little more than a week. People were a bit edgy. Some tried to fill the absence with wistful whistling:

Im getting very tired of this nervousness over the last weeks. I just want to inform you that decodes biggest assignment is to find the cure for cancer. I personally will give them two years to provide some solid numbers and I am sure that the will not fail me.

Long time Decode = $400[28]

Madscientist69 posted a message directed to everyone on every side—"longs, shorts, and naysayers"—that was noteworthy for its amalgamation of pessimism, realism, and optimism:

DeCODE and Market Reality

To Longs, shorts and naysayers:

1. There is a difference between good companies, good technologies, and good stocks,i.e.,exciting technology and a good biz plan don't always equal success.

2. The stock market is legalized gambling.

3. The institutions have become day traders.

4. Stock prices are manipulated by insiders.

Considering all of the above, deCode, with all its PR, from 60 Minutes to the Wall Street Journal is a reasonable risk. Mapping the Altz. and Sciz. genes, as well as partial ownership by one of the worlds largest drug companies makes for a combination which has a good chance of success.

Go long, don't go candyass.

The Mad Scientist[29]

Jabbiz came back with his sharp-edged pessimism: "LOL! One zero too much . . . the drop will be to $8–10 . . . even further?"[30] And indeed, by early January 2001, even before the expiration of the lockup period and the dip in share price that almost everyone expected, deCODE was trading at $7.775. Jabbiz, it would seem, was laughing all the way to Decodege's bank.

Some people had had enough and announced their decision to sell:

Dumping this stock.

I'm outta here. Long-term they'll never have enough cash. Burn, burn, burn. Folks in iceland should stick to fishing. A person can only take so many losses with a stock regardless of cash or partnerships. Hope everyone else does well.[31]

Others exhibited an interesting blend of blind optimism, genetic ignorance, and the kind of investment philosophy that made Microsoft what it is:

It really doesn't matter what DCGN falls to . . . it is the only game in town with the unique resources they possess. This investment will do extremely well over time.

Nowhere on earth is there another resouce with so much potential to shed light on human, and especially caucasian genes and genetic diseases. DCGN is the safest investment in BioTechs IMHO. Monopolies are always good investments.[32]

Still others were somewhere in the middle, displaying at least some convincing simulation of sophistication while they kept their stakes with deCODE. PaulaGem posted in late 2000:

OK, is this a reasonable picture?? . . .

We have the end of lockup coming in January (18th?), we have a major PR event coming in January (60 minutes). Is this coincidental? I think not.

We have a major institutional presence in this stock so we will probably NOT have a flood of selling when lockup ends.

I have also been watching the charts and this stock (and several other biotechs) seems to follow a pattern of going down on small sells and up on BIG buys. Somebody (bodies) likes it and wants more before the end of lockup.

Also I have observed twice (and I have only been following the stock for a couple of months) that there were HUGE buys (600,000 shares and 400,000 shares) in extended hours, these buys did not register properly on my real-time graphs and I suspect they would have to be from a significant player to show up this way.

Disclaimer, I am new to trading (although I have owned biotech stock for 10 years) and don't fully understand everything I see, but I find the movement of this stock to be educational!!!

I bought and 19, and sold out my original position 19–22, back in around 13, out and 15 3/4, and am now back in at 12 5/8 to 13 1/4. I did not believe this stock could go to 10–11 as it did.

I have every confidence in the company and the technology, but geez, I wish I understood this screwey market a little better.[33]

In a later post PaulaGem vouched again for the importance of the media to this economy:

I doubt you'll see your $4-$5 . . . biotech rally coming next week with TIME cover, and I think they've wisely timed the 60 minutes PR for end of lockup.

If so, they are real PRO's in the PR department and there will be more news to support the stock at end of lockup.[34]

XX

The much-anticipated *60 Minutes* piece finally aired in April 2001. I talked at some length with one of the producers, and a number of Mannvern-ders gave generously of their time and perspectives, as usual. When it aired, I think it's safe to say that the Mannvernders and my complicitous self all felt a bit disappointed. We were hoping for another Mike Wallace con-frontation with a slick corporate CEO, and we got Ed Bradley's face of difference extolling the virtues of genetic homogeneity. Not that there wasn't mention of the privacy concerns and such, which is exactly the kind of liberal democratic issue that *60 Minutes* loves to present. And not that harsher criticism would have transmitted any more clearly or reliably. What was noteworthy in the bulletin board responses was participants' ability to read the segment in multiple ways—one more volatility to play.

So one person could write to the Yahoo!Finance board: "DCGN getting slammed. 60 minutes making the company look unethical."[35] But other readings of the *60 Minutes* piece were put into play in this in-terpretive economy. Sometimes it depended on how you interpreted "unethical":

60 minutes made them look slightly unethical, but that is only because DCGN is creating a medical database that would be considered a breach of privacy in the US. It did however seem that there is great potential for breakthroughs profits. Maybe the exposure will help raise the stock price.[36]

It's only unethical, this post seems to be saying, because we think it would be unethical if it were being done in the United States—but it's not, be-cause it's being done in Iceland. See? In any case: good news, bad news, whatever—what really counts is sheer media exposure.

Another person wrote in:

The DCGN database will be encrypted with the best technology available. Don't let doubters mess up your mind. What has a patient to hide that appears on cam-era in front of millions and millions of people? Information is a two edged sword. You can use it for good things and bad things. If it is used for good, it is possi-ble that a cure can be found for some deadly diseases. Is that worth the risk? I was watching 60 minutes the other day, where they were talking about C225, a can-cer drug. People are willing to take in untested drugs to prolong their lifes. What is unethical about the DCGN database if it can help save lifes?

The only problem that DCGN is facing is the envy of the people that did not get the idea or did not have the money to make it come true or were not con-sulted at the right moment. That is the only thing that could be considered un-ethical about the database.[37]

And still others put an even better spin on it all:

there was alot of validation, legitimacy and value put in DeCode on this program too. Like the uniqueness of that medical database.

I thought it showed DeCode in a good light (even tho' they tried to debate the ethical question). This is a winner!![38]

But soon the ever-dour Jabbiz got in his two cents worth:

Sorry, but I predicted it drops to $5 when DCGN was at 18 . . . and now another -50% is needed.

Nothing wrong with a good idea that the company is working towards, but why public and in USA!! No US investors will get excited about this especially after 60minutes.[39]

Then, in a remarkable show of how cynicism can trump dourness, at least when it comes to the stock market, a self-described thirty-six-year-old married male and an "inventory analyst" from "deep in the heart of Dixie," responded directly to Jabbiz:

your wrong dude.

americans dont mind private intrusion as long as its profitable and at someone elses expense.

everybody wants better prisons,waste disposal,etc. just not in my backyard . . .

get it . . . these iclanders are the guinea pigs . . .

and they are perfectly ok with it . . .

if youre waiting for $3.00 share . . .

dont hold your breath. even in this bad market.[40]

In the end, however, undecidability ruled, and gambling and speculation remained the dominant mode. IceFresh will have the final word on early investing in deCODE over the Internet:

No volume today! Strange stock.

Must mean something the question is what?[41]

SameXDifference

> I caught the nine o'clock bus to Myvatn, full of Nazis who
> talked incessantly about Die Schönheit des Islands, and the
> Aryan quality of the stock "Die Kinder sind so reizend: schöne
> blonde Haare und blaue Augen. Ein echt Germanischer
> Typus." I expect this isn't grammatical, but that's what it
> sounded like.
>
> Auden and MacNeice, *Letters from Iceland,* 134

You don't have to be a Nazi to think that the Icelanders are all blonde-haired and blue-eyed. But neither did all Nazis believe that Icelanders were an *"echt Germanischer Typus"* — where *echt,* to expect a "grammatical" English translation, would "sound like" a thoroughly disseminated congeries of genuine, proper, honest-to-goodness, real, true, authentic, typical, bona fide, legit, lifelike, unfeigned, substantial, and/or *pure.* Same difference.

What Nazi was skeptical about Icelandic *echt*ness? Jón Baldvin Hannibalsson, Iceland's ambassador to the United States, gives one answer in a letter to the *Washington Post* in 1999 (just after the Health Sector Database legislation had passed). The ambassador was responding to an article in the *Post* by John Schwartz, "For Sale in Iceland: A Nation's Genetic Code":

Mr. Schwartz characterizes the Icelanders as a "largely blue-eyed, blond-haired populace." Elsewhere in the article he refers to "the original blend of ninth century Norse stock and Celtic seamen" as being "largely unchanged." Well, we gladly admit to our affinity with the Celts (the Irish, the Basque and the Breton), but they never looked particularly blond or blue-eyed to us. Icelanders are of a mixed Nordic-Gaelic origin, as recent medical and anthropological research has confirmed.

As a matter of fact, on the eve of World War II, Adolf Hitler's emissary in Iceland, Werner Gerlach, is on record for having been sorely disappointed at not finding the Fuhrer's master race in our country, where the Nazis imagined it had been preserved in isolation for centuries. No such luck. What he encountered was a tribe of tall, gray-eyed, auburn-haired and red-bearded storytellers, insolently lacking in respect for Teutonic self-delusions of grandeur.[1]

"Storytellers" is a fitting descriptor for the ambassador's fellow Icelanders; Egill, Halldór Laxness, Kári Stefánsson—I'm sure all would agree.

Notwithstanding protests like the ambassador's, throughout the disagreements and differences and debates over the HSD and deCODE there were at least two words that appeared everywhere: Iceland was "isolated" and its population was genetically "homogeneous." The media ate it up. And can you blame them? It seems so intuitively, obviously true—part of Iceland's exotic, Viking heritage. DeCODE investors who posted to online bulletin boards also clearly believed the "isolated," "homogeneous" story. Their baldest statements were sometimes creepy, as in this post to Yahoo!Finance from someone claiming to work for a company that was an "early leader" in the "business of scientific information management":

DCGN has a unique resource in its population; it is the purest race. They have a major advantage over their competitors.

I have shares in Celera, DCGN, LEON, as I believe that they are all solid long-term investments. I expect the prices to appreciate considerably in the future.[2]

Even when such statements sparked attempts to analyze the claims of homogeneity more critically, investors were clearly out of their league and had to seek scientific expertise, or at least trust in secondhand reports of scientific expertise.

you said:

>>DCGN has a unique resource in its population; it is the purest race. They have a major advantage over their competitors.<<

My understanding is that what you claim is a "major advantage" is actually a handicap; ie., because Icelanders are so "pure" (isolated) that many of the major genetic problems don't show up.

I believe that MYGN's population databases are far superior to DCGN's for that reason.

Can you offer any scientific proof to back up your assertion?

thanks in advance for any additional info

cheers

ps. I agree with you that genomics is going to be huge. I also agree the key investor's prospering in this future bonanza is to buy a basket of the right stocks in this sector. As you know, the difficulty is picking the right stocks[3]

Here "pure" is hedged by setting it in quotes, and a less charged supplemental term is offered, "isolated." MYGN is the stock symbol for Myriad Genetics, a Salt Lake City–based company that works with Mormon populations—long a mainstay of genetic research in the United States and extraordinarily useful for certain genetic studies, although the preferred description of Mormon genetics is "well-characterized" rather than "pure."[4] The slipperiness of these terms is worth bearing in mind: while it seems an almost natural slide from the shared phenotypic characters of blue eyes and blond hair apparent to a casual observer to the claim of "genetic homogeneity," things are hardly so simple.

But hold that thought as we stay for a bit longer with these online investors. They certainly do read the newspapers, which were publishing more and more articles on genomics and the populations that make it possible. The *Washington Post,* which covered genomics in Iceland in 1999, also reported on genomics in China in 2000, and one investor took note:

Some here have posted that Iceland is unique in having a homogenous population (not mongrelized). However, Iceland is not unique in that respect; see the long Washington Post article on an isolated area of China: . . .

"Because it was unusually homogenous and made medical research easier, the DNA in the local population's blood 'was more valuable than gold,' the lead Harvard researcher reportedly told colleagues. Ounce for ounce, that would prove a sound estimate." . . .

I believe that DCGN has a future, but I wait . . . for this stock to bottom out. Too much hype so far.[5]

Note the "promises," and their shards, that are said to be part of this national genomic story. Note, too, that other dangerous supplement to homogeneous: "not mongrelized." And yet this investor retains some degree of skepticism, believing the future of deCODE to be based on "too much hype."

Hype, I hope I have impressed upon readers, is a more volatile substance than is usually thought, and its complete eradication from genomics is neither possible nor desirable; I would hope that this investor is sophisticated enough to wait for "just enough hype." If hype cannot be tamed by a science or reason stripped of all speculative excess, "too much hype" nevertheless can and must be tempered by a careful, concerted effort to address this scientific question: casual phenotypic observations aside, what is the level of genetic variation, in terms of differences in DNA sequences, in the Icelandic population? And we might then go on to ask, what difference would any such differences make?

XX

Einar Árnason, the population geneticist whose service to Iceland's National Bioethics Commission ended with the NBC's dissolution, and who became a founder of and leading figure in Mannvernd, enters the story again. Among his dogged pursuits—kleptoparasitic skuas, U.S. Securities and Exchange Commission filings, international standards in informed consent procedures—none was as central to his scientific identity as the question of genetic variation—sameness and difference—in populations of organisms, from scallops to salmon to humans.

Thanks to my complicity with Mannvernd, I have watched Einar present his work on the heterogeneity of the Icelandic population several times. He usually began with a slide of quotes taken from the many articles about deCODE and Iceland:

"Natural born guinea pigs"

"the most homogeneous population on earth"

an "island so inbred that it is a happy genetic hunting ground"

a "largely blue-eyed, blond-haired populace"

"a nearly homogeneous population" . . . "carrying nearly the same genetic codes as the Viking explorers who settled here more than 1,100 years ago" . . . with "little immigration to muddy the genetic pool over the centuries"

These headlines and sound bites from the international press indicate the prevalence and power of the unspoken assumption about Icelanders, summed up most strikingly in the January 2000 cover of *Mother Jones* announcing an article critical of the deCODE project, but uncritically repeating deCODE's most tendentious and exoticist claim: Iceland is a homogeneous nation of blonde-haired, blue-eyed babes—and, presumably, hunks—which means they're genetically similar too.

Since Einar often followed that slide of headlines with a picture of Björk,

I traded him a slide I had made from my growing collection of Icelandic CDs for his headlines. Björk, Iceland's other famous media-hyped personality, released *Homogenic* in 1997, when deCODE had been legally incorporated but had yet to become a scientific, commercial, and political phenomenon. The "homogenic" title is coupled to a figure of Björk in the CD art who is not only *not* blond-haired and blue-eyed, but is utterly nonhomogeneous with anyone anywhere you might have seen. Not a single Viking-liking journalist ever flipped through their collection of CDs or recent *People* magazines in the airport and asked the opening question: What's with Björk? What makes us so sure that Icelanders are not only homogenic but, underneath their clothes and skin, genetically homogeneous?

XX

Years before the scientific studies on the Icelandic population (about to be discussed), and even before deCODE was incorporated, Kevin Kinsella of Sequana Therapeutics assumed he knew all he needed to know about the sameness of the Icelanders. Sequana, a company that no longer exists, even though it had once been called "one of the more aggressive DNA prospectors," had made an early splash in the genomic world by working with the population of another "isolated" island, Tristan de Cunha, isolating a gene apparently involved in asthma from blood donors there.[6] In 1995, Kinsella had discussions with Kári, then still at Harvard, about the possibility of Sequana undertaking a larger-scale gene-prospecting project in Iceland. Kinsella followed up on this conversation with a letter, which Kári later supplied to the Icelandic government as a kind of "proof of principle" document in support of his then-emerging plans for deCODE. Like many such documents, this letter eventually found its way to nongovernmental individuals, and from there to researchers like myself, Henry Greeley, and David Winickoff.[7]

One has to admire its baldness: "As we discussed, Iceland is perhaps the ideal genetic laboratory since there has been virtually no immigration (lots of emigration, of course); it is of manageable size (200,000+ inhabitants), is an island expected to have many founder effects, has high quality national healthcare—from which we can expect excellent disease diagnosis, has formidable genealogies and the population is Caucasian—of most interest to pharmaceutical companies."[8] This is "sameness" on a large scale: the scale of "race," a concept whose thorough problematization by recent genomics does not stand in the way of its rule-of-thumb use for making promises to Big Pharma.[9]

"What we would propose to do," Kinsella continued in the letter, "in partnership with you"—the project already revolves around, not a nation, nor a company, but Kári himself—

is sponsor a massive program to identify probands [affected individuals] in the entire Icelandic population, collect blood from the entire population, establish pedigrees . . . genotype members of the pedigrees, conduct linkage studies . . . and positionally clone the gene(s) of interest.

Sequana would establish in Iceland a massive genotyping facility, involving dozens of ABI machines. . . . We would require the full support of the Icelandic government and National Health Services. If all the ascertainment, enrollment, and phlebotomy [blood drawing] can be furnished by the Icelandic authorities, then the cost of doing this can be manageable. . . .

Your hard cost estimate of the project is $12 million. . . . We would calculate it much higher but it depends what you are counting. . . .

Sequana would obviously want the commercial rights to the gene discoveries, part of which we would be prepared to share with the Icelandic government to repay them for their financial commitment. In addition, we would see this resource as an ideal "laboratory" for ongoing pharmacogenetic studies during clinical trials of new small molecule drugs.

In my ethnographic collection of epithets used to describe Kári, which range from "charismatic" to "pathological," never once did anyone call him a fool. Some time soon after receiving this letter, Kári must have figured out that he needed a "partnership" with a California genomic company like he needed a *gjá* in his head. With some refinements to this prescient and bold sketch—Kári would make a more circumscribed argument about Icelanders than the "Caucasian" one, but the idea is the same—he went it alone.

Pay particular attention, before continuing our questioning of sameness and difference, to the last sentence quoted. In all the tumult and "debates" about what deCODE was promising to do in Iceland, the idea of using Iceland as a quote-unquote laboratory for clinical trials never came to the surface of public discussion. But it was there all along, a submerged current as cold as you can find.

XX

These days, the question of genetic sameness and difference is decided primarily by DNA sequence analysis. The same fast technologies—high-throughput sequencing, ever-enriching databases, venture capital, and so on—that produced changes in scientific and commercial realities and, more importantly, in *potentials and promises* of genomics in the last two decades have also transformed the study of population genetics.[10] Here we take a brief look into some of the technical details of population genetics as it attempts to answer the question of Icelandic homogeneity. In the process, we'll learn a few things about the scientific review process and about the process of science itself when it crosses not only with politics and business—with genomics, how could it not?—but with itself, as different scientists passionately defend radically different positions.

Previous chapters have described Einar Árnason drafting new procedures of informed consent for Icelandic genetic research, getting sacked along with the rest of the National Bioethics Committee when those procedures were deemed contrary to deCODE's interests, helping found Mannvernd and building an Internet archive of primary and secondary materials on the deCODE controversy for an international audience of scholars and regulators, and analyzing the financial aspects of deCODE through its U.S. Securities and Exchange Commission filings. We also saw him observing the behavior of kleptoparasitic birds, and we return now to his primary identity: Einar the population geneticist.

In November 1999, Einar and two colleagues, Hlynur Sigurgíslason and Eiríkur Benedikz, submitted a manuscript to *Nature Genetics* with the admittedly inflammatory title, "Genetic Homogeneity of Icelanders: Snake Oil or Restorative?" "Lately much has been made of the genetic homogeneity of the Icelandic population," the paper began, "in a grand scheme of pharmacogenomics promising to revolutionise drug discovery and drug treatment." This first sentence had two footnotes to other papers in the scientific literature, including one by deCODE's Jeffrey Gulcher and Kári Stefánsson. The manuscript went on to quote another scientific paper by Gulcher and Stefánsson, particularly its claim that "Iceland offers a powerful and rare resource in genomic research—a relatively homogeneous population," with a "gene pool [that] has not been mixed by immigration."[11] The manuscript then cited some of the claims from the popular press.

Einar and coauthors went on to present and analyze two different data sets, one consisting of eleven blood group and protein variation genetic loci from populations from Iceland, Ireland, Scotland, Denmark, England, and Norway, and another data set of mitochondrial DNA (mtDNA) variation in seventy-three randomly selected Icelanders. Details will follow, but for now we need only note their conclusion: "Our work thus provides not a shred of evidence for a great and special genetic homogeneity of Icelanders. Quite contrary, at the mtDNA level they are among the most variable Europeans probably due to admixture (6).

Three reviews came back in late January 2000. One reviewer argued that "the data do not really show what the authors claim very clearly" and that one of the tests run on the mitochondrial DNA was an insufficient test for the claims.[12] A second reviewer found "the analysis and comparisons to be straightforward," although this reviewer too said the chi-square test on the mitochondrial DNA was "not appropriate." But even though the "results are interesting and worth presenting," this reviewer concluded, "I do not think that the authors' argumentative and caustic tone will serve their cause very well," as it "makes it appear that the authors have a grudge to settle, and it detracts from the quality and credibility of their scientific findings."

A third reviewer found "no problems with the scientific part of the paper. It is quite clear that the amount of genetic variation in the Icelandic population does not deviate from that of other European populations." Yet this reviewer was "hesitant" to recommend publication: "There is nothing wrong with the data or conclusions, but I feel that they are not addressing a scientific debate, but rather a view upheld by the founders of Decode and that have been circulating in the public press." This reviewer confessed to being unable to find one of the scientific papers by Gulcher and Stefánsson, and he noted that the quotes from the popular press suggested that this was "not a purely scientific debate" and that the authors perhaps "should choose a different channel for their contribution." The *purity* of this debate about purported "purity" is thus put into question as well. "Is it the purpose of *Nature Genetics* to defuse such beliefs?" the reviewer asked in conclusion.

The three Icelandic population geneticists set about revising their manuscript. The "argumentative" and "caustic" doublet of "snake oil or restorative?" was changed—one might say purified—in their resubmitted manuscript of February 15, 2000, "Genetic Homogeneity of Icelanders: Fact or Fiction?" Other language was toned down, and the statistical analysis that had been critiqued by the reviewers was improved. More quotes from the scientific papers of Gulcher and Stefánsson were included, to make it clear that this *was* truly a scientific debate, even if an impure one that exceeded the boundaries of the scientific. The authors added an analysis of three hundred microsatellite DNA markers drawn from France's Généthon databank and again found the Icelanders to be at least as genetically heterogeneous, if not more so, than all of Europe combined. But they also departed from the "purely scientific" again, not by citing more quotes from the popular press, but by supplementing scientific analysis with history:

The claim that Iceland was isolated for 11 centuries is not supported by the work of historians. The rich fishing and whaling grounds around Iceland have drawn thousands of men to Iceland throughout the centuries. They were Norwegian, Swedish, Danish, British, German, Dutch, Flemish, French, Basque and American fishermen and merchants. Fortunes were made. Isolated, the Icelanders were not. Fishermen and merchants came ashore for varying lengths of time and survivors from frequent shipwrecks often would overwinter on farms. Despite stiff social, civil and church penalties (even death) against illegitimacy there are throughout the centuries records of babies resulting from liaisons between foreign men and Icelandic women. The extent of this has not been studied systematically by historians or geneticists, however, it would have resulted in gene flow to the Icelandic population.[13]

Aside from purifying "not a shred of evidence" to the logically equivalent "no evidence for a great and special homogeneity of Icelanders," the conclusions of the manuscript were exactly the same.

A month later, *Nature Genetics* wrote back, saying that the manuscript had been reviewed again by two of the initial reviewers, and that while "they feel the paper is improved, outstanding concerns remain." But in fact, one of the reviewers felt that "the authors have responded satisfactorily to my earlier comments" and asked only that they also address an analysis of mitochondrial DNA that had just been published in the *American Journal of Human Genetics,* since that paper reached a different set of conclusions about Icelandic homogeneity. This paper, whose lead author was Tómas Helgason and whose coauthors included Gulcher and Stefánsson, will be examined in a moment. This reviewer asked for no other changes.[14]

The first reviewer, however, felt that "the additions that have been made make the paper seem even more like a crusade against Decode. They question every assumption upon which that enterprise rests, generally by citing historical evidence about interbreeding and communications in the past, and the quality of population records, that are themselves as unsubstantiated and open to interpretation as the contrary assertions about isolation and the high quality of the genealogical record." (One could argue that, instead of "crusade," another term for the process of "question[ing] every assumption" might be "the scientific method." But this, of course, is not a purely scientific argument, but a rhetorical one.) "If the paper was focused on just the information in Table 1," this reviewer concluded, "and the arguments limited to the point about diversity made there, then it would be a contribution to the scientific debate about the prospects of mapping genes involved in common diseases in Iceland."

The purist views of referee one carried the day. The journal asked the authors to submit a "revised manuscript *that does not exceed 400 words, and includes Table 1 only*"; the emphatic italics are in the original. Gone was the historical supplement, gone were the long quotes from Gulcher and Stefánsson. The overall conclusion to the paper as it was finally published read, "Icelanders are among the most variable Europeans at the mtDNA level, probably due to admixture. Background linkage disequilibria are expected in admixed populations (under recent admixture even among loci on different chromosomes) and this may create difficulties (for example, false positives) for disease gene mapping. We therefore caution that before accepting the idea that the Icelandic population is ideal for gene discovery in complex disease, the assumptions be critically and independently examined."[15]

XX

"OK, it may be true that Icelanders don't all look alike," conceded the Stock Watch column at SmartMoney.com on July 10, 2000, only days before the long-delayed, much-anticipated deCODE initial public offering on NASDAQ. "But that doesn't mean you'd pick Reykjavík as the setting for a documentary called 'People of Color,' either."[16]

Nevertheless, Ann Snider's Stock Watch column went on to quote deCODE board member and venture capitalist investor, Jean-François Formela, in support of the scientific argument that the homogeneity of Icelanders was the difference that set deCODE apart from the pack of genomic companies that were then populating the IPO charts in large numbers. "DeCode has a special trick—a homogeneous population," Formela was quoted as saying. "The problems facing it are far lower than when research is done in the open population. The results are much more accurate and the process is less expensive." When Formela went on to cheerlead for Kári, reminding SmartMoney.com that "he came out of the battle with the government [sic!]" and was "meeting the milestones and delivering," the Stock Watch column concluded that "all he has to do now is convince U.S. investors that there's money to be made from Iceland's genetic purity."

If I say that the question of the genetic homogeneity of the Icelandic population requires further painstaking technical analysis, this does not mean that the outcome of such an analysis will be a number spit out at the end of a "purely scientific," machine-like process—"99.9% pure!"—with which every rational actor will be forced to agree. This would misunderstand how any science or technical analysis, including population genetics, works, and the kinds of answers such analysis produces. A leap—or crossing of a chiasmus, or access to a yet-to-arrive future—is necessary. The American scientist and philosopher Charles Sanders Peirce called this difficult-to-articulate procedure "abduction" and demonstrated that it was as essential to the operation of science as the other two components commonly agreed to constitute scientific reason, induction and deduction.[17]

But we can get by without understanding what Peirce meant by abduction. In the example we are about to look at, the term "assumption" plays the key role, and this, as the saying goes, is close enough to "abduction" for government work. Assumptions are vital to science—they are its promise—and this question of genetic homogeneity is no exception. One has to assume—take on, somewhere in one's reasoning apparatus—what has yet to arrive. Like any good investor, a scientist must, even if to a vanishingly small degree and with the greatest reluctance, speculate. Seeing how this actually works should help. Ready for a test of your sophistication, investors?

Three measures are relevant for assessing homogeneity or heterogeneity of populations from mtDNA sequence variation (Nei, 1987). The mean number of pairwise sequence differences, $\hat{\Pi} = n/(n-1) \Sigma p_i p_j \hat{\Pi}_{ij}$, which take into account the frequencies of different haplotypes, p, and the mutational differences between them, Π_{ij}, is a straightforward measure of diversity. Other estimators are the number of different haplotypes or lineages k and the number of segregating sites S in a sample of size n. Using assumptions of the infinite-alleles or the infinite sites models of the neutral theory the parameter θ, representing the effective population size N_e scaled by the mutation rate appropriate for the fragment μ, can be estimated from these basic statistics. The statistics θ_k and θ_s only depend on the sample size and the respective basic statistics, k and S.[18]

You can plainly see that this "straightforward measure of diversity" is not nearly as straightforward as the phrase "natural born guinea pigs." Yet these are the terms and equations with which the scientific question of the degree of homogeneity of the Icelandic population are addressed. Are we investors expected to be able to solve for Π? This investor can't. Even if we had the skills and time, there is more to the problem than that.

The quote above comes from an article that Einar published in 2003 in the *Annals of Human Genetics*, which bore an innocent title that neverthe-

less had its caustic edge: "Genetic Heterogeneity of Icelanders." This article was in large part a critical response to the article by Helgason, Gulcher,
and Stefánsson that Einar and colleagues had been instructed to consider
by the reviewer for *Nature Genetics*. This extensive article by Helgason and
coauthors, appeared in 2000 in the prestigious *American Journal of Human Genetics*. Given that three of its authors were employees of deCODE
(the Icelandic Helgason and another coauthor, Ryk Ward, were at Oxford
University), it's hardly surprising that Kári dismissed the work of Einar
and his colleagues and continued to speak of the special qualities of the Icelandic population that his own paper with Helgason appeared to uphold.

But the Helgason and colleagues paper spoke only indirectly to the
question of homogeneity—the word, in fact, never appears in the article,
which bears the title "mtDNA and the Origin of the Icelanders: Deciphering Signals of Recent Population History." Nor does this article even
cite its own coauthors' work: the earlier articles by Gulcher and Stefánsson that were supposedly the definitive, "purely scientific" literature that
Einar and his coauthors were supposed to focus on instead of the statements in the popular press (articles that were published in such insignificant venues that one reviewer could not even find copies) are *not
mentioned at all*. While at one point the Helgason and colleagues state that
"the Icelanders have been a small and isolated population throughout their
history (relative to most European populations)," and that "it can thus
be *assumed* [emphasis added] that virtually all mtDNA lineages observed
in the contemporary Icelandic population are descended from the original set of mtDNA lineages present in the female founders 1,100 years ago,"
the paper in fact has many divergent statements that are difficult to rec-
oncile with the claim of homogeneity:

Given the present comparative dataset, however, it is impossible to identify the
parental populations with certainty or to quantify admixture proportions between
them.
   Nonetheless, the Icelanders do harbor a considerable amount of mtDNA diversity, as is indicated by their gene-diversity and mean pairwise difference values,
which are among the highest in Europe for HVSI.[19]

The main thrust of this paper was less to defend homogeneity than it
was to describe an entire history, that began with a small population with
"low genetic diversity," which was also culled at various "bottleneck
points": the pneumonic plague in 1402–04, a smallpox epidemic in 1708,
famine caused by a volcanic eruption in 1784–85. Einar's *Annals of Human Genetics* article critiques this history and its purported effects on the

gene pool of the Icelandic population, in part by describing the role that "assumptions" must play when one is not measuring, but *modeling* a population like the Icelanders.

To return to the measures of homogeneity: If you compare π for the different populations of Iceland, France, Denmark and Germany, Einar and Helgason and his coauthors would agree that the number of pairwise differences is high for Iceland and thus seems to indicate a low degree of homogeneity or sameness. But Helgason and colleagues also "posit" that the female ancestors of Icelanders carried mitochondrial DNA sequences that had many DNA sequence differences, *and* the authors "prefer" to use the "number of haplotypes k and the accompanying θ_k statistic" that depends on *assuming* the infinite alleles model of the neutral theory (a population genetics theory)—at least this is what Einar argues. Furthermore, according to Einar, Helgason and coauthors "contend" that "k is a sensitive indicator of demographic events such as a recent bottleneck because rare haplotypes would then tend to be lost. A shortage of rare haplotypes could then be taken as evidence for a bottleneck or drift. Thus a low k and θ_k in Iceland are thought to be sensitive indicators of bottlenecks and recent demographic history of the Icelanders."[20] The higher k is, the higher θ_k is.

But with increasing sample size, k increases at a diminishing rate. This means that the k for Iceland can't simply be compared to the k for Denmark and France, because of different sample sizes. So Helgason and colleagues simulate, on the basis of the infinite alleles model, what would happen if you increased the Icelandic sample size to a "sampling saturation" point, that is, a point where you would have to increase the sample size by ten to get one new allele. "The inference, however," Einar continues, "is critically dependent on the model assumptions" (6).

Einar's paper concerns itself with three of these assumptions—parameters whose yet-to-be-established future values must be a matter of some speculation. One of these Einar simply characterizes as "debatable," and he just moves on. For even if that assumption is assumed to be correct, "there remain two major assumptions . . . namely, the assumption of selective neutrality and the assumption of steady state distribution" (6). Sparing the reader-investor more details, suffice it to say that Einar's paper goes on to raise serious doubts about these assumptions, using comparative data from studies of Norwegian and German populations. We can skip to the conclusion of this section of the paper: "The interpretation that there are fewer haplotypes in Iceland than in other countries due to a founder effect and genetic drift with a small effective female population size (Helgason *et al.* 2000b; Gulcher *et al.* 2000) is therefore unlikely. . . . The large number of polymorphic alleles in Iceland is thus contrary to expectations of a founder effect and drift. Admixture during or subsequent to the settlement of Iceland is a much more likely explanation" (7).

Let's be clear: we're dealing here not with certainties, but with the "much more likely." The lavaXland of genomics is rife with uncertainty, no matter where you are located.

Do you want more, investors? Do you think that more diligence is due?

Thus examining the primary data from the original sources, and avoiding the use of erroneous data such as those exemplified by data in Table 2, Iceland ranks among highly heterogeneous populations in Europe for $\hat{\Pi}$ and in the top half of distributions on all measures of heterogeneity or effective population size. This contrasts with previous inference of 'relative homogeneity' of Icelanders based on mtDNA (Helgason *et al.* 2000b; Gulcher *et al.* 2000; Helgason *et al.* 2001). (11)

Microsatellites represent another class of loci potentially useful for addressing these questions. Gulcher & Stefánsson (1998) reported that the Icelandic population 'is indeed more homogeneous as reflected in overall heterozygosity rates of microsatellite loci' because the heterozygosity rate of over 300 Genethon markers was 0.75 in Iceland compared to 0.79 in Europe as a whole. Previously, I (Árnason *et al.* 2000) pointed out that the Icelandic value was higher than the 0.70 for 5,264 loci spanning the entire genome in the French population (Dib *et al.* 1996). In reply Gulcher *et al.* (2000) objected to this comparison and stated that 'the 298 markers were specifically selected for gene mapping on the basis of high heterozygosity.' These are contradictory statements, however, for if the loci were specifically selected because of high heterozygosity they cannot give 'overall heterozygosity' because that implies a random selection of loci from the genome. (13)

Had enough now? Or should I go on to analyze the next scientific paper in this controversy's chain, another *Annals of Human Genetics* article by Helgason and company—literally, since by this time Helgason had moved from Oxford to deCODE. This iteration critiques Einar's critique and reasserts all the team's previous arguments.[21]

No? Well then, investors, I suppose it is time to take stock.

XX

"DNA Study Deepens Rift Over Iceland's Genetic Heritage," ran the headline of an article in *Nature* when Einar's 2003 study was published. In some ways the headline is a perfect description of the kind of chiasmic volatility we have just witnessed: no resolution, only a rift that continually plunges ever more deeply, probably abyssally. *Nature* cautiously condensed Einar's article to, "His results suggest that several characteristics of the mitochondrial DNA sequences vary as much in Iceland as they do in the rest of Europe." *Nature* also noted that "scientists at deCODE do not dispute Arnason's sequence data, but say that he has misinterpreted them." And anyway, the article concluded, "the company adds that Iceland's extensive genealogical data will aid the hunt for disease genes, whatever the genetic variation within the country's population proves to be."[22]

Homogeneous, heterogeneous: *whatever.* Same difference.

It's confounding. As always with chiasma, a greater degree of due diligence will be necessary. Due diligence, and some speculation. Both are necessary, once again, in this double bind.

Is that the same thing as saying that the rift only deepens? Yes.

No—it's different.

It made a difference to Kári and company to be able to say that the Icelandic population was different than others: it had a higher, even "unique" and "special," degree of genetic sameness. That population difference was what they said made deCODE different among the heavily populated genomic sector. Kári and company repeated this at every possible opportunity, years before anyone had even bothered to comparatively analyze Icelanders DNA. It made a difference to investors, who were looking for something different in a genomic company, to think that the genetic homogeneity of Icelanders was a scientific truth and not some PR ploy. It made a difference that investors could read these claims repeatedly, especially since none of them could do the real due diligence of examining the data, making careful assumptions, solving the equations, and mounting an interpretation. DeCODE held out the bait of a uniquely homogenous population, and journalists and investors in Iceland and the United States took it hook, line, and sinker, as they say in the fishing industry that still accounts for 70 percent of Iceland's foreign earnings. In multiple media stories, on investment Web sites, in deCODE's own registration statement with the U.S. Securities and Exchange Commission, the "unmuddied" quality of the gene pool was the big selling point that distinguished this otherwise undistinguished company from the genomic pack.

It's only now, when we know that Icelanders may not be so different from other populations after all, that Kári and company say this may not matter: *whatever—have we mentioned our beautiful Icelandic genealogies recently?*

And, as Helgason and company argue at the end of their article that I spared you from reading, "Putting aside theoretical arguments, the suitability of the Icelandic population for gene-mapping studies is now perhaps best judged by results; see, for example, Stefánsson et al. (2003), Hicks et al. (2002), Gretarsdottir et al. (2002), and Gudmundsson et al. (2002)."[23]

The references here are to published reports of newly discovered genes that deCODE claimed were associated with schizophrenia, late-onset idiopathic Parkinson's disease, some forms of stroke, and peripheral arterial occlusive disease. After years of publishing next to nothing but promising press releases announcing the achievement of "research milestones"—press releases that appear only to have made a difference to day traders poised to capitalize on the brief price fluctuations that followed—deCODE finally achieved some actual scientific publications reporting gene discoveries, or new associations between known genes and complex conditions. Does having published scientific findings make deCODE different from other genomic companies? Not at all. Does it suggest anything about the structure of the Icelandic gene pool? Not really—other companies working with other, presumably less homogeneous populations have had far more success. Don't trust me—do your own due diligence.

Does it say anything about what other kinds of stories can be told about other populations and the scientific prospects that stem from them? No. Estee Genokismus, the Estonian genomic company that copycatted de-CODE in a number of ways, argued that Estonia's more heterogeneous population would not only serve as a better platform for gene discovery, but would be a better proving ground for testing, marketing, and sales of future pharmacogenomics-based drugs because Estonia represented the actual genetic heterogeneity of "Caucasian populations" (see below) better than Iceland did.

And the more recent BioBank project, combining genetic analysis and medical records analysis for fifty thousand British citizens, also foregrounded the advantages of genetic heterogeneity: "The BioBank project is also expected to be more comprehensive than others because the UK population is descended from several waves of immigration and so is genetically highly heterogeneous. This means it contains more polymorphisms to investigate than do the relatively inbred [sic] populations of Iceland and Estonia, for example, although some overlap of results between studies is likely."[24]

Homogeneity, heterogeneity: same difference, different sales pitch.

Does it make a difference if you think the population that forms your commercial base is more homogeneous than it actually is? It does. One danger of presuming a greater degree of homogeneity than may actually exist in Iceland is an increased number of false positives in gene discovery experiments, as Joseph Terwilliger and Kenneth Weiss argued in the journal *Current Opinions in Biotechnology*.[25] So even the few gene discoveries that deCODE has managed to get into print must still withstand the test of time and the diligent scientific scrutiny it will bring; the scientific literature is littered with once-promising genetic findings that fade, quickly or slowly, into the rift of nonexistence. And even when a discovery sticks, a company still faces the fact that, at best, one out of ten of its discoveries will be developed into a drug ready for clinical trials. And then the drug might fail clinical trials, or might pass them but kill people on the street, or might work only for 27 percent of patients, or might cost too much, or . . .

Most of all, however, the actual genetic heterogeneity of Icelanders made a difference to Einar. And the fact that it was Einar making the arguments that I have favored here made a difference to me. An ungenerous reader will simply discount this as an effect of complicity, and it is impossible to argue with a lack of generosity. The fact is that I trust Einar. Or to put it differently: I promise you that Einar is a trustworthy individual and a trustworthy scientist. I would not make the same statement, or utter the same performative oath, about Kári. I have not done the due diligence to know if I would make the same statement about any of his coauthors and colleagues. But in addition to knowing Einar's reputation in the field of population genetics, I have watched the way he analyzes all sorts of data, from a wealth of DNA sequences to a wealth of disclosed financial transactions. He is relentlessly methodical and careful, and when he speculates or assumes or promises, as all good scientists must, he marks his assumptions and flags the rifts that must appear in any scientific work—"Here!"

So: are Icelanders as genetically heterogeneous as Einar argues, or as . . . well, *whatever,* as Helgason and colleagues argue? It should be clear where I have placed my investments.

PresumedXConsent

Someone on the Yahoo!Finance bulletin board—the disclosed information indicated only that he was thirty-two, single, male, and lived in the United States—posted a message on August 30, 2000, urging his fellow investors to buy the current issue of the scientific journal *Nature*: "U may be able to see about DCGN (deCODE genetics) in the current issue of Nature, 24th August, 2000. . . . It talks about: Iceland, its doctors, conflict of interests between deCODE and patients and how DCGN may be falsely showing their DCGN investor a nicer picture in their PR news in NASDAQ. Please buy this issue."[1]

Allison Abbott's *Nature* article, "Iceland's Doctors Rebuffed in Health Data Row," discussed how "the Icelandic Medical Association (IMA) has failed to reach agreement with the genomic company deCODE Genetics over Iceland's new national health sector database, which is to be run by the company. The dispute centres over the plan for automatic inclusion of patients' health records in the anonymized database." The IMA was insisting that informed consent was necessary for the database—people had to actively opt in—while deCODE continued to insist that the "presumed consent" the company had made sure was in the Health Sector Database legislation was sufficient. The talks went nowhere, and when discussions ended, deCODE and the IMA issued a joint press release in Icelandic, stating simply that the talks "had been concluded."[2]

DeCODE promptly made its own English translation, which was soon posted on the NASDAQ Web site. The chairman of the IMA noted "obvious inconsistency in the two versions," not surprisingly, since deCODE "did not seek our approval of their English version." Where the Icelandic joint press release had said the talks "covered the content and have been to the point," deCODE translated this with a more positive spin, saying the talks had been "both positive and productive."[3] Several days after de-CODE posted its versions of the press release, Iceland's state radio reported that the IMA had demanded that deCODE publish a correct translation. The original press release, the radio reporter noted wryly, was "short and appears simple to translate." When asked why he thought de-CODE's translation "suggested that the talks had been more fruitful" than was implied in the original, the IMA chair responded: "wishful thinking." Since "the conclusions of these negotiations might influence the price of shares [in deCODE]," continued the reporter, would the IMA demand that the deCODE translation be removed from the NASDAQ Web site (deCODE's IPO had occurred scarcely a month earlier) and a correct one posted? "The IMA is not in negotiations with deCODE in order to influence their share price," said the IMA chair, "nor to help or hinder anybody's business activities. But naturally we will demand that the correct version shall be published."[4]

Meanwhile, back on the Yahoo!Finance board, none of this mattered to the truly committed Icelandic deCODE investors:

I wouldn't be as concerned . . . and certainly not interpret the episode as it is portrayed in Nature. . . . The little "duel" staged in the media by the chairman of the IMA just before the general meeting, mostly one-sided though, if such a duel exists, was obviously just muscle-flexing meant for IMA-members to notice. . . . All indications, from the ministry of health, DC and IMA now point to renewed talks in the near future. An agreement, satisfactory to all parties concerned— company, investors, doctors, patients, government—are sure to be reached sooner than later.

What the few doctors passionately opposed to any dealings with DC (now why would that be?), have come to realize that Icelanders, like one of our recent posters on this board, do not understand why they should not take part in this venture for a better future. If not for them, then for their children. Icelanders in general, want their records included in the existing database, and help to build that database.

I would not put too much, if any, emphasis on this, but, then again, its only my opinion but I wanted to tell you if it might ease your feelings :) . . . but don't take my words on anything—do your own DD :-)[5]

Do your own due diligence: a mantra for the era of promising genomics. But no matter how much diligence you did, there would still be some debt due on the negotiation of this presumedXconsent.

Readers by this point know that I have taken liberties with the chiasmic construction that I take so seriously—"dogXwhale," for example. But this one takes the cake: presumedXconsent? There's no undecidability here, no blurred boundaries, no funny differential trafficking between these two acts, to "presume" and to "consent." They are fundamentally inconsistent. No matter how imperfect or bureaucracy-impaired the bioethical principle of "informed consent" might be, you have to admit that it utterly depends on some version of someone actually performing, orally or graphically, the speech act "I will," "I do," "I consent," or, most simply, "Yes." That speech act has to be performed and, in performing, does what it says. You create a future in which you have consented. Even the smallest nano-utterance, in the far corners of a legal or database architecture, of the contrary speech act "I presume" is enough to wipe out the place of the consenting subject. Presumed consent? That's no chiasmus, you say; that's doublespeak.

Yes. And no. I hope to show that consent always presumes, that there's always an element of unwillingness in every willing, that "full consent" is as much of a misnomer as "presumed consent." The better question is, where, in a database or a law, is the limit of consent and presumption placed?

XX

Icelanders are faced with only a more intense version of this volatile fissure that gapes beneath all our feet. What practices and concepts might improve our consenting relationships to biomedical futures about which we have vanishingly little information, but plenty of speculation?

For those volatile bodies[6] among us who don't have enough to read, transcripts of the public meetings of President Clinton's National Bioethics Advisory Commission (NBAC) are available on the Internet at what, in my opinion, is one of the scarier looking URLs out there, www.bioethics.gov. The urgent questions of what "informed consent" is and how it can be enacted are the subjects of days and days of discussion over months and years, with drafts upon drafts of reports and executive summaries and appendices that all remain, in the end, "advisory." Let's read only two microevents within this vast bioethical desert in which we're wandering.

In August 1999 the NBAC published its report, *Research Involving Human Biological Materials: Ethical Issues and Policy Guidance,* which discusses at length some of the difficulties that principles of informed consent face in a world become increasingly speculative and future-oriented. One of their recommendations reads:

Recommendation 9:

To facilitate collection, storage, and appropriate use of human biological materials in the future, consent forms should be developed to provide potential subjects with a sufficient number of options to help them understand clearly the nature of the decision they are about to make. Such options might include, for example:

a) refusing use of their biological materials in research,

b) permitting only unidentified or unlinked use of their biological materials in research,

c) permitting coded or identified use of their biological materials for one particular study only, with no further contact permitted to ask for permission to do further studies,

d) permitting coded or identified use of their biological materials for one particular study only, with further contact permitted to ask for permission to do further studies,

e) permitting coded or identified use of their biological materials for any study relating to the condition for which the sample was originally collected, with further contact allowed to seek permission for other types of studies, or

f) permitting coded use of their biological materials for any kind of future study.[*7]

(To note in passing: Not included in this list is any option like "g) claiming commercial rights to their biological materials and a 0.007 percent return on future licensing arrangements that might arise out of speculation based on using said materials." This absence marks a yawning chasm within a bioethical discourse where the principle of "autonomous individual choice" is supposed to trump everything and be the foundation for all other ethical principles.)

The asterisk at the end of this list of proposed consent-form options directs one to an enormously long footnote in the finest of print, in which three "Commissioners" articulate their disagreements about these options. Commissioner Capron thought that neither option e nor option f should be included on *any* consent form: since they "encompass future studies with unknown risks and benefit, neither adequate IRB [institutional review board] review nor informed consent is possible at the time when subjects are asked to provide consent for the future use of stored material." Commissioner Shapiro agreed with that reasoning, but only as applied to option f. But these commissioners were clearly in the minority on this issue of the volatile future.

Prevailing wisdom is represented by Commissioner Miike, who makes it clear that these are options, like on a menu, and he expects that individual researchers will choose among them what to include on their consent forms. He admits that option f is the "most controversial"; this is the option that deCODE employs, and indeed, most genomic concerns would like to opt for this "most controversial" option. It might seem that option f "contradicts" the "overall report, with its focus on consent as truly being informed," says Commissioner Miike, but one should look more carefully (65). In a clinical context, he suggests, when people's minds are likely to be preoccupied with some immediate treatment for their volatile body, it may be that we should not ask for such broad future consent, also called "prospective consent." But it is much more "reasonable" to ask for such consent—bioethicists, like the bioscientists they like to distinguish themselves from, are always going on about what is reasonable—in the context of long-term biomedical research divorced from an immediate need. I leave it to the reader to speculate on the diagram of forces that produce this particular form of reason that produces a particular form of a truncated future:

This general consent recommendation would seem to contradict the Commission's overall report. [This] report, however, addresses human biological materials collected both in research and clinical care settings. In the research setting, an extensive prospective consent form that includes the entire range identified in Recommendation 9 seems reasonable. Given the nature of current consent documents in the clinical care setting, however, I believe it is unreasonable to expect patients to deal with such a complicated consent form for permissible future research. . . . Patients, whose primary concern is treatment or diagnosis, cannot be expected to reasonably evaluate the diverse range of prospective consent choices as identified in Recommendation 9. Thus, for practical purposes, a general consent form must be used. . . . For participants in research projects who are asked to consent or decline to give permission for use of their tissues in future research projects, the range of consents identified in Recommendation 9 can be provided. . . . As for the specific language of the prospective research use, a complicated document will raise unnecessary concerns and would, I predict, lead to a significant decrease in the availability of such materials. . . . Any general consent would be reviewed when future research projects are undertaken: 1) to assess whether the consent is appropriate in view of the particular research project to be undertaken; 2) the practicability of contacting the tissue donor for updating that consent; and 3) designing the project to strengthen confidentiality and/or to ensure anonymity. Without a general consent option, I am concerned that consent forms in the clinical setting will become too complicated and patients will be overly concerned and opt not to sign. Even when the research will be minimal risk and not require informed consent, such biological materials will be forever lost to research. (65)

The second NBAC bioethics event pertains more to the scientific and economic culture in which such future-oriented research enterprises are located. In one of the NBAC's public meetings, bioethicist Jeffrey Kahn (whom we last saw channeled through CNN in "DistanceXComplicity") spoke about informed consent and the changes in the biomedical research environment since the days of the Belmont Report, which codified many consent processes and principles in the 1970s. Kahn spoke about a wide range of issues, including the change in social expectations in the United States, whereby clinical trials for experimental drugs or treatments had gone from being viewed with suspicion to being sought out as the "best" medical care available. His presentation left Stanford geneticist David Cox with two questions.

First, asked Cox, "why do you think it is that we have switched in this format from protecting people to everyone clamoring for the benefits? Where are those benefits and why has that come about? I have my own views but I would be very interested in yours." The second related question, Cox continued, was "if this is more in the context of explaining to people that they are partaking in a risky situation, [and] I actually think that that is exactly what the process is about, then why would anybody want to do it?"[8]

Kahn's answer was couched in terms of historical and social complexity: the 1980s and 1990s gave us a "mixed up" "cocktail" of AIDS activists demanding the reconfiguration of clinical trials and inclusion in them, women with breast cancer and other conditions similarly demanding greater attention to and direct involvement in research on women's health issues, and other large-scale changes in the culture of biomedical research. Having now collectively downed that cocktail, we have the "sort of sense that, you know, there are real benefits to be had in research and that is part of why it makes sense to be a research participant, rightly or wrongly" (276). Experimental biomedical research and its speculative treatments had become not only a normal part of the health care system, but a normal expectation.

Cox agreed with Kahn's narrative and analysis, but then added some of his own views. The geneticist Cox knew his own culture better than the bioethicist Kahn, or simply felt more at liberty to critique it in public:

I would have added one other thing: I think over the past 10 years the research community has become extremely adept at their own public relations . . . to the point where even they believe it. . . . And there is some truth to it but not on the time scale that it is represented. So it is long-term gains, not short-term gains. It is like the stock market. We should have some stock people actually doing this for us so that—so I really think that things have changed in my view. I think you are right but not because the process of consent has changed but because the players have changed and gotten—have changed sort of what the game is to get people to enroll. (277)

Scientists like David Cox can help all of us read the margins of organisms, of research communities, and of stock markets. He tells a brief story about indirect links, feedback loops, partial or emergent truths, compelling PR, and other nonlinearities that give rise to raised expectations among all participants in the game—the people taking drugs, the researchers that develop drugs, the people who invest in the corporations that make drugs. That's the game of promising genomics.

XX

The negotiations between deCODE and the Icelandic Medical Association never did become "positive," nor "productive." After the talks were broken off in August 2000, the chair of the IMA and Kári had two meetings; at the second of these, in early October, Kári was to have come with a proposal for how to handle the data in the Health Sector Database. He had none, but appears to have said he would provide it the next day. October went by: no proposal. November passed too: no proposal.

Finally, in December, the chair of the IMA wrote an impatient e-mail to the IMA board, copying it to the director general of public health (the official in charge of, among other things, the opt-out process). As the chairman of the IMA reported in a later letter to all IMA members,

Among other things [the chairman] wrote that it appeared that ÍE [deCODE] was in the thick of arranging contracts with the first health care institutions [for the acquisition of medical records] without regard for the talks with the IMA and without any assumption that the contracts might be conditional on the conclusions of those talks. It was, [the chairman] said, completely unnatural to sign agreements with health care institutions for the transfer of data from medical records, while talks were going on concerning the fundamental principles on which the transfer would depend. [The chairman] expressed the view that these developments could only harm the mutual trust that had been present in the talks in spite of disagreements.

Unexpectedly Kristján Erlendsson, an employee of ÍE, contacted the IMA the next day and suggested that talks should be resumed as soon as possible. On the 12th December the IMA received a letter from the head of ÍE, who announced that he [Kári] would not take part himself in the talks but had entrusted Kristján and professor Einar Stefánsson, who had also joined the staff of ÍE, with the negotiations. Two days previously Kári had spoken in a television programme in such a manner that we could be in no doubt about his real attitude to the talks. He had said that the IMA was formally not a party to negotiations, that it was good for one's image to be involved in these talks but it did not serve the interests of the IMA to reach an agreement.[9]

The letter discussed how Kári had then gone to the Icelandic media, telling the newspaper *Dagur* that "the ethics committee of the IMA considered a formal complaint against me because of some remarks that I made in a private conversation with someone from the IMA before some meeting or other that was held in March. It's frightfully hard to pursue reconciliation when the other party is so insincere that the talks lead to formal complaints. I have therefore felt forced to hold back somewhat from these talks and that is one reason why things have progressed so slowly."

The coyly characterized "someone from the IMA" was in fact the chairman, Sigurbjörn Sveinsson, who responded in the IMA's letter to all its members:

The head of ÍE is perfectly aware that the chairman of the IMA took a considerable personal risk in order to make the situation more bearable for the former in the light of the matter previously mentioned by him. The matter was not once mentioned as an obstacle to agreement and even less so as a reason for excessive delays from ÍE time and again. . . .

In the light of these events and other happenings in dealings with ÍE the chairman decided to cancel the talks due on 8th January and put the matter before the board for further consideration.

It is the opinion of the board that the basis for further talks is very weak and trust between the parties little if not in pieces. The agreement, that was their goal, would require complete mutual trust between the IMA and ÍE, since no individual or social institution is in the legal position to be able to oversee it or to ensure that it works. That trust unfortunately is not to be found. That is why the talks have ended.

The letter concluded on a stirring note: "It is natural and indeed most important that doctors make their opinions known in spite of those contracts that the health care institutions where they work might enter into. It is our social duty. If the administrators of health care institutions spurn our opinions under cover of the law, so be it. They will have to bear the consequences. Doctors will not be forced to participate in this regrettable act."

And there things stood: deCODE continued to make contracts with Icelandic hospitals and health organizations, presuming that "presumed consent" would be the basis for the Health Sector Database that was still, presumably, to be built. But all the while, a case was making its way through the Icelandic courts.

In one of its filings with the U.S. Securities and Exchange Commission, deCODE disclosed the following as one of the "risk factors" to its business plan:

CERTAIN PARTIES HAVE ANNOUNCED AN INTENTION TO INSTITUTE LITIGATION TESTING THE CONSTITUTIONALITY OF THE ACT

In February 2000, an organization known as The Association of Icelanders for Ethics in Science and Medicine, or Mannvernd, and a group of physicians and other citizens issued a press release announcing their intention to file lawsuits against the State of Iceland and any other relevant parties, including deCODE, to test the constitutionality of the Act. According to the press release, the intended lawsuit will allege that the Act and the IHD license involve human rights violations and will challenge the validity of provisions of the Act which allow the use of presumed consent for the processing of health data into the IHD and the grant of a license to operate a single database. deCODE believes that any such litigation would be without merit and intends to defend vigorously any such action in which we become a party. However, in the event that the Icelandic State by a final judgment is found to be liable or subject to payment to any third party as a result of the passage of legislation on the IHD and/or the issuance of the IHD license, our agreement with the Ministry requires us to indemnify the Icelandic State against all damages and costs incurred in connection with such litigation. In addition, the pendency of such litigation could lead to delay in the development of the IHD and the DCDP, and an unfavorable outcome would prevent us from developing and operating the IHD and the DCDP. This would have a material adverse effect on our business and financial condition.[10]

In April 2001, Ragnhildur Gudmundsdóttir sued the director general of public health in the Reykjavík District Court. Since Ragnhildur was a minor, the suit was formally brought by her mother, Birna Thórdardóttir, a tough-as-nails longtime activist (she took part in some of the anti-NATO demonstrations in the 1960s) and general thorn-in-the-side of the Icelandic state. Ragnar Adalsteinsson represented their case.

Ragnhildur's father, Gudmundur Ingólfsson, had died in 1991. Despite being dead for seven years, he was presumed to have consented to have his medical records placed in the database when the HSD Act passed in 1998. Since she had inherited half of his DNA, Ragnhildur requested that the director general of public health not transfer Gudmundur's medical records to the HSD. The director general refused her request, referring to wording in the HSD Act that there was "no provision for an individual to refuse to permit the transfer to the database of information about his/her deceased parents." So Ragnhildur was suing.

The case was soon dismissed. Ragnhildur appealed to the Icelandic Supreme Court. In November 2001, the Supreme Court reversed the lower court's verdict and ruled that the case should be heard, and the case proceeded in district court. In February 2002, the district court denied Ragnhildur's request that expert witnesses be allowed to testify:

The plaintiff (RG) asked that she be allowed to call expert witnesses in the field of computer science for reporting and answering questions and arguing that it can be shown that the health information that will be transferred to the health sector database will be personally identifiable. That this is especially relevant given the fact the Act allows for the interconnection of the health sector database with a database on genealogical data and a database on genetic data. The ruling states that since the prospective expert witnesses have not personally witnessed anything about the database they cannot be called as witnesses.[11]

This decision was appealed to the Supreme Court as well, but the higher court agreed with the decision. Ragnhildur would not be permitted to use computer scientists as expert witnesses; her attorney could present only oral arguments. On March 6, the district court ruled against Ragnhildur, contending that the information about her father that would be transferred to the HSD was not "personally identifiable" in a legal sense. This verdict, too, was appealed to the Icelandic Supreme Court, which finally handed down its ruling on November 27, 2003. Here are the two key paragraphs in the ten-page ruling:

Extensive information is entered into medical records on people's health, their medical treatment, lifestyles, social circumstances, employment and family. They contain, moreover, a detailed identification of the person that the information concerns. Information of this kind can relate to some of the most intimately private affairs of the person concerned, irrespective of whether the information can be seen as derogatory for the person or not. *It is unequivocal that the provisions of Paragraph 1 of Article 71 of the Constitution apply to information of this kind and that they guarantee protection of privacy in this respect* [emphasis added]. To ensure this privacy the legislature must ensure, *inter alia,* that legislation does not result in any actual risk of information of this kind involving the private affairs of identified persons falling into the hands of parties who do not have any legitimate right of access to such information, irrespective of whether the parties in question are other individuals or governmental authorities.

Article 7 of Act No. 139/1998 [the HSD Act] opens the possibility of a private entity, who is neither a medical institution nor a self-employed health service worker, obtaining information from medical records without the explicit consent of the person whom the information concerns. . . . The District Court . . . concluded that the so-called one-way encryption discussed in Item 5 of Article 3 of Act No. 139/1998, could be carried out so securely as to render it virtually impossible to read the encrypted information. . . . The annex to the operating licence issued to Íslensk erfdagreining ehf., mentioned earlier, which concerns the transfer of information to the Health Sector Database, appears to imply that only the identity number of the patient will be encrypted in the database and that the name, both of the patient and his family, together with the precise address will be omitted. It is obvious that information on these items is not the only information appearing in the medical records which could unequivocally identify the individual in question. In this regard, information concerning the age of a person, municipality of residence, marital status, education and profession, together with the specification of a particular disease, either all together or individually, might suffice. The law does not preclude the transfer of detailed information concerning these items into the Health Sector Database.[12]

In short, while one-way encryption might indeed work for an identity number, it was clear that much more information would be going into the database, information that collectively made a person identifiable. And as the decision went on to state, no one had ever clarified what kinds of information would be entered:

The provisions of Article 10 of Act 139/1998 discussed earlier do not specify what information from the medical records involving the personal identifiers of a patients which could be transferred into the Health Sector Database might be seen by a person receiving a response to a query submitted to the database. Nor are there any indications what overall picture could be gained in this respect from the connection of information from the Health Sector Database with databases containing genealogical information and genetic information, as discussed in the provisions. Instead, it is merely provided that steps should be taken in the processing of information to preclude linking of the information with identifiable individuals. . . . As mentioned earlier, no further plans are available concerning the actual implementation of this in the operation of the Health Sector Database.

Individual provisions in Act No. 139/1998 refer repeatedly to the fact that health information in the Health Sector Database should be non-personally identifiable. In light of the rules discussed above concerning the issues addressed in Articles 7 and 10 of the Act, however, the achievement of this stated objective is far from being adequately ensured by the provisions of statutory law.

At this point in the argument, one might think that deCODE's legal department or the director general of public health would simply start gearing up to write stricter, more explicit data guidelines. But this is where the Icelandic Supreme Court made it plain that it considered the problem not a regulatory one, requiring clearer standards and mechanisms, but a constitutional one:

Owing to the obligations imposed on the legislature by Paragraph 1 of Article 71 of the Constitution to ensure protection of privacy, as outlined above, this assurance cannot be replaced by various forms of monitoring of the creation and operation of the Health Sector Database, monitoring which is entrusted to public agencies and committees without definite statutory norms on which to base their work. Nor is it sufficient in this respect to leave it in the hands of the Minister [of Health] to establish conditions in the operating licence or appoint other holders of official authority to establish or approve rules of procedure concerning these matters, which at all levels could be subject to changes within the vague limits set by the provisions of Act No. 139/1998.

It was only left to gather all these arguments and verdicts into one summary statement: "Based on the above, it is impossible to maintain that the provisions of Act No. 139/1998 will adequately ensure, in fulfilment of the requirements deriving from Paragraph 1 of Article 71 of the Constitution, attainment of the objective of the Act of preventing health information in the database from being traceable to individuals."

Not only did Ragnhildur win her right to prohibit the transfer of her dead father's medical records to the proposed HSD, not only was she awarded 1.5 million krónur in court costs, but the HSD Act of 1998 was actually ruled unconstitutional.

Coverage of the verdict in *Nature* noted that the HSD had been "quietly put on ice in 2002 after the company was unable to reach agreements with regulators about what information the database would contain or with hospitals about who would pay for it." The article nevertheless quoted Kári as saying that deCODE was "still working with the government to put together the database," and the Ministry of Health insisted that the verdict did not invalidate the 1998 law: "The first issue for the government is to find a way to resolve the discussions according to what the law allows, and to everyone's satisfaction." So *Nature* rather optimistically characterized the HSD as "shelved." But for its final word, *Na-*

ture quoted "long-term critic Skúli Sigurdsson, a science historian affiliated to the University of Iceland, [who] predicts that the project will not
happen 'given the complexity of data mining and personal privacy issues,
and the tremendous inertia of health politics.'"[13]

XX

Just after the Icelandic Supreme Court verdict, in the waning winter days
of 2003, through those strange chiasmic ties described in an earlier chapter, Keiko was shelved too—or as most people would say, was dead. Keiko
had left his Westman Islands pen in the summer of 2002 and had followed
a fishing boat to Norway, the only nation to still hunt whales commercially—
an 870-mile journey that ended in Skålevikfjord.

Some local Norwegians were at first hostile, suggesting that the orca
be "put down"—orcas were, after all, as Susan Orlean put it so eloquently
in her *New Yorker* profile of Keiko, "blubbery fish-grinders that consume
commercial product by the ton."[14] The Norwegian Directorate of Fisheries made clear that killing the whale would not be an option. They hoped
he could be coaxed back to sea, but were preparing to relocate him to another fjörd if necessary.

Various Norwegian communities offered to give the celebrity whale a
home for the coming winter, although this hospitality was laced with the
knowledge that Keiko would be a boon for tourism. Keiko eventually
ended up in Taknes Bay, avoiding a bid by the Miami Seaquarium to "rescue" him from the wild.

But in December 2003, just two weeks after the Icelandic Supreme
Court decided that the HSD legislation was unconstitutional, Keiko was
dead as well, having succumbed to pneumonia there in Norway's Taknes
Bay. "Normal practice is to sink dead sea mammals in open sea," commented Olav Levke of Norway's Fiskeridirektoratet, the fishing regulatory agency, "but this is a special situation." The Free Willy–Keiko Foundation had pleaded with the agency to allow this named, celebrity dead
sea mammal to be buried; the Fiskeridirektoratet "evaluated several alternatives," Levke said, "but [we] agreed that this was the best thing to
do under the circumstances." For three hours in a heavy snowstorm, trac-
tors dug a thirty-foot-long, fifteen-foot-deep trench and buried Keiko—
"during the night," noted the local newspaper, "to keep it as private an
affair as possible."[15]

GenomicsXSlot Machines

"We as a community suffer from . . . political and commercial and scientific hype," mourned William Haseltine, CEO of Human Genome Sciences Inc., one of the earliest, largest, most successful, and most hyped genomic companies that lava-lamped their way into the U.S. bio-economy landscape in the 1990s. Haseltine—print media sources sometimes give "dazzle gene" as a pronunciation cue for their readers—was the keynote speaker at the World Genomics Symposium in September 2002, held that year in the Atlantic City Convention Center. At the conference Haseltine suggested that "the general perception is that the promises of genomics have largely been much greater than [the] reality" of genomics—an "understandable" perception, he admitted, although certainly not one he shared. And as a result of that perception, the "community" was now suffering on the dismal financial planes of the new millennium—venture capital dried up, investors disgruntled and impatient, the wave of alliances with Big Pharma crested.[1]

Haseltine seemed happy to lay a good deal of the blame on the leadership of the "public" Human Genome Project, who had prematurely announced "completion" and, worse, through "a series of long-term miscalculations," had misunderstood the needs of the pharmaceutical industry. The HGP had overemphasized and overproduced what Haseltine called "genetic genomics," privileging the reference sequence for the human genome, and had relied too heavily on using that sequence to isolate potential drug targets. That approach might be fine for "populations where there is a clear lineage"—Estonia was the example Haseltine used, but Iceland would have served just as well—but more "outbred" populations required what he called "expression genomics." Even so, the practical applications of understanding how all the genes in an individual's genome are expressed under various conditions were, Haseltine soberly concluded, "quite distant." Murmurs of begrudging agreement were reportedly heard throughout the convention hall.

"After hearing that dismal forecast," the reporter for Genome Web News concluded, "who could be blamed for skipping the rest of the conference to try his luck instead at the slot machines?"[2]

XX

When you play the slot machines in Atlantic City, you know that despite it being a game of chance, the game nevertheless has a well-defined structure: in the long run, the house always wins. But the gambler isn't playing a run anywhere near that long; luck and success can only be associated with a different speed. While investing in genomics isn't exactly parallel, since you always have the option of "going short" or "going long," in general, the house will have a structural advantage.

Mannvernd members were relentless in their careful efforts to understand the political-economic structures that deCODE helped build and operated within, an effort with which, as discussed in "PromiseXDisclosure," I was complicit. The disclosure requirements of the U.S. Securities and Exchange Commission and other market-regulating bodies are far from perfect—indeed, nowhere near perfectible, given the necessarily chiasmic relationship between disclosure and promise. But again, just as one can learn about intellectual property disputes and the events behind them from reading SEC documents, so one can glimpse how the sale of different kinds of deCODE shares, through different institutional machineries, resulted in flows of both cash and political power along definable channels—slots, if you will.

We return to 1999. The Health Sector Database legislation was passed by Iceland's majority conservative coalition in late 1998. The $200 million promise from Roche has been sworn, but is far from being in the bank. (Indeed, as later SEC filings by deCODE show, Roche paid only $74 million on this promise: $56 million in operating expenses, plus a very few "milestone payments" totaling $18 million.)[3] DeCODE's initial public offering on NASDAQ had not even been mentioned. Like all biotech startups with a high "burn rate" (in the neighborhood of $2 million per month), deCODE needed some cash. Where to get it? On the "gray market."

When I first heard people in Iceland talking about the "gray market," I was puzzled. I knew what a black market was, and I knew what a market was, but I had never thought about it as a "white market"—but then, as we've learned from critical race theorists, that's how "white" operates: by not needing to be explicitly stated as the "norm." But the gray market was a new one on me.

Leaving the gray market in a gray area for the moment, let's allow deCODE to disclose the basic elements of the story: "There is no public market for the Preferred Stock although some banking institutions in Iceland have been making a market for privately negotiated transactions among non-U.S. persons in the Series B preferred stock. Our stock transfer records indicate that approximately 10 million shares of Series B preferred stock were transferred during 1999 in approximately 7,000 transactions and approximately 1.1 million shares of Series B preferred stock were transferred during January 2000 in approximately 2,700 transactions. The majority of these transactions had an Icelandic financial institution as one of the counterparties."[4]

So in 1999, somewhere in the neighborhood of several thousand Icelanders bought ten million shares in their nation's darling company, mostly through some "Icelandic financial institution." (The SEC cared only that these investors were "non-U.S. persons," because a U.S. person would have to wait until the company had disclosed further business information for it to register its stock for sale through U.S. markets.) A total of $69,750,000 flowed from the bank accounts of Icelanders to the bank account of deCODE, the SEC documents show.

You might assume that the Icelandic financial institutions bought Series B shares from deCODE. Reasonable, but wrong. We must do our due diligence. Icelandic banks bought their shares from Biotek Invest SA. The "SA" stands for Societé Anonyme; it's a company in Luxembourg and, true to its name, that's pretty much all we know about it. It came into legal existence on June 29, 1999. On June 30, 1999, deCODE ("the Company") agreed to sell five million shares of Series B stock to Biotek Invest SA. ("the Purchaser"). DeCODE's subsequent March 2000 registration statement with the SEC provides the details:

A. On June 30, 1999 the Company and the Purchaser entered into a Stock Purchase Agreement pursuant to which the Purchaser agreed to purchase from the Company 5,000,000 shares (the "Series B Shares") of the Company's Series B Preferred Stock (the "Series B") at a price (the "Original Purchase Price") of US$7.50 per share.

B. Contemporaneously with the execution of the Stock Purchase Agreement, the Company and the Purchaser entered into an oral agreement pursuant to which they agreed that the Original Purchase Price would be increased to $15.00 per share (the "Adjusted Purchase Price"), with the amount in excess of the Original Purchase Price (the "Contingent Payment") to be payable only if the Purchaser were able to sell at least 50% of the Series B Shares at or above the Adjusted Purchase Price and if the trading price in the Icelandic market, as determined by agreement of the parties, remained at or above the Adjusted Purchase Price from the time of such resale to the end of 1999.

C. The Company and the Purchaser further agreed that if the Contingent Payment became payable, the Company would pay the Purchaser a commission of 7% on the aggregate Adjusted Purchase Price and the Purchaser would pay the Company interest at the rate of 6% per annum on the Contingent Payment from the date of closing of the transaction under the Stock Purchase Agreement (the "Closing Date"), to the date of payment of the Contingent Payment.

D. On August 8, 1999, the Closing Date, the Purchaser advised the Company that it had arranged for the sale of at least 50% of the Series B Shares at a price of $15.00.

E. On December 28, 1999, the Company and the Purchaser agreed that the trading price in the Icelandic market had remained at or above the Adjusted Purchase Price from August 8, 1999 through December 28, 1999 and that the Purchaser would pay the Contingent Payment plus interest but net of commission, on or before February 25, 2000.[5]

In other words, a day after the Luxembourg company was incorporated, deCODE sold it five million shares of Series B stock at $7.50 per share; at the same time, an "oral agreement"—while deCODE, like any U.S. corporation, is legally a person, one wonders what mouth it employs to make these kinds of spoken promises—was made that deCODE would be paid twice that amount if two conditions were met: the Luxembourg company had to sell at least half of the shares at $15, and the price in "the Icelandic market" could not go below $15 for the six months remaining in 1999.

These two conditions were not only met, they were exceeded: when I was in Iceland on January 13, 2001, the 6:00 P.M. radio news broadcast reported that six thousand Icelanders had bought stock in deCODE at prices between $30 and $65 per share on "the Icelandic market" before deCODE's July 2000 IPO. By comparison, at deCODE's IPO on NASDAQ in July 2000, the share price opened at $18, bubbled briefly to $27, and has never reached the opening price again.

XX

So what is a gray market? My advance man thought the best person to ask was Finnur Sveinbjörnsson, who in 2001 was president of the Icelandic Stock Exchange (ICEX). Trained as an economist, Finnur had worked for the Central Bank of Iceland early in his career, then for the Ministry of Commerce on issues related to the European Economic Area, and from 1995 to 2000 worked for the Bankers Association, a lobbyist organization. Those were years in which "the securities market changed quite a bit," he told me. "The securities departments in banks have grown tremendously, mostly because of the abolishing of foreign exchange controls, which meant that there was interest in foreign securities, and the banks responded. Also because there was appetite for corporate and local government bonds, and these entities responded by switching some of their financing away from traditional bank loans to the bond market. Furthermore many investors suddenly realized that there were more possibilities than just opening a savings account. They could invest in securities, both bonds and stocks, and get much nicer returns than previously. So there was basically an explosion, from both the supply and the demand side in the securities market."

There was also more money to invest. "Many individuals have become rich in this country," said Finnur. "The main source of wealth has been the quota system in fishing. There are a number of individuals who have sold their quotas and left this business, so they have gotten out of this business, and suddenly found themselves with considerable amounts of money in their hands. This money has to a large extent gone into the securities market. Furthermore, some of this increased activity has been financed through foreign money—money borrowed by Icelandic banks from overseas and lent to their local customers. Some individuals have borrowed and used the proceeds to speculate in the market."

So the broader Icelandic financial landscape was changing rapidly in the period before and during the deCODE years, and one feature of this new landscape was a more vibrant gray market. To understand what the Icelandic gray market was, Finnur explained to me, "it's probably best to look at a highly developed financial market like the U.S. for comparison. If companies in the U.S. want to raise money from the public, they must register with the SEC, and in order to do that, they must file a prospectus. So they must make certain information available to the public, about themselves and about the securities, including the main risk factors. Prior to this stage, they usually obtain funds from professional investors, sometimes through several rounds of financing prior to the IPO. And there are restrictions on the transferability of shares: if you raise money by selling shares to professional investors, such as venture capitalists, they cannot then turn around and sell shares to the public."

In Iceland, this was different. "There was an unclear, or gray, provision in the securities legislation," Finnur explained. "Apparently the legislation did not prevent professional investors from selling shares to the public without having to fulfill the stringent requirements of a public offering, as long as prospective buyers came to the investors asking for the shares—that is, active promotion and selling was clearly out of bounds but responding passively to demands was within limits." While the Icelandic financial institutions and professional investors that sold the shares to six thousand Icelanders may not have taken out ads in the newspapers, they did talk actively to journalists and played, like their foreign counterparts, a part in the securities hype of the late 1990s.

The number of shares bought by Icelanders was very high in the eyes of the Icelandic financial authorities, especially for securities so widely acknowledged as risky and requiring long-term financial strength to withstand likely losses. "The problem of the gray market was discussed thoroughly last winter and into the spring [1999–2000]," continued Finnur, "in a committee that the Ministry of Commerce set up with representatives from the market, from the stock exchange, from the ministry itself. This committee reviewed the legislation in our neighboring countries, and in the U.S., and came up with recommendations that were enacted by Althingi in the fall of 2000, thereby closing the legislative loophole that had allowed the gray market to develop."

With this explanation in mind, we can see more precisely the mechanisms behind deCODE's stock speculation: In a decidedly nonrisky deal, deCODE sold shares to a Luxembourg company with a sweetheart arrangement, promised orally, that if the share price stayed high, Biotek Invest SA would get a 7 percent commission. Biotek Invest sold the shares to Icelandic banks and securities companies, presumably for what is known as "a tidy profit." The Icelandic financial institutions, empowered through an "interpretation" of existing law—interpretation is never far from speculation—sold the shares to Icelanders eager to invest in "an Icelandic company" that they were told was uniquely positioned to understand and perhaps cure genetic diseases—a story told by Icelandic journalists with the encouragement of the Icelandic financial institutions, in newspaper stories and electronic media that would later be cited by anthropologists, bioethicists, and assorted others as evidence of a "democratic discussion." And the financial risks accrued at the bottom of this speculative chain, where six thousand Icelanders had their hands on a genomic slot-machine handle that they paid up to $65 to pull. The house wins again.

And Biotek Invest SA? It was liquidated in December 2000, having existed for barely a year and a half; assets of $5.25 million were transferred to an equally anonymous company called Damato Enterpises Inc. in Panama City, Panama. After the Luxembourg legal notices documenting this baroque story of globalization began coming to light in 2003, the Icelandic newspaper *DV* ran a headline on February 5, 2004, in huge, solid capital letters: "HVER FÉKK 400 MILLJÓNIRNAR FRÁ DECODE?" ("Who Received the 400 Million Krónur from deCODE?"). A small picture of Kári, rubbing his chin thoughtfully, had been inserted next to the question mark. Kári never responded.[6]

XX

"I'd never bought stocks before," Henrik Jónsson told James Meek, a reporter for the U.K. newspaper the *Guardian*. "I watched the TV news carefully and saw the stock prices rising consistently. You had stories in the media telling people how high Decode stocks were rising. My heart is crying."[7] Henrik had bought five million krónur worth of deCODE stock at $56 per share in the spring of 2000. Disabled in a traffic accident, Henrik invested nearly a quarter of the financial settlement he had fought to obtain from the insurance companies. The shares were selling at $6 when he returned to the National Bank of Iceland in 2002 to sell the shares they had sold him.

Meek collected numerous such stories when he was in Iceland in the fall of 2002. Perhaps the worst was that of the anonymous E., who had also bought in at the height of the exuberance in the spring of 2000, plunking down thirty million krónur—about $400,000—over three separate occasions. Some of the money he borrowed from the state-owned National Bank, from which he also bought the shares; in that case, E. mortgaged his house. He agreed to buy more from the Agricultural Bank and arranged another loan with the Bank of Iceland. A day later, the Bank of Iceland cancelled all its loans to buy shares, but the Agricultural Bank would not let E. off the hook. He spent the next month trying to arrange other financing, during which time the share price fell from $64 to $50, but the bank insisted he still pay $64. Meanwhile, the National Bank moved to foreclose on its loan. "I asked them if I could wait at least until the shares rose to $15. The lawyer from the bank said, 'You must know these shares won't go up.' I said, 'You sold me these shares, telling me they would go up to $100.' He said, 'If you're going to blame us you'd better pay up.'"

Meek also met with Kári while he was in Iceland and related some of these stories. "To come to the management of a company like ours and try to hold us responsible for the way in which shares have been traded in Iceland is somewhere between laughable and ridiculous," Kári told him:

We are not in the business of selling shares. We did not create a grey market in Iceland. We were not the ones who decided how this would be done. We sold a significant number of shares on the grey market because there was pressure on us to do that. There were people, politicians even, representing the left, who insisted we would have to sell shares in Iceland because they expected there would be great profits and they wanted Icelanders to share in that. All of a sudden the financial market turned sour.

I always insisted, when asked, that I would not comment on the wisdom of buying shares or the value of shares, and I always said people should not buy unless they had the backbone to suffer some losses.

Though I have been selective in quoting from deCODE's 200-plus-page SEC filing detailing the arrangement for the gray market shares, I assure you that I would have quoted, had it been in the filing, any statement like, "DeCODE ('the Seller') regrets having to make this lucrative arrangement with a Luxembourg company created just for this purpose of selling shares to the Icelandic banks, but we were pressured to do so by Icelandic leftists."

Icelandic Supreme Court attorney Hróbjartur Jónatansson offers what he says is a common-sense analysis of the Series B share selling, which Kári would no doubt dismiss as "a matter of speculation":

Without the Database Act the prospects for deCODE's future would be seriously jeopardized. The price of deCODE's stock has steadily increased since the enactment of the database bill. DeCODE's class B stock originally sold for five U.S. dollars per share. In March of 1999, however, deCODE stock sold for twenty-four U.S. dollars per share on the Icelandic stock market. Whether the decision to sell all of the stocks to domestic investors was a calculated move to gain a further endorsement for the proposed Database Bill, or whether deCODE just used the stock offering to raise capital for deCODE's operations is a matter of speculation. However, common sense suggests that the domestic investors concerned have definitely promoted the Bill with a view to giving their investment great value.[8]

Imagined statements and dissimulated shock aside, Icelanders appeared to have gotten the message of such promotion. "To financially untutored Icelanders," Meek wrote in the *Guardian*, "every TV appearance in which Stefánsson and his allies in government talked up the wonderful opportunities Iceland's genetic specialness presented was both reason to offer their blood for analysis and reason to dig into their pockets." Or as one television news figure told Meek, casting "leftists" in a slightly different role: "Ministers were showing up with Stefánsson whenever they had the chance. He was always in the company of the government elite. Of course, everyone got the impression this was foolproof. There were only a handful of left wing politicians shouting that something was wrong . . . at that time he had absolute control of the media."

The undersigned is usually skeptical about claims concerning the "absolute control of the media." But I swear, more than three of the Icelandic print and radio journalists I spoke with during the course of my research told me of their stories being killed or their jobs being threatened after a phone call from Kári to their supervisors. More than three of the U.S.-based journalists (as well as a bioethicist or two) with whom I have spoken told similar tales involving screaming and legal threats. But Meek is one of the only people to actually write about Kári's volatility. "Kári Stefánsson is an unusual man," he wrote. "He fits the cliché of being fiercely clever but he also has a tendency to lash out for no apparent reason, even at those who praise his firm. Three times in our difficult first interview in Reykjavík I try to quote to him people who have spoken well of Decode, only for him to interrupt and dismiss them all." Two days later, Meek returned for a second interview. Kári "apologise[d] for his temper the first time around, but still can't quite keep the lid on it." When Meek suggested "that the public sequencing had not cost $4bn, as he said, and that many scientists thought Craig Venter would not have reached his goal without using data from the public project, he explodes. 'I don't understand why I'm wasting my time talking to you when you haven't done your homework,' he says."

Meek is also one of the few reporters to reflect carefully on the media depictions of deCODE. "In Decode's heyday, journalists often described him [Kári] as resembling a Viking, as if that was understood to be a good thing," he observed, and then disarmed the trope by affirming it: "If a Viking is a brooding, grey-haired, 6ft 5in man with a nasty temper who wears tight T-shirts over a heavily muscled upper body, Stefánsson is a Viking."

XX

In December 2001, a class-action suit was brought against deCODE Genetics by the law firm of Milberg Weiss. This was hardly unusual at the time; over a thousand such securities fraud class-action suits were filed in the U.S. District Court of southern New York alone (where this particular suit was filed) in the wake of the market's collapse that year. Milberg Weiss, a law firm described as "dominat[ing] its field [securities class-action suits] to a degree that no private firm does in any other kind of litigation," accounted for a large number of these.[9] A cofounder of Milberg Weiss, William Lerach, would later bring a case against Enron. Lerach was among those who convinced President Clinton to veto the Private Securities Litigation Reform Act of 1995, a veto overturned by the Republican-controlled Congress. Indeed, according to one lawyer who lobbied for the PSLRA, "the whole idea behind the law was to destroy Lerach."

The complaint filed by Milberg Weiss was complex, but it centered on charges that deCODE and Kári Stefánsson, along with the co-lead underwriters of their IPO, Lehman Brothers and Morgan Stanley, had made "materially false and misleading statements" in their SEC prospectus and had "engaged in a pattern of conduct to surreptitiously extract inflated commissions" greater than the ones they had disclosed.[10] One mechanism by which this extraction occurred, claimed the suit, was that the "Underwriter Defendants agreed to allocate deCODE shares to those customers in the Offering in exchange for which the customers agreed to purchase additional deCODE shares in the aftermarket at pre-determined prices" (*Rubin v. deCODE*, 8).

Between January 1998 and December 2000, 460 "high technology and Internet-related companies" had come up for sale on the public markets; class-action suits against 309 of these, including deCODE, were consolidated for coordination and decision of pretrial motions and discovery, to be conducted by Judge Shira Scheindlin. The consolidated defendants, including Morgan Stanley, asked for dismissal of all the cases.

Judge Scheindlin's 238-page decision attempts to sort out the various complaints against the various underwriter defendants, deciding which complaints will be dismissed and on what grounds. The decision does not discuss the deCODE case directly, but the case is listed as one of those dismissed on the basis of "No Allegation of Motive" to violate Rule 10b-5, which prohibits market manipulation through devices such as tie-in agreements. In other words, even if Morgan Stanley and Lehman Brothers did use a tie-in agreement to require their customers to buy deCODE stock after the IPO, because no evidence was presented that they sold the stock after the IPO, the claim was dismissed. As Judge Scheindlin put it, "Mere ownership in the absence of profit-taking does not establish a motive that would support a 'strong inference that the defendant acted with the required state of mind.'"[11] Here again is a case in which intentionality, the ethical criteria based on what J. L. Austin called "an excess of profundity" (as discussed in "PromisesXPromises") in fact "paves the way for immorality"—or at least for getting out of court.

But the SEC can prevail where courts may not.[12] In a January 2005 settlement with the SEC, Morgan Stanley agreed to pay a $40 million civil penalty for "attempting to induce certain customers who received allocations of IPOs to place purchase orders for additional shares in the aftermarket." "These cases underscore the Commission's resolve," read the SEC's press release, "to ensure the integrity of IPO markets by prohibiting conduct that could artificially stimulate demand or higher prices in the aftermarket—whether or not there is manipulative effect."[13]

Some Morgan Stanley sales representatives referred to this practice, of their customers' buying in the immediate aftermarket, as fulfilling their "promises" or "commitments." In the action against Morgan Stanley, the SEC at one point used the deCODE case to illustrate how such promises took place: "In a third IPO, a sales representative e-mailed the syndicate manager, 'just for the record . . . despite a less than stellar allocation [a customer] was in buying decode in the aftermarket yesterday. As they said they would. Almost 200m at $28.' The syndicate manager responded, 'I am very aware of their aftermarket. Kudos to them and it will be remembered.'"[14]

XX

On March 25, 2004, Human Genome Sciences Inc.'s CEO William Haseltine pulled the arm of his genomic slot machine for the last time. Having "struggle[d] to successfully develop new drugs," HGSI announced that Haseltine was retiring from the company he had founded and that two hundred employees (20 percent of the company's employees) would be laid off. "It was believed that [genomic] research would lead to cures for all kinds of ailments," Reuters noted, "but the therapeutic solutions have proved to be slow going. While other companies have had sporadic breakthroughs, neither Celera nor Human Genome Sciences have successfully developed any of their own drugs so far."[15]

The lay-off trend had been growing by then for several years throughout the genomic sector. Incyte Pharmaceuticals had fired 400 people in November 2001. Craig Venter's Celera let 132 people go in April 2002. All told, the genomic sector downsized by more than 1,500 staff people between January 2001 and July 2002, and the industry began to reinvent (or just to *invent*) its strategy for making money through bioinformatics, whose promise had faded, or at least had receded to a more soberly regarded future.[16]

In September 2003 deCODE announced that Merck had made them a new promise: up to $90 million for deCODE's promising work on the genetics of obesity. DeCODE also announced, on the same day, that it would lay off two hundred employees to "accelerate the transition" to profitability. At least deCODE had managed to condense the doubled demands of reading the chiasmic future into one day's press releases.

The genomic economy was never again as ebullient as it was in this era of 1998–2001, an era that I have shamelessly punned, in an article on Venter's genomic company Celera, the Sell Era.[17] DeCODE, too, has been trying to reinvent itself in this changed economy—although its reinvention invites speculation that such revisioning was part of the plan all along. Recall from "SameXDifference" that in the 1995 letter from Kevin Kinsella of Sequana Therapeutics to Kári, Kinsella had talked of Iceland as "an ideal 'laboratory' for ongoing pharmacogenetic studies during clinical trials of new small molecule drugs."[18] Clinical trials are another hot spot of the biomedical research landscape, but one that is beyond the scope of this book.[19] But to cite one characterization of the situation that employs the language of promising in its necessary doublings: "Close to 80% of clinical trials fail to enroll the required number of patients in the time promised by investigators, and the problem promises only to get worse."[20] After many years in which Hoffmann-LaRoche was its only industry alliance, deCODE made alliances with Bayer, Vertex Pharmaceuticals, and Merck (which bought $10 million in deCODE stock) to run clinical trials using compounds developed by the pharmaceutical companies. Analysts at JPMorgan "estimate that clinical trials in Iceland could cost around a third ($3 million to $4.5 million) of those in the U.S."[21] These deals accompanied a rise in the value of deCODE shares, bringing them up from a low of $2 to the neighborhood of $8 in the spring of 2004.

And after years of producing almost no scientific publications of any kind, deCODE and its scientists can now point to a number of papers in respected journals, identifying a number of new genes involved in those monstrously complex conditions, type II diabetes, heart disease, and schizophrenia. A number of geneticists whose work and scientific opinions I respect have told me they believe these findings to be robust and as potentially significant as deCODE has said they are. You would not be wrong, scientifically or financially, to find the whole enterprise still promising.

EthicsXExpediency

In 1999, DeCODE printed a "code of ethics" in both Icelandic and English. It was written by "a group of deCODE employees," and the Ethics Institute of the University of Iceland is listed as "Advisors." No people are listed, just these collectivities. The twenty-page booklet with a heavy blue-paper cover was produced and mailed to the entire population Iceland, no small expense.

Skúli gave me the copy that came to his door. Its seven sections lay out a list of principles, numbered 1.5, 2.7, 3.3, and so on, creating an appearance of precision, order, and authority. It looks like a piece of legislation or some other legal document.

1.1 Objectivity and honesty are necessary ingredients of all research. No scientist will willingly distort the truth or present results in a manner likely to deceive.

1.4 No research on people or DNA samples from people will be conducted without a prior review of a Science Ethics Board.

2.5 If an employee inadvertently acquires knowledge about the identity of a participant in a research project he or she must remove the identity and maintain strict confidentiality. If needed, employees will remind their co-workers and collaborators of the rules and regulations that pertain to the handling of personal information at deCODE.

3.5 It is the goal of deCODE Genetics to attain amicable collaboration with healthcare providers in Iceland in order to promote research in biomedical sciences and to improve healthcare.

4.3 deCODE employees show prudence with regard to information about the company and its research projects and maintain confidentiality at all times.

6.1 Employees treat each other with respect and support one another profession-
ally. They discuss and critique each other's work freely, honestly, and constructively.

7.2 deCODE employees act responsibly when working with new chemicals, cell
lines or micro-organisms. They take special care in handling and disposing of waste
material.[1]

As is often the case with ethics, and particularly codes of ethical principles, there is not a single concrete noun in deCODE's principles that
signifies any specific historical, cultural, or institutional body or event;
there is only a homogeneous population of bland abstractions. Terms like
NASDAQ, European Data Protection Commission, Althingi, National
Bioethics Committee, Kári Stefánsson, cryopreservation unit, Health Sector Database, or Hoffmann-LaRoche are nowhere in the booklet. How
biosamples and bioinformation actually moves from person to clinic to
robotic assemblage to lab bench to database remains obscure. Anything
with a direct connection to actual events in and around Iceland, in other
words, is absent. The reader is dropped into a blank arctic whiteness—a
glacial ethics whose featurelessness offers no orientation.

Surely these Icelanders can come up with something a little more helpful?

XX

On one level, I sympathize with deCODE and the University of Iceland's
Ethics Institute: articulations of "ethics" will always begin inappropriately
and somewhat violently, and are never very satisfactory, because the word
"ethics" is catachrestic—an inappropriate name for an unnameable that
demands naming. Ethics is impossible, so even miserable failures should
not be scorned or ridiculed.

Such was my way of thinking when Skúli asked me to add a third public lecture, on ethics, to my September 1998 Icelandic publicity blitz—a
third lecture that, as fate would have it, Skúli had talked the University
of Iceland's Ethics Institute into sponsoring. I agreed to this out of obligation rather than enthusiasm. I agonized over it for weeks beforehand,
reading through countless articles and reports and books accumulated over
years of historical and ethnographic research on "the" ethical issues in genomics ("the" ethical issues being as accurate as saying "the" human
genome): informed consent, privacy of medical records and genetic tests,
patents and ownership, choice and autonomy, and so on. So much, so
urgent . . . so predictable, so numbing. Destined to failure anyway, I opted

for an experimental strategy built on what I would call "circumlocution-ary speech acts," an address styled to miss its mark.

Out of a combination of desperation and admiration, I decided to read to the Icelanders some literature by one of their own—from Halldór Lax-ness's *The Atom Station* that had enthralled me in the days before my first trip to Iceland. I read a section titled "Buying an Anemone" in a chapter named "Orgy." It must have taken fifteen minutes to get through the pas-sage, and I kept glancing up from the podium to see if the doctors and sci-entists and other Icelanders, many of whom I had been interviewing in previous days, were rummaging in their pockets for something to throw. Imagining the crowd's impatience, I kept trying to remind myself, *they're Icelanders, they've sat through far worse for far longer.* . . . I like to think it was worth it somehow—just as it's worth excerpting at length here.

The passage appears at the precise midpoint of the novel, and the middle—that interval between the proverbial rock and hard place—is al-ways the place of ethics. The chapter centers on a dialogue between Ugla, the "wise owl" from the north, and the organist, the bohemian-saint whom we last saw burning large sums of money.

The minister of Parliament and his wife have left town for a few days, leaving Ugla to watch after the three children, Arngrimur, Gudný, and Thordur. The kids, naturally, throw a party. Friends come, "the accepted ones and the secret ones," and then friends of the friends. A case of liquor arrives; later, platters of food. Valuable things are broken. There is jitter-bugging and singing, or rather a competition "to produce the weirdest sounds without words imaginable; never in my life had I heard in one single night such a medley of inarticulate human sounds. Then came the vomiting . . ." (Laxness clearly relishes reiterating and amplifying the highly dramatized vomit motif of the Icelandic sagas).[2]

Cleaning up the house the next day, Ugla is stopped and asked into conversation by Gudný, the fourteen-year-old girl who, in her cigarette-smoking, languid attitude of "infinite weariness," is "pure cinema." Gudný tells Ugla that she has been sleeping with "that damned Lingo," one of the boys at the party. Ugla is shocked and confused and feels somehow responsible. So she goes to the organist's house to ask him some ques-tions and get some ethical advice.

Buying an Anemone

"If everything starts tonight, the house filling up with people breaking still more crystal and vomiting on the carpets and ruining the veneer of the furniture, what am I to do? Call the police?"

"Why ask me, my dear?" said the organist.

"I don't know what to do," I said.

"In my house criminals and policemen sit at the same table," he said. "And sometimes clergymen too, what's more."

"It shocks me to see these drunken young devils," I said.

"Do not speak ill of the young in my hearing," he said, unaccountably switching to the formal mode of address, and completely serious. After a little thought he went on: "I imagined there was enough crystal in the world for those who read crystal. I for my own part take greater pleasure in a film of ice over a clear brook on an autumn morning."

"But what is one to do when those around one behave both wrongly and badly?" I asked.

"Behavioristically wrong?" he asked. "Biochemically badly?"

"Morally wrong and morally badly," I said.

"Morals do not enter into it," he said. "And there is no such thing as morality—only varyingly expedient conventions. What to one race is crime, is virtue to another; crime in one era is virtue in another; even a crime in one class of society is at the same time and in the same society virtue in another class. The Dobuans in Dobu have only one moral law, and that is to hate one another: hate one another in the same way that European nations used to do before the concept of nationalism became obsolete and east and West were substituted in its place. Amongst them, each individual is duty bound to hate the other as West is duty bound to hate East, amongst us. The only thing that saves the poor Dobuans is that they do not have such good weapons of destruction as Du Pont; nor Christianity, like the Pope."

"Are drunk as well as sober criminals to be allowed free rein, then?" I asked.

"We live in a rather inexpedient social system," he said. "The Dobuans are pretty close to us. But there is one consolation, and that is that man can never outgrow the necessity to live in an expedient social system. It makes no difference whether people are called good or bad; we are all here, now; there is only one world in existence, and in it there prevail either expedient or inexpedient conditions for those who are alive."

"Can I then come barging in here blind drunk and shoot your flowers?" I asked.

"Go ahead," he said, and laughed.

"Would that be right?" I asked.

"Alcohol produces certain chemical reactions in the living body and alters the functioning of the nervous system: you might fall downstairs. Jónas Hallgrímsson fell downstairs; some people think that thereby Iceland lost her finest poems—those which he had not yet composed."

"Of course he drank too much," I said.

"Do we think it makes much difference whether or not it was morally wrong of the man to take a drink so often? Perhaps he would not have fallen if he had only had ten drinks. Perhaps it was just the eleventh drink that felled him. Is it not just about as wrong morally to drink one drink too many as to remain out of doors for five minutes too long in the cold? For you might catch pneumonia. But both are inexpedient."

I went on contemplating this man.

"On the other hand it would deeply offend my aesthetic sense to see a beautiful north-country girl drunk," he added. "But aesthetics and morality have nothing in common: no one gets to heaven by being beautiful. The authors of the New Testament had no appreciation of beauty. On the other hand Mohammed said: 'If you have two farthings, buy yourself bread with the one and an anemone with the other.' Anyone is at liberty to break my crystal. And though my own rule is no drink, it is not a moral rule. On the other hand, I buy anemones."

After a moment's thought I began again: "Do you contend that it is right for a fourteen-year-old girl to shut herself in with a married man and perhaps come out again pregnant?"

He always gave a sort of titter when he thought something funny. "Did you say fourteen, my good girl?" he said. "Twice times seven: it is a downright twice-sacred number. But now I shall tell you about another creature that also counts in this case, except that it counts up to sixteen; it is a species of cactus that is said to grow in Spain. There the blessed plant stands, in those scorching Castilian uplands, and counts and counts with precision and care, yes, I am probably safe in saying with actual moral fervor, until sixteen years are up; and then blooms. Not until sixteen years have passed does it dare to bear this feeble red blossom which is dead tomorrow."

"Yes, but a child is a child," I said stubbornly; and to tell the truth I was becoming a little annoyed at having so frivolous an organist.

"Just so," he said. "A child is a child. And later the child stops being a child—without arithmetic. Nature asserts itself."

"I am from the country, and year-old ewe-lambs are never put to the ram."

"The lambs of year-old ewe-lambs are not usually much good for slaughtering," he said. "If mankind were reared for the slaughterhouse, to be sold by the pound, your point of view would be valid. It is a common saying in Iceland that the children of children are fortune's favorites."

"Is one then to believe every damned stupid proverb there is?" I said, and was now a little angry.

"Look at me," he said. "Here you see one of fortune's favorites."

It was the same as always: all conventional thinking turned into crude exaggeration, and universally-accepted notions into vulgarity, when one was talking to this man. My tongue tied itself in knots, for I felt that anything further I said in this direction was bound to cause him unpardonable offence—this man who had the clearest and most gentle eyes of any man.

"Was it wrong that I should come into being? That my mother should give birth to me the summer after she was confirmed?" he asked. "Was it bad? Was it wicked?"

Something flashed into my mind and I kept silent. He went on watching me. Did he expect me to reply? At last I said in a low voice, the only thing I could say: "You are so far ahead of me that you are almost out of sight; and I hear you as if on the long distance telephone from the other end of the country."

"She was a clergyman's daughter," he said. "Christianity has robbed her of all peace of soul. For these few decades of a whole lifetime she has lain awake most nights to beg forgiveness of the enemy of human life, the god of the Christians; until Nature now in her mercy has deprived her of memory. You may be thinking, perhaps, that those who believe in such a bad god must become bad themselves, but that is not so; man is more perfect than God. Although this woman's doctrine, in which she was brought up from childhood, told her that all men were lost sinners, I have never heard her censure any man with so much as half a word. All her life is symbolized on the only words which she knows in her dotage, when she has forgotten all other words: Please do; and, God bless you. I think she has been the poorest woman in Iceland; but nevertheless for half a century she has kept open house for all Iceland; and most especially for criminals and harlots."

I was silent for a long time, until I looked up at him and said, "Forgive me." And he patted me on the cheek and kissed me on the forehead.

"I am sure you understand now," he said with an apologetic smile, "why I am always stung if I hear views that reflect on my mother; and on me; on my existence as a living being." (105–9)

In this passage there is no easy appeal to either a stable nature or a stable culture. The metaphors never translate perfectly, and they sometimes contradict each other. Nature, culture, and the relationships between them are unsettled—ever-unstable equilibria, in François Jacob's terms—and that should be simultaneously risky, confounding, and exhilarating. If "nature asserts itself," as the organist says—biochemically, mathematically, sheepishly—so too does something called culture, and one is left with only a series of questions about how fourteen-year-old girls and year-old ewe lambs and Spanish cacti and a specific culture's sexual morals might be made to hang together. *Should* be made to hang together, but for the sake of "expediency."

Ugla arrives at no resolution, only a persistent return to questioning. The organist responds to Ugla's stubborn, pressing, practical questions obliquely, even frivolously, and who doesn't share Ugla's annoyance? This guy, this vehicle of the anthropologist's knowledge of other cultures that was spreading all over the immediate postwar world, is no help at all. He exaggerates, he vulgarizes, he ties her tongue in knots until there's only one thing she can say: you are far away, very distant . . . but I hear you, through the technological circuit. But maybe there's some excess value in the exchange itself, something that escapes the restricted economy of give and take.

How does one keep an open house? Does a nation that is an open house invite an American military base in? Or a giant multinational corporation, "your own" business founded by one of "your own" scientists, that wants to go fishing for promised disease genes and their promising therapies? How does one have an open house and still have a necessary measure of privacy? Where does the domestic end and the foreign begin? How does one treat strangers? And perhaps most importantly, what will be expedited, for whom, and with what effect?

If this seems like a funny way of talking about ethics, I won't argue with you. But I am confident that sending these few pages of Laxness's book to every Icelandic household in the nation (most of which have shelves already full of his work) would have been a far more interesting, entertaining, and productive use of money than sending deCODE's code.

XX

"Man is that animal species that rides a pony and has a God," Ugla's father tells her while she is home in the north, waiting to have her baby. Ugla asks him what God he is referring to. "To explain God would be to have no God, my little one," her father replies. So it's not a Lutheran God, Ugla surmises. No, her father answers, "we who work our farms up in the valleys of Iceland do not much care what Gods are thought up by Germans and preached with murder by Danes." Maybe he's talking about "the late Papal God," she continues. Better than the Lutheran one, but still no, her father replies. Is he then suggesting that the new church they are building (with funds from the Althingi, courtesy of the minister) be dedicated to Thor, Odin, and Frey? "Be blessed for naming them," Ugla's father responds, "but still it is not they." Bringing this little lesson in negative theology to its formal conclusion, her father finally announces: "Our god is that which is left when all Gods have been listed and marked No, not him, not him" (148–9).

There will be no grounding of an ethics in a god for Laxness, a convert to Catholicism who studied for the priesthood in the 1920s. Whatever ethics might be, it's far more associated with "nature" of "life" than with any of the gods nameable in language. Biochemistry has more to do with ethics, in Laxness's view, than any theological or even humanist exegesis. "There is only one world in existence," was the chord struck by the organist, "and in it there prevail either expedient or inexpedient conditions for those who are alive."

This elevation of "expediency" to a kind of ethical principle intrigued me, and it kept reoccurring in *The Atom Station,* often in tandem with biochemical references. Later in the novel, for example, Ugla asks her minister for a day-care center: "Why does Parliament and the Town Council not want my children to have a nursery like your children? Are my children not chemically and physiologically as good as your children? Why can we not have a society which is just as expedient for my children as it is for your children?" (139).[3]

"Expedient" is a concept full of folds. If the older senses imparted to expediency were not exactly equivalent to "ethical," they were at least not far removed. As the *Oxford English Dictionary* defines it:

Expedient: A. 1. Hasty, 'expeditious', speedy. Also, of a march: Direct. 2. Conducive to advantage in general, or to a definite purpose; fit, proper, or suitable to the circumstances of the case. B. *n.* 1. Something that helps forward, or that conduces to an object; a means to an end.

If "ethical," centered on slow deliberation, is somehow in tension with speed, it seems that "expedient" may be less so. But "expedient" began acquiring more negative senses, as the *OED* explication continues with "3. In depreciative sense, 'useful' or 'politic' as opposed to 'just' or 'right'." The *OED* quotes John Stuart Mill's 1861 treatise *Utilitarianism* here: "The expedient, in the sense in which it is opposed to the Right, generally means that which is expedient for the particular interest of the agent himself." Where, then, does one cross the line, or cross the cross, between the ethically suitable and the expediently politic?

XX

Genomic biobanks and databases are not only here to stay, they're here to develop and swell and mutate. The genomic ecology is simply too rich and too developmentally canalized for anything else to happen. So we will have to experiment with new expedient solutions.

David Winickoff offers one set of possibilities.[4] As a student at Harvard Law School, Winickoff spent a summer in Reykjavík working closely with Mannvernd on legal and regulatory issues related to the Health Sector Database. He brought Einar Árnason, Pétur Hauksson, and the Supreme Court attorney Ragnar Adalsteinsson to lead a seminar at Harvard Law School on the HSD and international law, and more recently he coauthored an article with his father that describes structuring biobanks as charitable trusts, which would be more expedient for the people whose tissues are in biobanks than are most prevailing models, including deCODE's.

"The charitable trust is a promising legal structure," the Winickoffs note, "for handling such a set of obligations, for promoting donor participation in research governance, and for stimulating research that will benefit the public."[5] Their use of the descriptor "promising," intentional or not, is apt: the Winickoffs propose a structure whose effects are not fully known, but that seem worth experimenting with in order to more expediently handle the kinds of promissory relationships and commitments that inhere in biobanks: "These large sets of tissue and blood samples and health data have profound medical, legal, ethical, and social implications for privacy, individual and group autonomy, and benefits to communities. In the United States, a number of biotechnology companies are amassing samples—millions of them, in some cases—in private tissue banks. Many of these companies act as brokers of tissue and of health data for a wide range of researchers. Although this brokering has sparked ethical concerns, the role of academic medical centers as suppliers for these private 'biobanks' has received little attention" (1180).

The Winickoffs extol the charitable trust as "an elegant and flexible legal model that has a number of advantages over private biobanks." Flexibility is a particularly important criterion for the volatile territories of promising genomics. While "private biobanks may be forced to sell off their inventory in the event of bankruptcy," charitable trusts have a greater degree of flexibility that gives them "the advantage of longevity." That kind of longevity will be more expedient for researchers interested in undertaking long-term or cross-generational studies than it would be for those seeking a quick reward. In addition, "charitable trusts accord well with the altruism that characterizes gifts of tissue." And the charitable trust model is not necessarily incompatible with "market-based solutions," since "biotechnology and pharmaceutical companies that want tissue or data from a hospital could be partners with the tissue bank in order to help fund it" (1180).

In summary, the Winickoffs argue that

the charitable trust is an alternative that has clear ethical, legal, and scientific advantages. It can accommodate and foster the altruism, good governance, and benefit to the public that are necessary for the success of such a project over the long term. In addition, the tissue trust can comply with increasingly stringent rules about privacy and informed consent without losing its value as an information-rich genomic resource. Moreover, the channels for public participation and communication provided by a charitable trust would forestall the political battles that have stymied biobanking endeavors such as the Icelandic Health Sector Database and the Framingham genome project. Based on the principle that genomic biobanking is both a scientific and a social endeavor, the charitable-trust model can foster a level of cooperation among teaching hospitals, researchers, and donor communities that will ensure responsible and fruitful use of research material. (1183–84)

EverythingXNothing

To breed an animal with the right to make promises—is not
this the paradoxical problem nature has set itself in relation to
man? And is it not man's true problem?

Nietzsche, *"Birth of Tragedy"* and *"Genealogy of Morals,"* 57

"The Big Con," linguistic anthropologist David Maurer pointed out in
his classic 1940 book of the same name, flourished in that period after
World War I and before the Great Depression when, as in more recent
times, "every man believed himself a potential millionaire."[1] Such a belief made every man a potential "mark," and those marks would find themselves roped into various Big Cons, like the wire or the rag, or short cons,
like the hype, otherwise known as the flop or simply the sting, not to be
confused with the slide, the push, or the boodle worked by lowly circus
grifters. There was a definite hierarchy to cons. The Big Con was the domain of people such as Pretty Willy, Slobbering Bob, Barney the Patch,
Queer-Pusher Nick, Lilly the Roper, and many Kids—the High Ass Kid,
the Square Faced Kid, the Hashhouse Kid, the Seldom Seen Kid, and the
Sanctimonious Kid, to name only a few.

As Maurer knew from his years of talking with these men, the belief
that one could become a millionaire was only enough to rope in a mark;
getting the mark to stay and play, and sometimes even to play again for
a larger sum, required something more. It required a certain kind of structure, a structure of undecidability—which is to say, a structure marked
by volatility, by not-structure—although this structure had to hold only

for a limited period of time. A con worked because of an undecidable quiver, a rapid oscillation between the con game and the square deal and between the con artist and the businessman. A quiver so fast as to hold fast, an oscillation so rapid that the word "between" loses its sense, and an *indiscriminateness* kicks in:

> If fifty [con men] were selected and mixed indiscriminately with a group of successful business and professional men, all the correlations and statistics of a Hooton or a Lombroso would not set them apart; and, if a census of opinions upon politics, ethics, religion, or what-not were taken from the entire group, not even a Solomon could separate the sheep from the goats on the basis of their social views. If confidence men operate outside the law, it must be remembered that they are not much further outside than many of our pillars of society who go under names less sinister. They only carry to an ultimate and very logical conclusion certain trends which are often inherent in various forms of legitimate business. (178–79)

These "trends" that the con man and the professional man alike capitalize on have been gestured toward in this book through names as numerous and colorful as those held by Slobbering Bob and his companions: volatility, speculation, chiasmus, promise, anticipation, hype, hope, becoming, the future, and the *á-venir* or *de-venir* of certain French theorists like Disseminating Jacques or the Plateau Kid. These "trends"—the swerving, drifting, veering that seems to be an emergent effect of every structure[2]—hold sway at all times, from the Roaring Twenties to the Screaming Nineties, from horse races to genome races, from the Big Con to Big Pharma, and from the United States to Iceland. To give yet one more name to this volatile trend inherent in any economy, which the con man simply pushes to its limits, let's conjure that old stand-by of deconstruction and call it the "pharmakon."

A naming of the unnameable that inhabits every name, the pharmakon is that trend that rends the subject in the half-time of a present out of joint with the future. The pharmakon undecides a future, opens the fissure that never quite separates the all-too-imaginable future from the inconceivable yawning unspeakable emptiness outside the now. The pharmakon is the gift-poison that volatilizes contemporary genomics and its futures on its multiple plateaus—scientific, economic, and cultural. The pharmakon is the chiasmus, the X that crosses and crosses out, writing and erasing everything—and nothing.

The pharmakon is, or makes possible, the promise.

Promising Genomics has traveled this confounded ground to produce an ethnography of promises as they operated in and through genomics in Iceland and the United States. Like many chapters at the end of books, this one negotiates the chiasmus that asks a writer to say both everything—summing up the entire book—and nothing—what could there possibly be to add if the book has done its job and fulfilled its promise?

Since everything and nothing are not in themselves inviting options, let's begin with something in between, however crude and reductive it may be: one. *Promising Genomics* might be thought of as a response to one overarching question, "How do you tell the difference, if there is one, between a pharmakon and a pharma con?" Or in the condensed form that sophisticated investors in Iceland, the United States, and other hot spots of the globalizing life-sciences business would have started asking themselves in the final years of the twentieth century, "DeCODE Genetics: pharmakon or pharma con?"

This is a question that the undersigned has kept open, at least nominally, trying to respect its extreme volatility, if not its formal undecidability. Can it be answered now? Can the volatility be quelled? Is there a response that would not draw on speculation?

XX

At dinner with the Mannvernd crew one night, we discussed the figure of the con artist in our various national literatures and mythologies. I offered up the 1962 film *The Music Man* as a possible allegory for genomics in lavaXland. The Icelanders were not familiar with it. I explained how the opening segment of the film establishes the structure for the entire plot: traveling salesmen on the economy-expanding train, traders in real goods (the anvil salesman figures heavily in the plot) who bemoan the effects the Music Man's con game has had on their reputations, even as they establish the disruptive force of language—"waddayatalk, waddaya-talk, waddayatalk?"—joining its rhythm to that of the technology that conveys them to their distant markets. Iceland's position in an Interneted global economy in the late twentieth century was only slightly less marginal than a railroaded Iowa's was in early twentieth-century America.

I tried to summon up an image of a young Icelandic version of a lisping Ron Howard singing about how Hoffmann-LaRoche's pharmacogenomics division, rather than the Wells Fargo Wagon, was bringing "thomething thpecial / jutht for me." Any half-decent lyricist could adapt the famous "Trouble!" song-and-dance number to work for Reykjavík rather than River City: "Oh yes we got genes / right here in Reykjavík

City / With a capital G / that rhymes with P / that stands for Gene Pool!" Kári would have to be played by someone a bit more menacing than Robert Preston, but still capable of seduction, plotting, and careful timing— "milestone payments . . . milestone payments" has the same hypnotic rhythm as "fifteen minutes . . . fifteen minutes" that the Music Man uses to time his seduction of the librarian (played by Björk in the Icelandic version, of course), to be quickly followed by his departure on the next train out of town, one step ahead of the mob with tar and feathers . . .

The novels of Halldór Laxness harbor more than a few con artists, as we've seen, so the members of the Mannvernd crew had their own literary analogs to try out. One of their favorites was Gardar Hólm, from Laxness's *The Fish Can Sing*—Hólm is an Icelandic opera singer of global fame, judging by the postcards and letters he sends back from metropolises all over the world. Bankrolled by a powerful and successful businessman, Gardar fails to show up for his big homecoming concert because he can't carry a tune in a bucket—his career is a complete fabrication, the postal messages of his success having been mailed from the scattered corners of the world by traveling Icelanders.

And of course there was Two Hundred Thousand Pliers in Halldór Laxness's *The Atom Station*, as we've seen—he of the Figures Faking Federation, also known as the joint stock company Snorredda, also known as the prime minister. Kári as Two Hundred Thousand Genes is an easy substitution—or at least Twenty-Nine Thousand Genes, per the more recent estimates of the total number of genes in a human genome.

Most would regard such a telling as too speculative. The legal scholar Henry Greely, for example, has written an article about Iceland and deCODE Genetics that is, by and large, quite critical of the enterprise for reasons that I suspect many readers would agree with: the exclusive license and twelve-year monopoly on the Health Sector Database, the flaunting of international standards of informed consent, and so on. I want to read where Greely's article locates the limit of reading—the line beyond which lies speculation, a currency that Greely prefers not to traffic in: "A thorough skeptic, noting the difficulties of creating successful biotechnology drugs—or biotechnology companies—might suggest that the database act was a way to increase the share value of deCODE so that, when it went public, the venture capitalists and other early owners would make money. DeCODE's infrastructure and ongoing research in Iceland would seem to make this implausibly elaborate as a scam."[3]

Indeed. But a good scam, as anyone from Slobbering Bob to the Sanctimonious Kid would testify, requires the *most* elaborate mechanisms one can muster. What kind of mechanism other than the most elaborate one could even hope to work at all within the teeming confines of the multiple chiasma that volatilize all the doublings this book has traversed? Elaborateness alone at least is no reason to rule out, as "implausible" and too speculative, the possibility that the entire deCODE-Iceland baroque pharmakonic gene machine was nothing but a pharma con—or at least, no matter what else deCODE may turn out to be, was *also* a pharma con. No skeptic, to return to Greely's vocabulary, can be thorough enough, and speculative possibilities will always remain.

But if you have read *Promising Genomics* as building a case for deCODE as scam —if you think the undersigned has given only an accounting of deCODE as an "implausibly elaborate" Ponzi scheme—then I have failed. The main intent here has not been to burst virtual bubbles with the pins of skepticism or realism, or to debunk hype, or to expose Kári as the Keiko Kid. As I hope to have shown over and over again—for while bubble- and hype-bursting is an instantaneous affair, showing is always a matter of repetition—something more than that bubble bursting is necessary for genomics.

One answer to the question, "How do you tell a pharmakon from a pharma con?" is that there's no telling without speculating. "It's the real thing" and "It's a big con" are both speculative statements. Any sophisticated investor can tell you that. Another response is that all things genomic, including deCODE, are pharmakonic—doubled and disseminated, such that the possibility of a con can never be ruled out but always remains, haunting. But perhaps the best response is to insist that, in asking if deCODE is a pharma con, I have posed an unproductive question. Because that question produces only one possibility: a final and thus inappropriate settlement of a chiasmus.

So let's try another question: how should we read genomics' promises?

XX

The genomic industry itself knows full well that it's an inescapably volatile and speculative endeavor. And given that it's the scientists and other professionals who make their living in this industry that know more about it than any of us, it's not surprising that they have perhaps the keenest awareness of genomics' unsettling and ultimately unsettled chiasma.

In the April 2002 issue of *Genome Technology,* the trade magazine ran a humorous last-page piece, as it does each month, that mimicked the once-popular matchbook campaign, "You, too, can be an artist!" But the promise hawked here assured the anonymous "you" that "You, too, can speak genomics!!!" (figure 10). This "unique, interactive, and fun" learning course—"held at TROPICAL RESORTS near many leading genomics conferences"—promised to prepare attendees to "work in GENOMICS or POST-GENOMICS business development or marketing!" by providing them—you!—with "a dynamic, interactive SPEAK GENOMICS! vocabulary lesson!" Among the most important words to learn in this new vocabulary:

PIPELINE: Theoretically, products that are in the works. Realistically, a fictional tube full of the waste products from the hot air you have blown at your venture capitalists to get them to fund your operation.

ROBUST: It might work. As in, our technology platform is robust. *Ant.* Exploratory, experimental, innovative. As in, our technology is innovative, experimental, i.e., we have no idea if it will ever work.

VALIDATE: Manufacture some hard data PDQ to show that your company and its products aren't a total joke.

PRESENTATION: A ritual that occurs in a darkened, slightly freezing hotel ballroom in which first a computer malfunctions, then a series of Powerpoint slides accompany a few feeble jokes and a somewhat melodic lullaby of somnolence-producing numeric recitations.[4]

The speculative, pharmakonic quality of *any* genomic enterprise, not just Icelandic ones, is only too evident to industry insiders. And there's something funny about that. (Unless you're about to default on the second mortgage the state bank sold you so you could exercise your patriotism and buy stock in a nationalist enterprise.) And there's something necessary about that. Promising can't be reduced to either empty hype or to formal contract, but occupies the uncertain, difficult space in between. Without promising, science, business, and thought itself would all die, unable to break out of the bounds of the known or the presently possible. Genomics, like much else, has to be promissory.

This book matches that matchbook: "You, too, can read genomics!" is its pitch. To read genomics is to read promises, and this required reading is always a doubled one. To read promises is to read chiasma, in all their volatility. To read chiasma is to keep one's house open to mania, hype, and speculation, while seating people around a table set with fundamentals, disclosures, calculations. To read promising genomics, then, is to throw yourself, without reserve, into both speculation and due diligence.

It doesn't matter whether we could finally decide that deCODE was a con or the greatest corporation ever. Reading promising genomics isn't

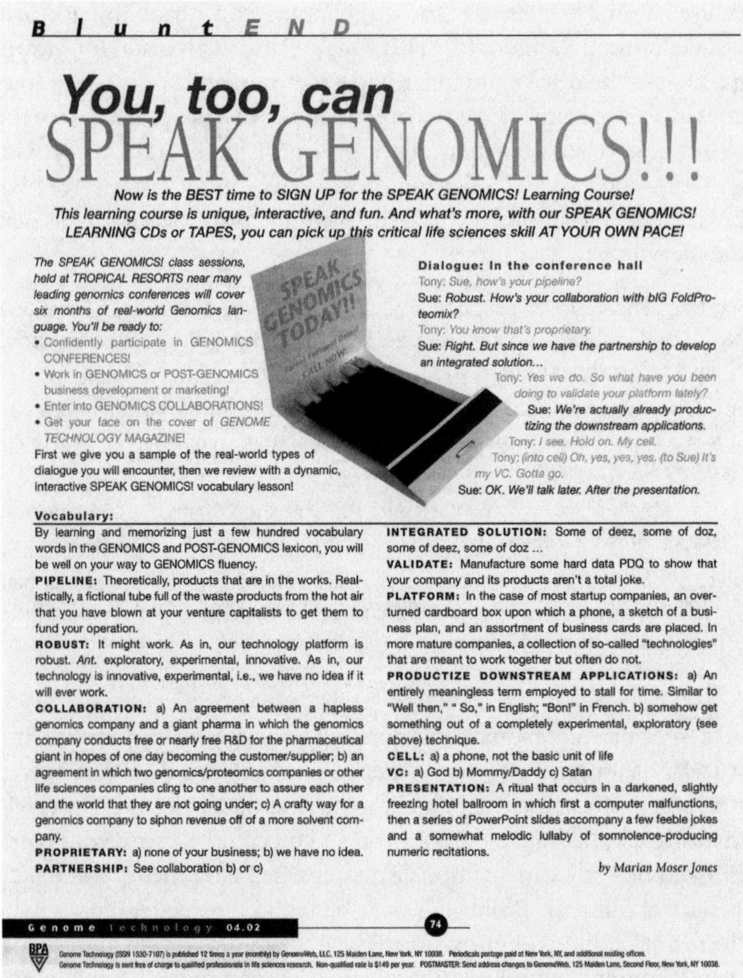

FIGURE 10. "You, Too, Can Speak Genomics!!!" Text by Marian Moser Jones, in *Genome Technology*, April 2002. Reprinted with the permission of *Genome Technology* (www.genome-technology.com).

a matter of *knowing* what "is" the case; promising runs on what can't be known. It's like asking, "Did he really mean that promise?" As we saw J. L. Austin first argue, the speech act "I promise . . ." does not, and *should* not, depend on *knowing* the true intention of the speaker. You can't know that, and you don't need to know that to follow the real consequences that flow as a result of the utterance. Or it's like asking, "Is money real?"

and expecting the yes or no answer that the question sets up. Halldór Laxness helped us dispense with those false alternatives in the case of counterfeitXmoney. What matters is the circulation, the effects, the action set in motion by the volatility of the chiasmus. What matters is the flowering, the excessive and ephemeral.

DeCODE, too, poses an undecidable question. What matters are the effects, the finite relations, the specific forces that constituted the events surrounding deCODE. These events can be diagrammed, with due diligence. This book is that diagram. Is deCODE a con? What can I tell you? Here's where the counterfeitXmoney came from, here's how it ended up in Panama via Luxembourg, here's how it went from the banks to six thousand Icelanders, temporarily, and thence to deCODE. Here's how online investors made decisions about things they didn't or couldn't know. Here's how presumedXconsent functioned in a larger set of biomedical and bioethical machines. Here's how the force of celebrity had multiple effects in the late-1990s economy. Here are the papers announcing genomic discoveries that have been published in peer-reviewed scientific journals

In every case of chiasmic undecidability, due diligence is the demand. Democratic debate about genomics? How exactly does this thing called democracy work in this particular country, in these particular years, with these particular individuals and institutions? And where does the science of genomics find itself entangled with a political economy becoming global (a becoming long coming)? At a time in which ever-present financial speculation and risk has been heightened through particular mechanisms of law and a proliferating pack of investors, you want me to buy shares in *what*? I'll just take a look at some of these details that another part of the law requires you to disclose . . .

Diagramming and due diligence, like ethnography, demand prolixity and specificity. Due diligence demands a nonXgovernmental organization, like Mannvernd, that establishes an archive, that undertakes the difficult and always necessary act of public education, that pursues questions and actions through every possible channel while dredging out some new ones. And due diligence must be accompanied by speculation.

Speculation: what more can be said about this concept?

XX

Speculation, this speculation thus would be foreign to
philosophy or metaphysics. More precisely, speculation would

represent the very thing which philosophy or metaphysics guard themselves from, which philosophy or metaphysics consist in guarding themselves from, maintaining with it a relation without relation, a relation of exclusion which signifies simultaneously the necessity and the aporia of speculation. And it is within the "same" word—speculation—that the translation is to find its place, between the philosophical concept of speculation in its dominant, apparently legitimate determination, the determination granted to the elementary consensus of the philosophical tradition, and the concept that is announced here. This latter has been able to be the other's other by inhabiting it, by letting itself be excluded without ceasing to work upon it in the most domestic fashion. . . .

What to do with this inconceivable concept? How to speculate with this speculation? . . . What is it that fascinates under this heading? And why does it impose itself at the moment when it is a question of life death, of pleasure-unpleasure, and of repetition?

Jacques Derrida

We're going to have to learn to live with increasing volatility.

Dennis Purcell, global head
of life sciences, Chase
H&Q, San Francisco

Dennis Purcell gets points for brevity.[5] He's got a knack for getting right to the point in the chummy first-person plural, not repeating himself, not piling question upon question, not scattering his infinitives all over the place with complex phrases and paradoxes networked in between, but efficiently packing them together on iambic feet: to have, to learn, to live. A global head of life sciences needs that kind of skill.

But brevity can't be the only virtue in an era in which organisms like us are apprehended by billion-character genetic informational sequences, downloaded and uploaded with increasing frequency, and always supplemented by a growing list of equally prolix annotational practices that refer and connect to protein studies, gene expression studies in particular tissues at particular times, clinical findings, and many other conceptual-empirical nodes on an ever-denser network on the way to a promised "systems biology." Doubled epigraphs for a fissured terrain demanding doubled readings and doubled writings will be a minimum requirement for learning to live with increasing volatility.

No surprise, then, that if you were net-searching for genomic investment advice in today's market, wondering about the status of speculation there, you would find only doubled readings that require yet another round of some kind of speculation. On the one hand, the *Motley Fool* provides the nonexuberant, sober, post-bubble, post-genomics advice: "There's no reason why the average investor, one with a casual interest in stocks, should be invested in biotechnology companies. None. It doesn't make sense, from a risk-reward perspective, for the average investor to make big bets in a debate waged by scientists, doctors, and researchers, if you're investing money you don't want to lose. . . . You can only pay so much for promises."[6]

That would appear to be due diligence speaking, silencing speculation. But the *Fool*'s bottom-line advice—"You can only pay so much for promises"—is nevertheless haunted by the open question: *just how much would that be?*

Or, taking your Internet investing advice not from the *Motley Fool* but from *Red Herring:*

What's an investor to do? Believe the unbelievable. "Like never before," says Mr. Deleage. Certainly cancer victims have little else to do; same with parents of premature babies, men with testicular cancer, and women with breast cancer. It was not so long ago that these maladies meant certain death. Biotechnology has changed that one-way course, if only by a few precious degrees. What human being would not want to be a part of that? Surely the naive and the perplexed can be forgiven for their enthusiasm about what this industry is capable of in the next 25 years.[7]

This axiom, "Believe the unbelievable," unleashes speculation and enthusiasm, but is still haunted by its own spectral question: *just how much naiveté and perplexity can be forgiven?*

I have tried in this book to diagram rather than resolve the tangle of recombinant forces that occur within these genomic sites, the simultaneous "necessity and the aporia of speculation," in which futures fold into presents. If they have been diagrams of due diligence, they have also been diagrams of speculationXspeculation, that inconceivable and unworkable concept that never ceases to work—diagrams, since *clear and globally applicable* rules for separating the "good" speculation from the "bad" are too much to ask. SpeculationXspeculation, that relation without relation, is the essential if disavowed force inhabiting biological, economic, and political reason and inhabiting biological, economic, and political activity. It inhabits us and we inhabit it, and there would be no life—and no life sciences—without it. Unsettled settlement that we are going to have to learn to live.

To have to learn to live?

Maybe global head of life sciences Dennis Purcell has been reading
Derrida in his spare time. In the opening "Exordium" to *Specters of Marx*,
Derrida takes up exactly this speech act, "to learn to live":

Someone, you or me, comes forward and says: *I would like to learn to live finally* . . .
    To learn to live: a strange watchword. Who would learn? From whom? To teach
to live, but to whom? Will we ever know? Will we ever know how to live and first
of all what "to learn to live" means? . . .
    By itself, out of context—but a context, always, remains open, this fallible and
insufficient—this watchword forms an almost unintelligible syntagm. Just how
far can its idiom be translated moreover?[8]

The translator's note here reads, "Not very far because 'apprendre à
vivre' means both to teach how to live and to learn how to live" (177).
Another chiasmus, linking teacher and student, writer and reader.

Is that not impossible for a living being? Is it not what logic itself forbids? To live,
by definition, is not something one learns.
    And yet nothing is more necessary than this wisdom. It is ethics itself: to learn
to live—alone, from oneself, by oneself. Life does not know how to live otherwise. And does one ever do anything else but learn to live, alone, from oneself,
by oneself? This is, therefore, a strange commitment, both impossible and necessary, for a living being supposed to be alive: "I would like to learn to live." (xviii)

This strange, "impossible and necessary" commitment is shared by
Ugla. In the final pages of *The Atom Station*, Ugla returns to Reykjavík,
leaving her newborn Gudrún at her family's home in the north until she
can manage "to fix myself up." She calls her former employer and Parliament minister from a phone booth in the public square. He asks her what
her plans are. "I want to become a person," is her response. "A person
amongst persons. I know it's laughable, contemptible, disgraceful, and
revolutionary that a woman should not wish to be some sort of slave or
harlot; but that's the way I'm made."[9]
    The minister meets her and brings her to a small clandestine apartment
that he keeps in the city. As they continue talking, Ugla again tells him
that she feels she has become "nothing but a longing to become a person, to know something, to be able to do something for myself" (182).

"Is there anything more ludicrous than a penniless girl from the north who says
she is going to become a person?" I said.
    "All that you ask for, you shall have," he said. . . .
    "By the way," I said, "where do these words come from?"
    "I wrote them when I learned the truth," he replied. (180)

The minister's nonanswer is left standing. They are words he had written to her before, and he again makes it clear that he is prepared to give her anything, to forsake everything, to move to Patagonia, "the land of the future in the middle of the present." It's the present of the Cold War where, he says, "the battlefield covers all lands, all seas, all skies; and particularly our innermost consciousness. The whole world is one atom station." The decision, he says, is hers (183).

They each go to sleep separately, but Ugla soon wakes and steals away in the early morning hours. Eventually she ends up at the organist's house. Over an elaborate breakfast, the organist tells her what has become of her child's father, the self-conscious policeman. Inspired by Two Thousand Pliers's F.F.F. corporation, the self-conscious policeman started the Northern Trading Company. "He thought it would be enough to float a dummy company like the Northern Trading Company and have dealings with a dummy millionaire like Pliers," reported the organist. While the organist warned him that "if someone wants to steal in a thieves' community, he must steal according to the laws; and he should preferably have taken part in making the laws himself," this advice was to no avail. The self-conscious policeman ended up in jail, said the organist, although "his methods were near enough to general business practice to make it debatable whether to convict him would not be an insult to some of our upper class citizens" (197).

It would take only a hundred thousand krónur to free him, the organist tells Ugla. She hardly needs to tell him that she has nowhere near that amount of money, but she has nevertheless made up her mind: "He is the father of my little Gudrún, and whether he goes to prison or not he is my man." The organist "smiled warily and looked at [her] distantly. 'Búi Árland . . . your Member of Parliament and former employer, would soon write you out a check for that amount." Ugla, without ever saying anything, makes it clear that she will do no such thing (198).

At this point the organist unwraps one last large parcel that has been sitting on the breakfast table full of food. It contains stacks of bank-notes. "Help yourself," the organist tells Ugla. "Is that real money?" she asks. "Hardly. At least I did not manufacture it myself. But bring your case over here just the same." When Ugla demurs, the organist shrugs and heads for the fireplace. Having once witnessed the organist's willingness to carry the potlatch through, Ugla stops him and accepts the money. As she is stuffing it into her suitcase, he snips all the blooms from every plant in his house, presents her with the resulting bouquet of flowers, embraces her in farewell, and tells her not to bother returning to the house looking for him; he has sold it and is moving. When Ugla asks where he is going, he replies, "The same road as the flowers" (199–200).

On her way to the prison, Ugla passes by the cathedral and finds herself in the midst of an "ultra-distinguished" funeral. An ornate coffin, holding either the bones of the Nation's Darling, Portuguese sardines, or Danish clay—Laxness gives his readers no choice but to speculate—is being carried by the prime minister and the other "overlords of the country," including Búi Árland. Ugla is suddenly struck:

> "All that you ask for, you shall have." Somehow I had never been able to place it until now, when an old Christian text which I had learned as a child flashed into my mind again: "All these things will I give thee, if thou wilt fall down." . . .
>
> I looked for the quickest way to escape from this square, pressed my bouquet closer to me, and took to my heels. What point would there have seemed to be in living if there had not been these flowers? (201–2)

XX

It is a time of speculating in volatile bioeconomies, volatile life sciences, volatile concepts, and volatile bodies.[10] Wonderful—let a thousand speculations bloom. As long as it is also a time of due diligence, utter honesty, painstaking effort, and extreme care. LavaXland. What seems to be called for is the equivalent of some kind of hedge fund or straddle that would allow us to take radically different positions in the genomic economy. What's needed is an analytic adroitness, a tolerance for contradictions and paradoxes, the personal stamina and institutional infrastructure for sustained critical involvement, and an ability to juggle laughter and outrage.

Then and only then would we have become a person, the animal Nietzsche heralded—not the promising animal (we're already that, in spades), but the animal with *the right to make promises*. We're going to have to learn to live as that animal of paradox and promise. It will require some lively combination of exuberance, caution, speculative excess, attention to fundamentals, and ineradicable but hopefully modest risk, whose precise titration as yet—and may always—escapes us. As economic theorist Charles Kindleberger summarizes the paradox and dilemma of regulating financial speculation, "'Too little, and too late' is one of the saddest phrases in the lexicon not only of central banking but of all activity. 'Too much, too early' is not an evident improvement. Enough at the right moment is better than either. But how much is enough? When is the right time?" The person to whom those questions are addressed "faces dilemmas of amount and timing. . . . As for timing, it is an art. That says nothing—and everything."[11]

Forward Looking

Certain statements in this document are forward looking. These may be identified by the use of forward-looking words or phrases such as "anticipate," "promise," "expect," "speculate," "chiasmus," "market," "genome," "democracy," "should," "want," "must," "law," "ethics," "know," "based on," "grounded in," "structure," "is," "was," "will be," "gene," "genetic information," "we are going to have to learn to live with increasing volatility," among others. These forward-looking statements are based on the current expectations of the author, who sometimes does business as The Undersigned Inc. These statements involve, at minimum, risk and uncertainty, because they relate to events and depend on circumstances that will occur in the future. The morphology of writingXthought itself provides a safe-harbor for such forward-looking statements. In order to comply with the terms of the safe harbor, The Undersigned Inc. notes that a variety of factors could cause actual results and experience to differ materially from the anticipated results or other expectations expressed in such forward-looking statements. The risks, uncertainties, infelicities, exigencies of time, lapses of attention, and other ineradicable contingencies that may affect the operations, performance, development, and results of *Promising Genomics* or any other product of The Undersigned Inc. include but are not limited to (1) early stage of operations; (2) there being no precedent for The Undersigned Inc.'s writing plan; (3) the need to manage rapid growth; (4) the uncertainty of successful integration of subsidiary operations; (5) the uncertainty of sequencing strategy; (6) the uncertainty of the successful operation of new technologies and machine-like operations;

(7) the uncertainty of polymorphism data; (8) the sheer multiplicitous existence of polymorphism data; (9) anticipated future losses and the uncertainty of operating results; (10) a high dependence on selected key writers; (11) the uncertain protection of intellectual property and proprietary rights; (12) the adverse effect of public disclosure of The Undersigned Inc.'s writing products; (13) the highly competitive business climate; and (14) other factors that might be described from time to time in The Undersigned Inc.'s future filings with its readers.

Notes

Ch 1. LavaXLand

1. Roche, "Roche and DeCode Genetics Inc."

2. For a bibliography of over four hundred publications on deCODE Genetics, there is no better source than Skúli Sigurdsson, "Bibliography for Studying the HSD deCODE Controversy," www.raunvis.hi.is/~sksi/kit.html (accessed December 2007).

3. Gibbs, "Natural-Born Guinea Pigs," 24.

4. Bill on a Health Sector Database (submitted to Parliament at 123rd session, 1998–99), Mannvernd, www.mannvernd.is/english/laws/HSD.bill.html (accessed August 2002). This online version of the bill was circulated later in the summer of 1998 by the Ministry of Health and is slightly different from the March version, but the later text provides the bestsummary sense of what was at stake. All quotations of the legislation are from this later version.

5. Richard Doyle provides multiple diagnoses of how the future infects bodies and flesh in his book *Wetwares*.

6. See, for example, Mark C. Taylor's *Nots*.

7. The chiasmus "can always, hastily, be thought of as the thematic drawing of dissemination"; "everything passes through this chiasmus, all writing is caught in it." Derrida, *Truth in Painting*, 166.

8. Quoted in Auden and MacNeice, *Letters from Iceland*, 59.

9. Kunzig, "Blood of the Vikings," 97.

10. Auden and MacNeice, *Letters from Iceland*, 19.

11. The phrase "experimental moment" needs elaboration. George Marcus writes that ethnography needs to become experimental: inventive, risky, searching, and at pains to probe a whole range of fissures, including those that punctuate anthropology's own concepts, methods, and texts. Ethnography becomes, in Marcus's words, a "strategy of engagement" oriented toward "finding where

the 'fissures' are—that is, finding those concepts, methods, ideas, practices, and life experiences within the culture of the mainstream, about which there is self-doubt and uncertainty" and "understanding these potentially self-critical cultural formations . . . ethnographically, in their own terms and expressions." Marcus, "Critical Cultural Studies as One Power/Knowledge," 213.

12. Laxness, *Under the Glacier,* 18.

13. Eyfjörd et al., "deCODE deferred," 496.

14. See Derrida, *Specters of Marx,* on the *á-venir* of democracy.

15. *Nature Biotechnology,* "Keep the Story Straight," 491.

16. In "Postgenomics? A Conference at the Max Planck Institute for the History of Science in Berlin," Thieffry and Sarkar provide a summary of the conference, at which "many participants . . . agreed that the promise of genetic medicine had been exaggerated to the public" (226).

Ch 2. FriendXAdvance Man

1. Fortun and Sigurdsson, "'So Human a Brain' ."

2. Articles for which I was a "source" include Crenson, "National Treasure or Black Hole?"; MacPherson, "Tapping Iceland's Genetic Jackpot"; and Meeks, "Decode Was Meant to Save Lives."

3. Skúli's own publications on the topic include Sigurdsson, "Yin-Yang Genetics, or the HSD deCODE Controversy." An ongoing work—a bibliography of nearly everything published on these events—is available at his Web site, www.raunvis.hi.is/~sksi/hsd_dec.html (accessed July 2006).

4. Pálsson and Rabinow, "The Iceland Controversy," 92.

Ch 3. FastXFast

1. *American Heritage Dictionary*, 4th ed. (Boston: Houghton Mifflin, 2000).

2. Seabrook, "Why Is the Force Still With Us?" 40.

3. Pennisi, "Academic Sequencers Challenge Celera," 1822.

4. See M. Fortun, "Human Genome Project and the Acceleration of Biotechnology"; and M. Fortun, "Projecting Speed Genomics."

5. Quoted in M. Fortun, "Projecting Speed Genomics," 33.

6. CIBA Foundation, *Human Genetic Information,* 30.

7. U.S. Congress, Senate Committee on Energy and Natural Resources, *Workshop on Human Gene Mapping,* 12.

8. U.S. Congress, Senate Subcommittee on Energy Research and Development, *Human Genome Project,* 91–92.

9. Eric Lander, interview with author, December 19, 1990, quoted in M. Fortun, "Projecting Speed Genomics," 32.

10. U.S. Congress, Senate Committee on Energy and Natural Resources, *Workshop on Human Gene Mapping,* 47.

11. Edwards, "How the Elephants Dance Part 1."

12. Quoted in Erickson, "Incyte Serves Up Information," 36.

13. Ibid., 39.

14. J. O. Hamilton, "How SmithKline and Incyte Became Lab Partners," *Signals Magazine*, December 22, 1997, www.signalsmag.com/signalsmag.nsf (accessed December 2007).

15. Millennium Pharmaceuticals, U.S. Securities and Exchange S-1 Registration Statement, May 8, 1996, www.sec.gov/Archives/edgar/data/1002637/0000950 135–96–001935.txt (accessed December 2007).

16. The Institute for Genomic Research (TIGR), "TIGR/HGS Funding Relationship Reaches Early Conclusion," press release, June 24, 1997, www.tigr.org/news/pr_06_24h_97.shtml (accessed December 2007).

17. "Research Institute Posts Gene Data on Internet," *Business Today,* June 25, 1997, www.businesstoday.com/archive/topstories/gene25.htm (accessed November 1998).

18. Keller, *Refiguring Life,* 6–7.

19. Donna Haraway, *Simians, Cyborgs, and Women: The Reinvention of Nature* (New York: Routledge, 1991), 44.

20. Margaret Mead, quoted in *Time,* September 4, 1954, quoted in Marshall McLuhan, *Understanding Media* (New York: Routledge, 2001), 30.

Ch 4. CounterfeitXMoney

1. Rotman, *Signifying Nothing,* 89–90.

2. Derrida, *Specters of Marx,* 163.

3. Soros, "Theory of Reflexivity." The subsequent Soros quotation is also from this source.

4. Hamilton, "Mapping Out Stocks for the Genome Gold Rush."

5. Laxness, *Atom Station,* 21–22. On the links that connect the excesses of tobacco with those of gift giving, as part of an extended telling of the counterfeitXreal chiasmus and the disseminated effects produced in and out of that volatile fissure, one of which is time, see Derrida, *Given Time.*

6. Maurer, *Mutual Life, Limited,* 2005.

Ch 5. KáriXdeCODE

1. See Andrews, "U.S. Seeks Patent on Genetic Code, Setting Off Furor."

2. See ibid.; M. Fortun, "Projecting Speed Genomics"; Roberts, "OSTP to Wade into Gene Patents Quagmire"; Roberts, "NIH Gene Patents, Round 2"; and Veggeberg, "Controversy Mounts Over Gene Patent Policy."

3. Preston, "Genome Warrior," 72. For more on Celera, see M. Fortun, "Celera Genomics."

4. And in Venter's case, that binding up turned out to be quite literal: it later

became known that, contrary to previous statements, the genome that Celera sequenced was Venter's own.

5. Preston, "Genome Warrior," 80.

6. Specter, "Decoding Iceland," 44–45.

7. Ernir Snorrason, "Assault on Democracy," *DV,* November 7, 1998, trans. Mannvernd, www.mannvernd.is/english/news/07.11.1998_vidtal_ernir_snorrasone.html (accessed September 16, 2002).

8. See C. Keller, "Die Isländer, unsere Labormäuse."

9. See Hodgson, "Genetic Heritage Betrayed or Empowered?"; and Hodgson, "deCODE Looks Forward."

10. Specter, "Decoding Iceland," 44.

11. deCODE Genetics, "Non-Confidential Corporate Summary," 17.

12. Laxness, *Under the Glacier,* 10.

Ch 7. HistoryXFable

1. Kellogg, introduction to *The Sagas of Icelanders*, lii.

2. Laxness, *Under the Glacier,* 87.

3. Kunzig, "Blood of the Vikings," 90–92.

Ch 8. KeikoXK.Co.

1. The chronology of events surrounding Keiko (and associated quotations unless otherwise noted) were taken from the Oregon Coast Aquarium Web site, www.aquarium.org/keiko (accessed July 8, 2003).

2. According to the U.S. State Department: "Iceland left the International Whaling Commission (IWC) in June 1992 in protest of an IWC decision to refuse to lift the ban on whaling, after the IWC Scientific Committee had determined that the taking of certain species could safely be resumed. That year, Iceland established its own commission—which the U.S. does not recognize—along with Norway, Greenland, and the Faroes for the conservation, management, and study of marine mammals. Since then, Iceland has not resumed whaling but has asserted the right to do so." U.S. State Department, "Background Notes: Iceland," October 1999, www.state.gov/www/background_notes/iceland_9910_bgn.html (accessed January 20, 2003). Iceland rejoined the IWC, with reservations, in June 2001. For some history of the IWC and the refusal by Iceland, Norway, and Japan to comply with its directives, see the IWC Web site, www.iwcoffice.org. Historian of science Karen Oslund discusses the unique "mystique" of whales, in Iceland as elsewhere, in her article "Protecting Fat Mammals or Carnivorous Humans?"

3. Air Force Link, www.af.mil/news/Sep1998/n19980910_981367.html (accessed June 18, 2001).

4. Leonard, "Keiko Discovers What 'Hammer' Time Is All About."

5. Muldoon, "Keiko May Be Moved."

6. "Keiko Leaves the Nest," *Iceland Review Daily News,* August 13, 2002, http://icelandreview.com (accessed August 13, 2002).

Ch 9. TrustXGullibility

1. Auden and MacNeice, *Letters from Iceland,* 117.

2. See M. Fortun, "For an Ethics of Promising," for another statement of this.

3. For an example of this defense of democracy-by-the-numbers approach, see Pálsson and Rabinow, "The Iceland Controversy."

4. Bogi Anderson, e-mail to author, December 7, 1999.

5. Ethics Council of the IMA (ECIMA) comments on the HSD bill, Mannvernd, www.mannvernd.is/english/news/02.11.1998_ethics_committe.html (accessed December 2007). The ECIMA was chaired by Tómas Zoëga, one of the signatories to the *Nature Biotechnology* letter (Eyfjörd et al., "deCODE deferred") that had first made the HSDXdeCODE controversy public at the international level. Zoëga, whose family came to Iceland from Spain via Denmark, is a psychiatrist at the National University Hospital who could hardly be construed as "antigenetic"; as part of various national and international research collaborations, he has coauthored a number of articles on the genetics of schizophrenia.

6. Specter, "Decoding Iceland," 51.

7. Ethical Council of the IMA comments on the HSD bill, Mannvernd, www.mannvernd.is/english/news/02.11.1998_ethics_committe.html (accessed December 2007).

8. "Report of the University of Iceland Medical School's Committee on Medical Databases, Summary," Mannvernd, www.mannvernd.is/english/articles/10.12.1998_medschool_comittee__on_database.html (accessed December 2007).

9. Mannvernd summarized these critiques; see "Comments on the 31 July 1998 Version," Mannvernd, www.mannvernd.is/english/articles/29.11.1998_comments_on_july_draft.html (accessed December 2007).

10. "The Health Committee of Althing Concludes Its Examination of the Bill on the Health Sector Database," Mannvernd, www.mannvernd.is/english/articles/30.11.1998_health_comittee.html (accessed December 2007).

11. "No Information about Patients Unless They Permit," Mannvernd, www.mannvernd.is/english/news/06.12.1998_44_general_practioners.html (accessed December 2007).

12. Páll Pálsson, opinion piece, *Morgunbladid,* December 5, 1998, excerpted on the Mannvernd Web site, www.mannvernd.is/english (accessed December 2007).

13. Roche, "Roche and DeCode Genetics Inc."

14. Specter, "Decoding Iceland," 50.

15. Laxness, *Atom Station,* 22–23

16. "The Status of the Bill on the Health Sector Database in Iceland and the Controversy Surrounding the Proposed Legislation and on deCODE Genetics, the Government's a priori Candidate for the Monopoly," Mannvernd, www.mannvernd.is/english/news/status.html (accessed December 2007).

Ch X. PromisesXPromises

Epigraphs: McCaffery, "Reason to Avoid Biotech Stocks"; Drews quoted in Licking et al., "Move Over, Dot-Coms"; Firn, "Takeovers Cure for German Biotechs"; Risch, "Searching for Genetic Determinants in the New Millennium," 848; Wong, "Judgment Day Is Here for Biotechs"; Enserink, "Physicians Wary of Scheme to Pool Icelanders' Genetic Data," 891; member of the Althingi, interview with author, March 18, 2000.

1. Taylor, *Nots,* 41.

2. For a treatment of the ethical, textual, and biological strands of meaning spun by *entrelacement*, see Derrida's piece devoted to Levinas, "At This Very Moment in This Work Here I Am," in *Re-Reading Levinas,* ed. Robert Bernasconi and Simon Critchley (Bloomington: Indiana University Press, 1991), 11–48.

3. Felman, *Scandal of the Speaking Body,* 3–4.

4. Austin, *How to Do Things with Words,* 9–10.

5. Derrida, *Monolingualism of the Other,* 67.

6. Derrida, *Specters of Marx,* 75.

7. See Hannah Arendt, *The Human Condition* (Chicago: University of Chicago Press).

8. Greenspan, "Economic Volatility."

9. Felman, *Scandal of the Speaking Body,* 74.

Ch 10. DistanceXComplicity

1. Michel Foucault, "For an Ethic of Discomfort," in *Power: Essential Works of Foucault 1954–1984,* vol. 3, ed. James D. Faubion (New York: New Press, 2000), 443–48.

2. Durrenberger, *Icelandic Essays,* ix–x.

3. Jeffrey Kahn, "Attention Shoppers: Special Today—Iceland's DNA," CNN .com, February 1999, www.cnn.com/HEALTH/bioethics/9902/iceland.dna/template.html (accessed December 18, 2002).

4. It almost goes without saying that certain CNN practices are similar to those CNN questions of deCODE—collecting and marketing personally identifiable and non-personally identifiable information, with an "opt out" clause for those who would decline this valuable service. As CNN's privacy statement makes clear, "The information we collect in connection with our online forums and communities is used to provide an interactive experience. We use this information to facilitate participation in these online forums and communities and, from time to time, to offer you products, programs, or services. . . . We sometimes use the non-personally identifiable information that we collect to improve the design and content of our site and to enable us to personalize your Internet experience. . . . Although we take appropriate measures to safeguard against unauthorized disclosures of information, we cannot assure you that personally identifiable information that we collect will never be disclosed in a manner that is inconsistent with this Pri-

vacy Notice. . . . Certain AOL Time Warner sites may disclose personally identifiable information to companies whose practices are not covered by this privacy notice (e.g., other marketers, magazine publishers, retailers, participatory databases, and non-profit organizations) that want to market products or services to you. If a site shares personally identifiable information, it will provide you with an opportunity to opt out or block such uses. For instructions on how to opt out from such disclosures, please click here." "CNN Privacy Statement," CNN, www.cnn.com/privacy.html (accessed December 18, 2002).

5. Specter, "Decoding Iceland," 49.

6. See Rose, *Commodification of Bioinformation;* and Greely, "Iceland's Plan for Genomics Research."

7. See Merz, McGee, and Sankar, "'Iceland Inc.': On the Ethics of Commercial Population Genomics."

8. Marilyn Strathern, foreword in Rose, *Commodification of Bioinformation,* 4.

9. Pálsson and Rabinow, "Iceland: The Case of a National Human Genome Project," 18.

10. K. Fortun, *Advocacy after Bhopal.*

11. M. Fortun, "Experiments in Ethnography and Its Performance," Mannvernd, February 12, 2000, www.mannvernd.is/english/articles/mfortun.html (accessed December 2007).

12. Hafstein, "Honesty and Trust."

13. Jóhannesson, "Are Icelandic Politicians for Sale?"

14. See M. Fortun, "Mediated Speculations in the Genomics Futures Market."

15. On the logic of rumor, see Ronell, "Hitting the Streets: *Ecce Fama.*"

16. Philipkoski, "Genetics Scandal Inflames Iceland." She also noted that "deCODE's S-1 filing also did not reference certain expenditures, according to [Bogi] Andersen. For example, about a year ago, an article in *Dagur* reported that the company purchased a building to serve as its headquarters from a company called Hans Petersen, which is owned by the family of the prime minister's wife, Ástríður Thorarensen. Thorarensen is a shareholder and a member of the board of directors of Hans Petersen. The purchase price was kept secret at the time, and the transaction is not cited in the S-1 filing."

17. Ibid.

18. See Crenson, "National Treasure or Black Hole?"; MacPherson, "Tapping Iceland's Genetic Jackpot"; and Meek, "Decode Was Meant to Save Lives."

19. "The historian of science Mike Fortun (Rensselaer Polytechnic Institute) recalls: 'In 1998 two heroes returned simultaneously to Iceland accompanied by tremendous media spectacle; Keiko, the whale from the film "Free Willy," and Kári, the CEO of deCODE.' He adds: 'I was then already on the ground in Iceland and the similarity between the staging of the two events was quite striking.'" Langenbach, "Island: Kafkaeskes Gen-Fischen," 37.

20. "'For me this is not at all an "Icelandic Saga,"' says Skúli Sigurdsson (University of Iceland, Reykjavík), 'but a bureaucracy which, as in the case of Kafka, manhandles its citizens.'" Langenbach, "Island: Kafkaeskes Gen-Fischen," 37.

21. Arnst, "An Icelandic Saga about Privacy and DNA."

22. Pálsson and Rabinow, "Iceland: The Case of a National Human Genome Project," 14.

23. Sigurdsson, "Yin-Yang Genetics, or the HSD deCODE Controversy," 112.

24. Billings, "Iceland, Blood and Science."

25. On what Mannvernd calls the "Ousting of the National Bioethics Committee," see www.mannvernd.is/english/news/imj.nbc.html#editorial (accessed December 2007).

Ch 11. NonXGovernmental Organization

1. See MacPherson, "Tapping Iceland's Genetic Jackpot."

2. See Rose, *Commodification of Bioinformation,* for an opening in this direction.

3. MacPherson, "Tapping Iceland's Genetic Jackpot."

4. deCODE Genetics, "Non-Confidential Corporate Summary," 4.

5. deCODE Genetics, *deCODE Genetics Inc.: The Population-Based Genomics Company, Corporate Profile June 1999,* 25.

6. deCODE Genetics, U.S. Securities and Exchange Commission Form 10-Q, for the period ending June 30, 2000, p. 17, www.sec.gov/Archives/edgar/data/1022974/0000893220-00-000955.txt (accessed December 2007).

7. Anderson, "DeCODE Proposal for an Icelandic Health Database."

8. Anderson, "Comments on the Security Targets for the Icelandic Health Database."

9. Arnardóttir, Björgvinsson, and Matthíasson, "The Icelandic Health Sector Database," 347.

10. That "justice is always deferred" defers a much more complicated and volatile argument concerning the deconstructibilty of the law and the undeconstructibility of justice and how the "force of law" plays at the limit between the two. I have been guided in my thinking on this by numerous sources, beginning with Derrida, "Force of Law: The Mystical Foundation of Authority"; Cornell, *Philosophy of the Limit;* and Cornell, *Transformations: Recollective Imagination and Sexual Difference.*

11. McPhee, "Cooling the Lava," 136, 179.

12. Einar Árnason and P. R. Grant, "The Significance of Kleptoparasitism during the Breeding Season in a Colony of Arctic Skuas *Stercorarius parasiticus* in Iceland," *Ibis* 120 (1998): 41–42.

13. The letter from deCODE is available at Mannvernd, www.mannvernd.is/english (accessed December 2002).

14. The Ministry of Health and Social Security letter is available at Mannvernd, www.mannvernd.is/english (accessed December 2002).

15. Einar's letters are available at Mannvernd, www.mannvernd.is/english (accessed December 2002).

16. The text of the interview with the director general of pubic health reads: "It was discussed that it would be attempted to ensure the participation of a representative of patients in the committee. It was pointed out to me that there were so many different associations of patients and it could be difficult to reach an agree-

ment about their representative. Instead the road was taken to let the Director General of Public Health nominate one member and that member could be partly looked at as a representative of patients. I do not think that it makes the most difference who appoints the committee but rather who is appointed. The people who have now been chosen for the committee are all good people, independent and trustworthy and I am confident that they will do their work with diligence." *Icelandic Medical Journal* 85 (1999): 724–25, available at Mannvernd, www.mann vernd.is/english/news/imj.nbe.html (accessed December 2007).

Ch 12. IcelandXWorld

1. The primacy of the "and" is stressed by Gilles Deleuze: "The whole of grammar, the whole of the syllogism, is a way of maintaining the subordination of conjunctions to the verb to be, of making them gravitate around the verb to be. One must go further: one must make the encounter with relations penetrate and corrupt everything, undermine being, make it topple over. Substitute the AND for IS. A *and* B. The AND is not even a specific relation or conjunction, it is that which subtends all relations, the path of all relations, which makes relations shoot outside their terms and outside the set of their terms, and outside everything that could be determined as Being, One , or Whole. The AND as extra-being, inter-being. Relations might still establish themselves between their terms, or between two sets, from one to the other, but the AND gives relations another direction, and puts to flight terms and sets, the former and the latter on the line of flight which it actively creates. Think *with* AND, instead of thinking IS, instead of thinking *for* IS: empiricism has never had another secret." Deleuze and Parnet, *Dialogues,* 57.

2. Hjálmarsson, *History of Iceland,* 180.

3. Quoted in Pálsson, "Human-Environmental Relations," 63.

4. Lockhart and Winzeler, "Genomics, Gene Expression and DNA Arrays," 830.

5. Weinstein, "Fishing Expeditions," 628.

6. Kaiser, "Population Databases Boom," 1160.

7. See, for example, Hilary Rose's analysis of Sweden's Uman Genomics in Rose, "An Ethical Dilemma."

8. Wallace, "Opportunity, Not Exploitation: Valuing the Icelandic Genome."

9. Sigurdsson, "Electric Memories and Progressive Forgetting," 135.

10. Quoted in Hjálmarsson, *History of Iceland,* 117.

11. Björnsdóttir, "Public View and Private Voices," 102.

12. Hjálmarsson, *History of Iceland,* 130.

13. Gudjonsson, "BBC Interview."

14. Laxness, *Atom Station,* 72.

15. Strauss, "It May Be Small, But Reykjavík Rocks Big Time."

16. If genomics was the most contentious topic debated by the Althingi in the late 1990s, the legalization of beer was the most contentious topic debated by the Althingi in the late 1980s; see Gunnlaugsson, *Wayward Icelanders,* chapter 3.

17. Laxness, *Atom Station,* 152.

18. Hjálmarsson, *History of Iceland,* 103.

19. Quoted in Jónas Hallgrímsson, *Selected Poetry and Prose*, tr. and ed. Dick Ringler (Madison: University of Wisconsin–Madison General Library System, 1999), http://digital.library.wisc.edu/1711.dl/Jonas (accessed December 2007).

20. Laxness, *Atom Station,* 60–61.

Ch 13. PublicXPrivate

1. Slud, "Boom Time for Biotech."

2. Steve Flaks quoted in Gillis, "Putting 'Buy' in Biotech," E1.

3. See Licking et al., "Move Over, Dot-Coms."

4. See O'Brien, "Fund Manager Sees Biotech Bubble."

5. Fisher, "Biotechnology Rally Continues."

6. McGarry, "Biotech Stocks Push Key Index Up 12%."

7. "International Large-Scale Sequencing Meeting," *Human Genome News* 7.6 (April–June 1996), www.ornl.gov/sci/techresources/Human_Genome/publicat/hgn/v7n6/19intern.shtml (accessed December 2007).

8. Gillis, "Putting 'Buy' in Biotech," E-1.

9. See Boyce and Coghlan, "Your Genes in Their Hands."

10. Williams, "Listen Up, Genomics Day Traders!"

11. Bloomberg News, "Biotech Stocks Rally as Clinton Clarifies Policy."

12. Pender, "Biotech Stocks Make for a Thrill Ride."

13. Turner, "Dresdner's Biotech Fund Springs Back to Health."

14. Luskin, "Genome Gnomes Cause Market Mayhem." Subsequent Luskin quotations are also from this source.

15. *Nature Biotechnology,* "Accidental Death of a Bubble," 469.

16. "What Does It Mean to Be a Genomics Company in a Post-genomics Era?" BioSpace.com, www.biospace.com/articles/biogenomics.cfm (accessed January 15, 2001).

17. The term "story stocks" dates to around 1994, when "certain stocks for which an intriguing argument could be made—called story stocks—began responding largely to chat-room comment and newsletter hype." That, at least, is the intriguing argument made by Browning, "False Negatives," A1.

18. Shiller, *Irrational Exuberance*.

Ch 14. Open FutureXSafe Harbor

1. See Fortun and Fortun, "Due Diligence and the Pursuit of Transparency."

2. U.S. Securities and Exchange Commission, "Concept Release and Notice of Hearing: Safe Harbor for Forward-Looking Statements." The quotations immediately following are from this document unless otherwise indicated.

3. *Marx v. Computer Sciences Corporation,* 507 F.2d 485 (9th Cir. 1974).

4. U.S. Securities and Exchange Commission, "Concept Release and Notice

of Hearing: Safe Harbor for Forward-Looking Statements." The SEC also noted "more extreme positions" taken by some courts, which ruled that "soft," "puffy" statements "upon which no reasonable investor would rely" would not be actionable unless they were worded in the language of a guarantee.

5. Ibid. The footnote to this passage refers to two documents to substantiate the SEC's historical argument: R. Eccles and S. Mavrinac, "Improving the Corporate Disclosure Process" (working paper, Harvard Business School, Boston, 1994) and "Your Company's Most Important Asset: Intellectual Capital," *Fortune*, October 3, 1994, p. 68.

6. U.S. Securities and Exchange Commission, "Concept Release and Notice of Hearing: Safe Harbor for Forward-Looking Statements."

7. *Washington Post*, "Override the Securities Bill Veto," A18. This editorial was inserted in the *Congressional Record* by advocates of the legislation.

8. Quoted in U.S. Securities and Exchange Commission, "Concept Release and Notice of Hearing: Safe Harbor for Forward-Looking Statements." In another example of the mass media being aimed at the reading and citational practices of a few readers, this editorial too was included in the *Congressional Record*.

9. Protected corporations in federal courts, at least. One effect of the PSLRA was to create a rush to file suits in various state courts, a problem addressed by the Securities Litigation Uniform Standards Act of 1998, which preempts class-action suits being filed in state courts; see Lerach, "The Private Securities Litigation Reform Act of 1995 — 27 Months Later," Lerach also states that "there is little doubt now that Congress legislated [the PSLRA] on the basis of erroneous data in 1995" (601). But that's a different story.

10. See, for example, Perino, "What We Know and Don't Know about the Private Securities Litigation Reform Act of 1995," testimony before the Subcommittee on Finance and Hazardous Materials of the Committee on Commerce, U.S. House of Representatives, October 21, 1997, available from Stanford Law School, Securities Class Action Clearinghouse http://securities.stanford.edu/research/reports/19971021.html (accessed July 2, 2000).

11. Weiss and Moser, "Enter Yossarian."

12. Branson, "Securities Litigation in State Courts," 518–19

13. Rosen, "The Statutory Safe Harbor for Forward-Looking Statements," 656–57. Rosen continues in this passage to rely on the reasonable investor: "I would submit that, however anomalous the result may seem on the facts of a particular case, this result is correct as a matter of policy as well. The theory of the Act — like that of much prior case law — is that no reasonable investor could rely on a forward-looking statement in light of specific attendant risk disclosures, so a prediction that is adequately hedged with concrete cautionary language simply is not material" (657).

Ch 15. ManiaXFundamentals

1. Herrera, "Talkin' 'Bout My GENEration."

2. Garber, *Famous First Bubbles*, 6.

3. Alan Greenspan, quoted in ibid., 7.

4. Galbraith, *Short History of Financial Euphoria*, 1.

5. Kindleberger, *Manias, Panics and Crashes*, 27. J. L. Austin claims the name "expositives" for such speech acts, although he admits that these are "difficult to define. They make plain how our utterances fit into the course of an argument or conversation, how we are using words, or, in general, are expository. Examples are 'I reply', 'I argue', 'I concede', 'I illustrate', 'I postulate'. We should be clear from the start that there are still wide possibilities of marginal or awkward cases, or of overlaps." Austin, *How to Do Things with Words*, 152.

6. Although Derrida and deconstruction are usually credited with the insight that all grounds are already undermined, the argument is also one made by Gilles Deleuze: "The world of the ground is undermined by what it tries to exclude, by the simalcrum which draws it in only to fragment it. . . . An entire multiplicity rumbles underneath the 'sameness' of the Idea." Gilles Deleuze, *Difference and Repetition* (New York: Columbia University Press, 1994), 274.

Ch 16. PromiseXDisclosure

1. "Hype" is often intensified as "mere hype" in the same way that "promise" is always open to the intensification of "empty promise." But "hype" is itself an interesting word with uncertain but probably hybrid origins, with an open-ended meaning that depends, not surprisingly, on the more general economy of language into which it is inserted and analyzed, and in which it operates. What "hype" *is* must be speculated on, an operation that thus partakes of the rhetoric of hyperbole itself. In the *American Heritage Dictionary,* for example, one finds a disdainful set of tropes for both "hype" and "hyperbole":

hype 1. Excessive publicity and the ensuing commotion: *the hype surrounding the murder trial.* 2. Exaggerated or extravagant claims made especially in advertising or promotional material: *"It is pure hype, a gigantic PR job"* (Saturday Review). 3. An advertising or promotional ploy: *"Some restaurant owners in town are cooking up a $75,000 hype to promote New York as 'Restaurant City, U.S.A.'"* (New York). 4. Something deliberately misleading; a deception: *"[He] says that there isn't any energy crisis at all, that it's all a hype, to maintain outrageous profits for the oil companies"* (Joel Oppenheimer). —hype *tr.v.* hyped, hyping, hypes. To publicize or promote, especially by extravagant, inflated, or misleading claims: *hyped the new book by sending its author on a promotional tour.* [Partly from *hype,* a swindle (perhaps from hyper-) and partly from hype(rbole).]

hy • per • bo • le *n.* A figure of speech in which exaggeration is used for emphasis or effect, as in *I could sleep for a year* or *This book weighs a ton.* [Latin *hyperbolē,* from Greek *huperbolē,* excess, from *huperballein,* to exceed : *huper,* beyond; see HYPER- + *ballein,* to throw;

But the *Random House Dictionary* expects and/or produces a different economy of signification and meaning:

Hype: 1. to stimulate, excite, or agitate (usually fol. by up): *She was hyped up at the thought of owning her own car.* 2. to create interest in by flamboyant or dramatic methods; promote or publicize showily . . . 3. to intensify (advertising, promotion, or publicity) by ingenious or questionable claims, methods, etc. (usually fol. by *up*) 4. to trick; gull . . . 5. exaggerated publicity; hoopla. 6. an ingenious or questionable claim, method, etc. . . . [1925–30, *Amer.*; in sense "to trick, swindle," of uncert. orig.; subsequent sense perh. by reanalysis as a shortening of HYPERBOLE]

Hyperbole is also given a slightly different set of inflections, in which both speaker and recipient are assumed to be more critically equipped, as *already expecting or anticipating* the hyperbolic effects:

Hyperbole: 1. obvious and intentional exaggeration. 2. an extravagant statement or figure of speech not intended to be taken literally, as "to wait an eternity."

2. Each of these different operations might be gathered under a name like "conceptual leveraging." I have learned to trace the productive limits of various forms of truth seeking—platonism, the Hegelian *Aufheben,* philosophy more generally, psychoanalytic theory, and literature, among others—from the extensive, disseminated writings of Jacques Derrida. Derrida, *Post Card: From Socrates to Freud and Beyond,* is a valuable starting point for coming to terms with the disjunctions that bind and separate truth and speculation in any system of writing.

3. Grose, New Icelandic Saga," 43.

4. See the "GenomicsXSlot Machines" chapter for further detail on Iceland's "gray market."

5. See "SameXDifference" and also Árnason, Sigurgislason, and Benedikz, "Genetic Homogeneity of Icelanders: Fact or Fiction?"

6. deCODE Genetics press release, March 9, 2000.

7. deCODE Genetics, U.S. Securities and Exchange Commission S-1 Registration Statement, March 8, 2000, www.sec.gov/Archives/edgar/data/1022974/00 00950123–00–002076.txt (accessed December 2007). All quotations from deCODE's SEC S-1 filing are from this source.

8. See Fortun and Fortun, "Due Diligence and the Pursuit of Transparency," and Maurer, *Mutual Life, Limited.*

9. Mannvernd letter to U.S. Securities and Exchange Commission, Division of Corporate Finance, March 31, 2000, in author's possession. Subsequent Mannvernd quotations are also from this letter.

Ch 17. Yahoo!XFinance

1. deCODE Genetics, U.S. Securities and Exchange Commission Form 10-Q, for the period ending June 30, 2000, p. 33, www.sec.gov/Archives/edgar/data/10 22974/0000893220–00–000955.txt (accessed December 2007).

2. Message posted to Raging Bull: deCODE genetics Message Board, July 19, 2000, http://ragingbull.lycos.com/mboard/boards.cgi?board=DCGN&read=117 (accessed January 10, 2001).

3. Casinomom, message posted to Raging Bull: deCODE genetics Message Board, July 18, 2000, http://ragingbull.lycos.com/mboard/boards.cgi?board=DC GN&read=96 (accessed January 10, 2001).

4. Casinomom, message posted to Raging Bull: deCODE genetics Message Board, http://ragingbull.lycos.com/mboard/boards.cgi?board=DCGN&read=206 (accessed January 10, 2001).

5. Casinomom, message posted to Raging Bull: deCODE genetics Message Board, July 18, 2000, http://ragingbull.lycos.com/mboard/boards.cgi?board=DC GN&read=70 (accessed January 10, 2001).

6. Message posted to Yahoo! Message Boards—deCODE genetics, Inc. (DCGN), August 28, 2000, http://messages.yahoo.com/bbs?.mm=FN&board= 1600905257&tid=dcgn&sid=1600905257&action=m&mid=94 (accessed January 10, 2001).

7. Message posted to Yahoo! Message Boards—deCODE genetics, Inc. (DCGN), August 31, 2000, http://messages.yahoo.com/bbs?.mm=FN&board=1600905257 &tid=dcgn&sid=1600905257&action=m&mid=106 (accessed January 10, 2001).

8. Decodege, message posted to Yahoo! Message Boards—deCODE genetics, Inc. (DCGN), August 8, 2000, http://messages.yahoo.com/bbs?.mm=FN& board=1600905257&tid=dcgn&sid=1600905257&action=m&mid=26 (accessed January 10, 2001).

9. Decodege, message posted to Yahoo! Message Boards—deCODE genetics, Inc. (DCGN), August 9, 2000, http://messages.yahoo.com/bbs?.mm=FN& board=1600905257&tid=dcgn&sid=1600905257&action=m&mid=29 (accessed January 10, 2001).

10. Decodege, message posted to Yahoo! Message Boards—deCODE genetics, Inc. (DCGN), August 10, 2000, http://messages.yahoo.com/bbs?.mm=FN& board=1600905257&tid=dcgn&sid=1600905257&action=m&mid=40 (accessed January 10, 2001).

11. Message posted to Yahoo! Message Boards—deCODE genetics, Inc. (DCGN), August 9, 2000, http://messages.yahoo.com/bbs?.mm=FN&board= 1600905257&tid=dcgn&sid=1600905257&action=m&mid=32 (accessed January 10, 2001).

12. Message posted to Yahoo! Message Boards—deCODE genetics, Inc. (DCGN), August 10, 2000, http://messages.yahoo.com/bbs?.mm=FN&board= 1600905257&tid=dcgn&sid=1600905257&action=m&mid=38 (accessed January 10, 2001).

13. Flunked_biology101, message posted to Yahoo! Message Boards—deCODE genetics, Inc. (DCGN), August 16, 2000, http://messages.yahoo.com/bbs?.mm= FN&board=1600905257&tid=dcgn&sid=1600905257&action=m&mid=52 (accessed January 10, 2001).

14. Ribozyme, message posted to Yahoo! Message Boards—deCODE genetics, Inc. (DCGN), August 17, 2000, http://messages.yahoo.com/bbs?.mm=FN& board=1600905257&tid=dcgn&sid=1600905257&action=m&mid=53 (accessed January 10, 2001).

15. Message posted to Yahoo! Message Boards—deCODE genetics, Inc. (DCGN),

August 18, 2000, http://messages.yahoo.com/bbs?.mm=FN&board=1600905257& tid=dcgn&sid=1600905257&action=m&mid=55 (accessed January 10, 2001).

16. Message posted to Yahoo! Message Boards—deCODE genetics, Inc. (DCGN), August 18, 2000, http://messages.yahoo.com/bbs?.mm=FN&action=m&board=1600905257&tid=dcgn&sid=1600905257&mid=58 (accessed January 10, 2001).

17. deCODE Genetics and Roche press release, August 18, 2000, www.decode.com/news/releases/item.ehtm?id=3626 (accessed January 10, 2001).

18. NASDAQ Charts, deCODE Genetics, http://charting nasdaq.com/ext/charts.dll?2–1-14–0-0–5120–03NAooooooDCGN=&SF:4|5-WD=484-HT+395—XTBL (accessed December 2007).

19. Message posted to Yahoo! Message Boards—deCODE genetics, Inc. (DCGN), August 18, 2000, http://messages.yahoo.com/bbs?.mm=FN&board=1600905257&tid=dcgn&sid=1600905257&action=m&mid=63 (accessed January 10, 2001).

20. Message posted to Yahoo! Message Boards—deCODE genetics, Inc. (DCGN), August 18, 2000, http://messages.yahoo.com/bbs?.mm=FN&board=1600905257&tid=dcgn&sid=1600905257&action=m&mid=64 (accessed January 10, 2001). It's worth noting, however, that press releases don't always work their forward-looking magic. A deCODE-Roche press release announcing the achievement of another milestone—the putative mapping of a "gene" for osteoporosis to some "small" chromosomal region—did nothing for the stock value later that year. In fact, shares dipped from $18.875 on November 14, 2000, when the numbingly unspecific press release was released, to $13.563 on November 22.

21. Jabbiz, message posted to Yahoo! Message Boards—deCODE genetics, Inc. (DCGN), August 28, 2000, http://messages.yahoo.com/bbs?.mm=FN&board=1600905257&tid=dcgn&sid=1600905257&action=m&mid=90 (accessed January 10, 2001).

22. Message posted to Yahoo! Message Boards—deCODE genetics, Inc. (DCGN), September 19, 2000, http://messages.yahoo.com/bbs?.mm=FN&board=1600905257&tid=dcgn&sid=1600905257&action=m&mid=153 (accessed January 10, 2001).

23. Message posted to Yahoo! Message Boards—deCODE genetics, Inc. (DCGN), October 16, 2000, http://messages.yahoo.com/bbs?.mm=FN&board=1600905257&tid=dcgn&sid=1600905257&action=m&mid=181 (accessed January 10, 2001).

24. Message posted to Yahoo! Message Boards—deCODE genetics, Inc. (DCGN), October 11, 2000, http://messages.yahoo.com/bbs?.mm=FN&board=1600905257&tid=dcgn&sid=1600905257&action=m&mid=164 (accessed January 10, 2001).

25. Reyjo2, message posted to Yahoo! Message Boards—deCODE genetics, Inc. (DCGN), October 11, 2000, http://messages.yahoo.com/bbs?.mm=FN&board=1600905257&tid=dcgn&sid=1600905257&action=m&mid=166 (accessed January 10, 2001).

26. Message posted to Yahoo! Message Boards—deCODE genetics, Inc.

(DCGN), October 13, 2000, http://messages.yahoo.com/bbs?.mm = FN&board = 1600905257&tid = dcgn&sid = 1600905257&action = m&mid = 176 (accessed January 10, 2001).

27. Partyspoiler, message posted to Yahoo! Message Boards—deCODE genetics, Inc. (DCGN), October 15, 2000, http://messages.yahoo.com/bbs?.mm = FN&board = 1600905257&tid = dcgn&sid = 1600905257&action = m&mid = 179 (accessed January 10, 2001).

28. Message posted to Yahoo! Message Boards—deCODE genetics, Inc. (DCGN), October 25, 2000, http://messages.yahoo.com/bbs?.mm = FN&board = 1600905257&tid = dcgn&sid = 1600905257&action = m&mid = 200 (accessed January 10, 2001).

29. Madscientist69, message posted to Yahoo! Message Boards—deCODE genetics, Inc. (DCGN), October 24, 2000, http://messages.yahoo.com/bbs?.mm = FN&board = 1600905257&tid = dcgn&sid = 1600905257&action = m&mid = 197 (accessed January 10, 2001).

30. Jabbiz, message posted to Yahoo! Message Boards—deCODE genetics, Inc. (DCGN), October 28, 2000, http://messages.yahoo.com/bbs?.mm = FN&board = 1600905257&tid = dcgn&sid = 1600905257&action = m&mid = 235 (accessed January 10, 2001).

31. Message posted to Yahoo! Message Boards—deCODE genetics, Inc. (DCGN), January 10, 2001, http://messages.yahoo.com/bbs?.mm = FN&board = 1600905257&tid = dcgn&sid = 1600905257&action = m&mid = 261 (accessed January 10, 2001).

32. Message posted to Raging Bull: deCODE genetics Message Board, December 27, 2000, http://ragingbull.lycos.com/mboard/boards.cgi?board = DCGN&read = 567 (accessed January 10, 2001).

33. PaulaGem, message posted to Raging Bull: deCODE genetics Message Board, December 9, 2000, http://ragingbull.lycos.com/mboard/boards.cgi?board = DCGN&read = 561 (accessed January 10, 2001).

34. PaulaGem, message posted to Raging Bull: deCODE genetics Message Board, January 10, 2001, http://ragingbull.lycos.com/mboard/boards.cgi?board = DCGN&read = 580 (accessed January 10, 2001).

35. Message posted to Yahoo! Message Boards—deCODE genetics, Inc. (DCGN), April 22, 2001, http://messages.yahoo.com/bbs?.mm = FN&board = 1600905257&tid = dcgn&sid = 1600905257&action = m&mid = 370 (accessed July 2, 2001).

36. Message posted to Yahoo! Message Boards—deCODE genetics, Inc. (DCGN), April 22, 2001, http://messages.yahoo.com/bbs?.mm = FN&action = m&board = 1600905257&tid = dcgn&sid = 1600905257&mid = 371 (accessed July 2, 2001).

37. Message posted to Yahoo! Message Boards—deCODE genetics, Inc. (DCGN), May 14, 2001, http://messages.yahoo.com/bbs?.mm = FN&board = 1600905257&tid = dcgn&sid = 1600905257&action = m&mid = 381 (accessed July 2, 2001).

38. Jabbiz, message posted to Yahoo! Message Boards—deCODE genetics, Inc. (DCGN), April 23, 2001, http://messages.yahoo.com/bbs?.mm = FN&action = m&board = 1600905257&tid = dcgn&sid = 1600905257&mid = 373; (accessed July 2, 2001).

39. Message posted to Yahoo! Message Boards—deCODE genetics, Inc.

(DCGN), April 23, 2001, http://messages.yahoo.com/bbs?.mm=FN&action=m& board=1600905257&tid=dcgn&sid=1600905257&mid=375; (accessed July 2, 2001).

40. Message posted to Yahoo! Message Boards—deCODE genetics, Inc. (DCGN), April 25, 2001, http://messages.yahoo.com/bbs?.mm=FN&action=m& board=1600905257&tid=dcgn&sid=1600905257&mid=377 (accessed July 2, 2001).

41. IceFresh, message posted to Raging Bull: deCODE genetics Message Board, February 27, 2001, http://ragingbull.lycos.com/mboard/boards.cgi?board =DCGN&read=595 (accessed July 2, 2001).

Ch 18. SameXDifference

1. Jón Baldvin Hannibalsson, letter to the editor, *Washington Post,* January 25, 1999, available at Mannvernd, www.mannvernd.is/english/news/jon.baldvin .WP.ensk.html(accessed March 31, 2004).

2. Message posted to Yahoo! Message Boards—deCODE genetics, Inc. (DCGN), December 7, 2000, http://messages.yahoo.com/bbs?.mm=FN&board =1600905257&tid=dcgn&sid=1600905257&action=m&mid=246 (accessed January 10, 2001).

3. Message posted to Yahoo! Message Boards—deCODE genetics, Inc. (DCGN), December 9, 2000, http://messages.yahoo.com/bbs?.mm=FN&board =1600905257&tid=dcgn&sid=1600905257&action=m&mid=250 (accessed January 10, 2001).

4. One of the founders of Myriad Genetics, Mark Skolnick, was one of four authors of the 1980 scientific paper that first laid out some of the fundamental ideas and techniques for using recombinant DNA technologies to map the genomes of humans and pull out genes implicated in disease. Myriad can also boast Nobel laureate Walter Gilbert as one of its directors. Myriad has alienated a number of scientists in the breast cancer genetics community, however, through its rush to isolate and patent the BRCA-1 gene. See Sarah Zielinski, "BRCA1 Discovery Led to Patent Debate, Genetic Screening," *Journal of the National Cancer Institute* 96 (July 7, 2004): 986.

5. Message posted to Raging Bull: deCODE genetics Message Board, December 29, 2000, http://ragingbull.lycos.com/mboard/boards.cgi?board=DCGN &read=574 (accessed January 10, 2001). The *Washington Post* article referred to is "In Rural China, a Genetic Mother Lode: Harvard-Led Study Mined DNA Riches; Some Donors Say Promises Were Broken," www.washingtonpost.com/ wp-dyn/articles/A26797-2000Dec19.html.

6. Marshall, "Gene Prospecting in Remote Populations."

7. See Greely, "Iceland's Plan for Genomics Research," and Winickoff, "Genome and Nation" for additional discussion of this letter.

8. Kevin Kinsella, letter to Kári Stefánsson, May 26, 1995, copy in possession of the author, also cited in Winickoff, "Genome and Nation." Subsequent quotations from this letter are from the author's copy.

9. For summaries of how genomics has fissured, if not completely voided, racial

categories, see Shields et al., "The Use of Racial Categories in Genetic Studies of Smoking Behavior"; Wilson et al. "Population Genetic Structure of Variable Drug Response"; and Haga and Venter, "FDA Races in Wrong Direction."

10. See Chakravarti, "Population Genetics—Making Sense Out of Sequence."

11. Einar Árnason, Hlynur Sigurgíslason, and Eiríkur Benedikz, "Genetic Homogeneity of Icelanders: Snake Oil or Restorative?" November 15, 1999, p. 3, manuscript provided to the author by Einar Árnason.

12. Quotations from the reviewers are from *Nature Genetics,* letter and reviews sent to Einar Árnason, January 24, 2000, provided to the author by Einar Árnason.

13. Einar Árnason, Hlynur Sigurgíslason, and Eiríkur Benedikz, "Genetic Homogeneity of Icelanders: Fact or Fiction?" February 15, 2000, p. 5, manuscript provided to the author by Einar Árnason.

14. Quotations from the second review are from *Nature Genetics,* letter and reviews sent to Einar Árnason, March 22, 2000, provided to the author by Einar Árnason.

15. Árnason et al., "Genetic Homogeneity of Icelanders: Fact or Fiction?" 374.

16. This and subsequent quotations are from Ann Snider, "Mining the Icelandic Genome," Stock Watch column, SmartMoney.com, July 10, 2000, www.smart money.com/stockwatch/index.cfm?story=200007101 (accessed December 2007).

17. For more on Charles Sanders Peirce, the abductive process, and the gaps, leaps, and twists that inhabit the sciences and their methods, see M. Fortun, "Human Genome Project and the Acceleration of Biotechnology."

18. Árnason, "Genetic Heterogeneity of Icelanders," 6.

19. Helgason, Sigurdardottir et al., "mtDNA and the Origin of Icelanders," 1012.

20. Árnason, "Genetic Heterogeneity of Icelanders," 6.

21. Helgason, Nicholson et al., "A Reassessment of Genetic Diversity in Icelanders."

22. Abbott, "Iceland's Doctors Rebuffed in Health Data Row," 819.

23. Helgason, Nicholson et al., "A Reassessment of Genetic Diversity in Icelanders," 296.

24. Mitchell, "UK Launches Ambitious Tissue/Data Bank Project," 529.

25. Terwilliger and Weiss, "Linkage Disequilibrium Mapping of Complex Disease: Fantasy or Reality?"

Ch 19. PresumedXConsent

1. Message posted to Yahoo! Message Boards—deCODE genetics, Inc. (DCGN), August 30, 2000, http://messages.yahoo.com/bbs?.mm=FN&board= 1600905257&tid=dcgn&sid=1600905257&action=m&mid=103 (accessed January 10, 2001).

2. Abbott, "Iceland's Doctors Rebuffed in Health Data Row," 819.

3. Quoted in ibid.

4. Icelandic State Radio, news hour at noon, August 23, 2000, transcript avail-

able at Mannvernd, www.mannvernd.is/english/news/eIMA.ruv2308.html (accessed December 2007).

5. Message posted to Yahoo! Message Boards—deCODE genetics, Inc. (DCGN), September 1, 2000, http://messages.yahoo.com/bbs?.mm=FN&board=1600 905257&tid=dcgn&sid=1600905257&action=m&mid=119 (accessed January 10, 2001).

6. In *Volatile Bodies: Toward a Corporeal Feminism,* Elizabeth Grosz lays some of the foundations for an understanding of bodies as volatile chiasmas. "Volatile bodies" is Grosz's name for a biological flesh that is, as a matter of fact, both inside and outside at once, contiguously, like a Möbius strip.

7. National Bioethics Advisory Commission, *Research Involving Human Biological Materials: Ethical Issues and Policy Guidance,* vol. 1 (Rockville, MD: National Bioethics Advisory Commission), 64–65, http://bioethics.georgetown.edu/nbac/ hbm.pdf (accessed December 2007).

8. National Bioethics Advisory Commission, *41st Meeting of the National Bioethics Advisory Commission,* vol. 2, 273–74.

9. Quotations are from Icelandic Medical Association board to association members, January 23, 2001, English translation by Mannvernd, www.mannvernd .is/english/news/IMA_terminates.html (accessed December 2007).

10. deCODE Genetics, U.S. Securities and Exchange Commission S-1 Registration Statement, March 8, 2000, p. F14, www.sec.gov/Archives/edgar/data/ 1022974/0000950123-00-002076.txt (accessed December 2007).

11. Mannvernd, summary of Reykjavík District Court ruling of February 13, 2002," available along with original verdict in Icelandic at Mannvernd, www.mann vernd.is/english/lawsuit.html (accessed December 2007).

12. All quotations from the Supreme Court decision are from *Ragnhildur Gudmundsson v. The State of Iceland,* Icelandic Supreme Court, no. 151/2003, November 27, 2003, English translation by Mannvernd available with Icelandic original at Mannvernd www.mannvernd.is/english/lawsuit.html (accessed December 2007).

13. Abbott, "Icelandic Database Shelved as Court Judges Privacy in Peril," 118.

14. Orlean, "Where's Willy?" 45.

15. Nina Berglund, "Keiko Secretly Buried On Shore," *Aftenposten,* December 15, 2003, www.aftenposten.no/english/local/article691382.ece (accessed December 30, 2007).

Ch 20. GenomicsXSlot Machines

1. Quoted in Burke, "Haseltine Says Biopharma, Duped by HGP, Should Turn to Expression Genomics."

2. Burke, "Haseltine Says Biopharma, Duped by HGP, Should Turn to Expression Genomics."

3. Roche's payments can be gleaned from deCODE's 10-K statement filed with the SEC for fiscal year 2001, when a new agreement was negotiated with Roche and the first one terminated. See Skúli Sigurdsson, "Springtime in Iceland and

$200 Million Promises," April 20, 2002, www.raunvis.hi.is/~sksi/e_web.html (accessed July 2005).

4. deCODE Genetics, U.S. Securities and Exchange Commission Form 10–12B/A, June 20, 2000, p. 4, www.sec.gov/Archives/edgar/data/1022974/0000 893220-00-000774.txt (accessed December 2007). Series A preferred stock is the stock owned by venture capitalists; Series C stock is the stock owned by Roche; the Series B stock sold to Icelanders came in part from a repurchase of Series A and C stocks and a repurchase of 333,333 shares of Kári's common stock.

5. deCODE Genetics, U.S. Securities and Exchange Commission S-1 Registration Statement, March 8, 2000, exhibit 10.32, p. 6, www.sec.gov/Archives/edgar/data/1022974/0000950123-00-002076.txt (accessed December 2007).

6. Skúli first faxed me the legal notices about the Luxembourg company in the fall of 2003, having received them anonymously. Mannvernd also received them anonymously and packed the documents together with excerpts from deCODE's SEC filings, annotated the whole bunch, and made sure they got to Icelandic reporters.

7. Quotations from the *Guardian* article are from Meek, "Decode Was Meant to Save Lives."

8. Jónatansson, "Iceland's Health Sector Database," 53.

9. This and the subsequent quotation are from Toobin, "The Man Chasing Enron," 87, 88.

10. This and the subsequent quotation are from *Linda Rubin v. deCODE Genetics, Inc., Lehman Brothers, Inc., Morgan Stanley & Co. Incorporated, Kári Stefánsson, and Axel Nielsen*, doc. no. 01-cv-11219, filed December 6, 2001, in U.S. District Court, Southern District of New York, pp. 2, 8.

11. *Opinion and Order in re: Initial Public Offering Securities Litigation*, Shira A. Scheindlin, USDJ, U.S. District Court, Southern District of New York, doc. no. 03–01555, February 19, 2003. p. 165.

12. For a discussion of the SEC's strategies in such cases where legal proceedings may not be viable, or may simply take too long, see the interview with a former SEC lawyer in Fortun and Fortun, "Due Diligence and the Pursuit of Transparency."

13. U.S. Securities and Exchange Commission, "SEC Sues Morgan Stanley and Goldman Sachs for Unlawful IPO Allocation Practices," press release, January 25, 2005, www.sec.gov/news/press/2005-10.htm (accessed July 2006).

14. *SEC v. Morgan Stanley*, No. 1: 05 CV 00166 (Complaint), January 25, 2005, U.S. District Court, District of Columbia, , pp. 21–22, available at U.S. Securities and Exchange Commission, www.sec.gov/litigation/complaints/comp 19050.pdf (accessed July 2006).

15. Reuters, "Human Genome Founder to Retire, Company Cuts Jobs," Medscape.com, March 25, 2004, www.medscape.com/viewarticle/472494?mpid=26745 (accessed March 30, 2004).

16. *GenomeWeb News*, "Genomics Sector Has Fired More Than 1,500 Staff Since January 2001," *GenomeWeb News*, July 8, 2002, www.genomeweb.com/issues/news/120591-1.html (accessed December 2007).

17. See M. Fortun, "Celera Genomics."

18. Kevin Kinsella, letter to Kári Stefánsson, May 26, 1995, copy in possession of the author, also cited in Winickoff, "Genome and Nation."

19. See Petryna and Kleinman, *Global Pharmaceuticals: Ethics, Markets, Practices.*

20. Wolpe, "Not Just How, but Whether: Revisiting Hans Jonas," viii.

21. Fletcher, "Genomics Companies Shop Around for Chemical Expertise," 138.

Ch 21. EthicsXExpediency

1. deCODE Genetics, *Code of Ethics.*

2. Laxness, *Atom Station*, 101.

3. There are a number of rich themes in *The Atom Station* that would take too long to fully explicate, but that deserve comment. For example, the assertion of chemical and physiological sameness is a trope worth extending. An ethics of biological sameness is one of the greatest unfulfilled promises of genomics, the dream being that once every recognizes that 99.99 percent of "our" DNA is the "same," racism and al other forms of prejudice and inequality will be swept away, groundless.

This powerful promise of sameness takes place most clearly in a later scene in the novel. One night walking home, Ugla comes upon Cleopatra, a prostitute who is another frequenter of the organist's house. She is bleeding from the head and sobbing. Ugla asks what happened. "They beat me up and threw me out," Cleopatra responds. Who? asks Ugla. "Who but Icelanders? . . . They didn't want to pay. . . . It was all right while there were Yanks. But now there are only a few strays left and they all have something steady, so I have to start scratching around like when I was a girl, and going home once again with Icelanders who take snuff and beat you up and refuse to pay. . . . Dear darling Americans, Jesus let them come with the atom bomb quick."

Ugla is at first put off by this kind of venom, but she "started thinking a bit, and came to the conclusion that this girl's blood and tears were of the same chemical composition as that of other girls, and so I invited her home with me to stay the night" (131–32).

Having placed ethics under the banner of biochemistry, Laxness does the same, in effect, for all human interactions: "Words themselves say least of all, if in fact they say anything; what really informs us is the inflection of the voice (and no less so if it is restrained), the breathing, the heart-beat, the muscles round the mouth and eyes, the dilation and contraction of the pupils, the strength or the weakness in the knees, as well as the chain of mysterious reactions in the nerves and the secretions from hidden glands whose names one never knows even though one reads about them in books; all that is the essence of a conversation—the words are more or less incidental" (176).

4. Those interested in making claims about the "Harvard mafia" that became critics of deCODE and the Health Sector Database would be sure to include Winickoff in that grouping. One godfather of that "mafia" would be Richard

Lewontin, population geneticist colleague of Einar Árnason and writer of the letter to the *New York Times* that became a focus of Pálsson and Rabinow's ire. Another godfather would be historian of science (and my thesis advisor) Everett Mendelsohn; as a Harvard Law School student, Winickoff was a teaching assistant for one of Mendelsohn's hugely popular lecture courses, just as my advance man and I had once been.

5. Winickoff and Winickoff, "Charitable Trust as a Model for Genomic Biobanks," 1180.

Ch 22. EverythingXNothing

1. Maurer, *Mutual Life, Limited,* 175.

2. *Webster's Revised Unabridged Dictionary* supplies a geological sense for "trend" that aligns with my fissure metaphors: "trend 2. (Geol. & Mining) A dislocation caused by a slipping of rock masses along a plane of facture; also, the dislocated structure resulting from such slipping."

3. Greely, "Iceland's Plan for Genomics Research," 108n1.

4. Jones, "You, Too, Can Speak Genomics!!!" 74.

5. Section epigraphs: Derrida, "To Speculate—On 'Freud,'" in *The Post Card,* 277; Dennis Purcell quoted in Dorey, "Biotechnology Becomes the New Dot Com," 140.

6. McCaffery, "The Reason to Avoid Biotech Stocks."

7. Herrera, "Talkin' 'Bout My GENEration."

8. Derrida, *Specters of Marx,* xvii.

9. Laxness, *Atom Station,* 175.

10. See Grosz, *Volatile Bodies.*

11. Kindleberger, *Manias, Panics and Crashes,* 220.

Bibliography

Abbott, A. "DNA Study Deepens Rift Over Iceland's Genetic Heritage." *Nature* 421 (February 13, 2003): 678.

———. "Icelandic Database Shelved as Court Judges Privacy in Peril." *Nature* 429 (May 13, 2004): 118.

———. "Iceland's Doctors Rebuffed in Health Data Row." *Nature* 406 (August 23, 2000): 819.

Anderson, R. "Comments on the Security Targets for the Icelandic Health Database." www.ftp.cl.cam.ac.uk/ftp/users/rja14/iceland-admiral.pdf (accessed December 30, 2007).

———. "The deCODE Proposal for an Icelandic Health Database." October 20, 1998. www.cl.cam.ac.uk/~rja14/iceland/iceland.html (accessed December 30, 2007).

Andrews, E. L. "U.S. Seeks Patent on Genetic Code, Setting Off Furor." *New York Times,* October 21, 1991, A1.

Arnardóttir, O. M., D. T. Björgvinsson, V. M. Matthíasson. "The Icelandic Health Sector Database." *European Journal of Health and Law* 6.4 (1999): 307–62.

Árnason, E. "Genetic Heterogeneity of Icelanders." *Annals of Human Genetics* 67.1 (2003): 5–16.

Árnason, E., H. Sigurgislason, and E. Benedikz. "Genetic Homogeneity of Icelanders: Fact or Fiction?" *Nature Genetics* 25 (August 2000): 373–74.

Arnst, C. "An Icelandic Saga about Privacy and DNA." *Business Week,* March 27, 2000, p. 109.

Auden, W. H., and L. MacNeice. *Letters from Iceland.* 1937. London: Faber and Faber, 1965.

Austin, J. L. *How to Do Things with Words.* Cambridge, MA: Harvard University Press, 1962.

Billings, P. "Iceland, Blood and Science." *American Scientist* 87 (May-June 1999): 199.

Björnsdóttir, I. D. "Public View and Private Voices." In *The Anthropology of Iceland*, ed. G. Pálsson and E. P. Durrenberger, 98–118. Iowa City: University of Iowa Press, 1989.

Bloomberg News. "Biotech Stocks Rally as Clinton Clarifies Policy." *Boston Globe*, April 6, 2000, E2.

Boyce, N., and A. Coghlan. "Your Genes in Their Hands." *New Scientist*, May 20, 2000, p. 15.

Branson, D. "Securities Litigation in State Courts: Something Old, Something New, Something Borrowed . . ." *Washington University Law Quarterly* 76.2 (Summer 1998): 509–36.

Browning. E. S. "False Negatives." *Wall Street Journal*, February 25, 2000, A1.

Burke, A. "Haseltine Says Biopharma, Duped by HGP, Should Turn to Expression Genomics." *GenomeWeb News*, September 19, 2002. www.genomeweb.com/issues/news/120781–1.html (accessed December 2007).

Chakravarti, A. "Population Genetics—Making Sense Out of Sequence." *Nature Genetics Supplement* 21 (January 1999): 56–60.

CIBA Foundation. *Human Genetic Information: Science, Law, and Ethics*. New York: John Wiley and Sons, 1989.

Cornell, D. *The Philosophy of the Limit*. New York: Routledge, 1992.

——. *Transformations: Recollective Imagination and Sexual Difference*. New York: Routledge, 1992.

Crenson, M. "National Treasure or Black Hole?" *Pittsburgh (PA) Post-Gazette*, March 25, 2001, C3.

deCODE Genetics. *Code of Ethics*. Reykjavík: deCODE Genetics, 1999.

——. *deCODE Genetics Inc.: The Population-Based Genomics Company, Corporate Profile June 1999* (Reykjavík: deCODE Genetics, 1999).

——. "Non-Confidential Corporate Summary." Reykjavík: deCODE Genetics, 1998.

Deleuze, G., and C. Parnet. *Dialogues*. 1977. New York: Columbia University Press, 1987.

Derrida, J. "Force of Law: The Mystical Foundation of Authority." *Cordoza Law Review* 11.5–6 (1990): 920–1045.

——. *Given Time: I. Counterfeit Money*. Chicago: University of Chicago Press, 1992.

——. *Monolingualism of the Other; or, The Prosthesis of Origin*. Palo Alto, CA: Stanford University Press, 1998.

——. *The Post Card: From Socrates to Freud and Beyond*. Chicago: University of Chicago Press, 1987.

——. *Specters of Marx: The State of the Debt, the Work of Mourning, and the New International*. New York: Routledge, 1994.

——. *The Truth in Painting*. Chicago: University of Chicago Press, 1987.

Dorey, E. "Biotechnology Becomes the New Dot Com." *Nature Biotechnology* 18 (February 2000): 140.

Doyle, R. *Wetwares: Experiments in Postvital Living*. Minneapolis: University of Minnesota Press, 2003.

Durrenberger, E. P. *Icelandic Essays: Explorations in the Anthropology of Modern Life.* Iowa City: Rudi Publishing, 1995.

Edwards, M. "How the Elephants Dance Part 1." *Signals Magazine,* 1997. http://recap.com/signalsmag.nsf/EEFF75EF4BC76142882567290060DB96/26B8214 EACB049E28825682B00835C96?OpenDocument (accessed August 3, 2003).

Enserink, M. "Physicians Wary of Scheme to Pool Icelanders' Genetic Data." *Science* 281 (August 14, 1998): 890–91.

Erickson, D. "Incyte Serves Up Information." *In Vivo: The Business and Medicine Report,* May 1996, pp. 35–38.

Eyfjörd, J. E., H. M. Ögmundsdóttir, G. Eggertsson, and T. Zoëga. "deCODE Deferred." *Nature Biotechnology* 16 (June 1998): 496.

Felman, S. *The Scandal of the Speaking Body: Don Juan with J. L. Austin, or Seduction in Two Languages.* Stanford, CA: Stanford University Press, 2002.

Firn, D. "Takeovers May Be Cure for German Biotechs." *Financial Times,* June 15, 2000, p. 35. www.ft.com (accessed June 15, 2000).

Fisher, L. M. "Biotechnology Rally Continues." *New York Times,* February 18, 2000.

Fletcher, L. "Genomics Companies Shop Around for Chemical Expertise." *Nature Biotechnology* 22.4 (February 2004): 137–8.

Fortun, K. *Advocacy after Bhopal: Environmentalism, Globalization, and New World Orders.* Chicago: University of Chicago Press, 2001.

Fortun, M. "Celera Genomics: The Race for the Human Genome Sequence." In *Encyclopedia of Life Sciences.* Chichester, U.K.: John Wiley and Sons, 2006.

———. "Experiments in Ethnography and Its Performance." Mannvernd, February 12, 2000. www.mannvernd.is/english/articles/mfortun.html (accessed December 2007).

———. "For an Ethics of Promising, or: A Few Kind Words about James Watson." *New Genetics and Society* 24.2 (2005): 157–73.

———. "The Human Genome Project and the Acceleration of Biotechnology." In *Private Science: The Biotechnology Industry and the Rise of Contemporary Molecular Biology,* ed. A. Thackray, 182–201. Philadelphia: University of Pennsylvania Press, 1998.

———. "Mapping and Making Genes and Histories: The Genomics Project in the United States, 1980–1990." PhD diss., Harvard University, 1993.

———. "Mediated Speculations in the Genomics Futures Market." *New Genetics and Society* 20.2 (2001): 139–56.

———. "Projecting Speed Genomics." In *The Practices of Human Genetics: International and Interdisciplinary Perspectives,* ed. M. Fortun and E. Mendelsohn, 25–48. Dordrecht, The Netherlands: Kluwer, 1999.

Fortun, M., and H. J. Bernstein. *Muddling Through: Pursuing Science and Truths in the 21st Century.* Washington, DC: Counterpoint, 1998.

Fortun, M., and K. Fortun. "Due Diligence and the Pursuit of Transparency: The Securities and Exchange Commission, 1996." In *Paranoia within Reason: A Casebook on Conspiracy as Explanation,* ed. G. E. Marcus, 157–93. Chicago: University of Chicago Press, 1999.

Fortun, M., and S. Sigurdsson. "'So Human a Brain': Ethnographic Perspectives on an Interdisciplinary Conference." In *So Human a Brain: Knowledge and Values in the Neurosciences,* by A. Harrington, 325–37. Boston: Birkhäuser, 1992.

Galbraith, J. K. *A Short History of Financial Euphoria.* Ed. W. S. Rukeyser. Knoxville, TN: Whittle Communications, 1990.

Garber, P. M. *Famous First Bubbles: The Fundamentals of Early Manias.* Cambridge, MA: MIT Press, 2000.

Gibbs, W. W. "Natural-Born Guinea Pigs." *Scientific American,* February 1998, p. 24.

Gillis, J. "Putting 'Buy' in Biotech." *Washington Post,* February 25, 2000, E1.

Greely, H. T. "Iceland's Plan for Genomics Research: Facts and Implications." *Jurimetrics* 40.2 (2000): 153–91.

Greenspan, A. "Economic Volatility." Remarks at a symposium sponsored by the Federal Reserve Bank of Kansas City, Jackson Hole, WY, August 30, 2002. Federal Reserve Board. www.federalreserve.gov/boarddocs/speeches/2002/2002 0830/default.htm (accessed August 31, 2002).

Grose, T. "The New Icelandic Saga." *Time,* September 29, 1997, pp. 42–43.

Grosz, E. *Volatile Bodies: Toward a Corporeal Feminism.* Bloomington: Indiana University Press, 1994.

Gunnlaugsson, H., and J. F. Galliher. *Wayward Icelanders: Punishment, Boundary Maintenance, and the Creation of Crime.* Madison: University of Wisconsin Press, 2000.

Guthjonsson, V. "BBC Interview." 2004. www.bbc.co.uk/music/features/iceland/ fraebbb.shtml (accessed June 25, 2004).

Hafstein, S. J. "Honesty and Trust." Mannvernd, December 11, 1998. www.mann vernd.is/english/news/dagur.um.greidslur.ensk.html (accessed December 15, 1998).

Haga, S. B., and J. C. Venter. "FDA Races in Wrong Direction." *Science* 301 (July 25, 2003): 466.

Hamilton, D. "Mapping Out Stocks for the Genome Gold Rush." TheStreet.com, July 13, 2000. www.thestreet.com/stocks/biotech/999201.html (accessed December 2007).

Helgason, A., G. Nicholson, K. Stefánsson, and P. Donnelly. "A Reassessment of Genetic Diversity in Icelanders: Strong Evidence from Multiple Loci for Relative Homogeneity Cause by Genetic Drift." *Annals of Human Genetics* 67.4 (2003): 281–97.

Helgason, A., S. Sigurdardottir, J. R. Gulcher, R. Ward, and K. Stefánsson. "mtDNA and the Origin of Icelanders: Deciphering Signals of Recent Population History." *American Journal of Human Genetics* 66 (2000): 999–1016.

Herrera, S. "Talkin' 'Bout My GENEration." *Red Herring,* April 15, 2001. www.her ring.com/home/6456 (accessed May 3, 2001).

Hjálmarsson, J. *History of Iceland: From the Settlement to the Present Day.* Reykjavík: Iceland Review, 1993.

Hodgson, J. "deCODE Looks Forward as Database Law Passes." *Nature Biotechnology* 17 (February 1999): 127.

———. "A Genetic Heritage Betrayed or Empowered?" *Nature Biotechnology* 16 (November 1998): 1017–19.

Jacob, F. *The Logic of Life: A History of Heredity.* New York: Random House, 1982.

Jóhannesson, V. "Are Icelandic Politicians for Sale?" Mannvernd, November 2, 1999. www.mannvernd.is/english/articles/forsale.html (accessed December 15, 2003).

Jónatansson, H. "Iceland's Health Sector Database: A Significant Head Start in the Search for the Biological Grail or an Irreversible Error?" *American Journal of Law and Medicine* 26.1 (2000): 31–67.

Jones, M. M. "You, Too, Can Speak Genomics!!!" *Genome Technology,* April 2002, p. 74.

Kahn, J. "Attention Shoppers: Special Today—Iceland's DNA." CNN.com, February 1999. www.cnn.com/HEALTH/bioethics/9902/iceland.dna/template.html (accessed December 18, 2002).

Kaiser, J. "Population Databases Boom." *Science* 298 (November 8, 2002): 1158–61.

Keller, C. "Die Isländer, unsere Labormäuse." *Das Magazin,* October 3, 1999, pp. 13–24.

Keller, E. F. *Refiguring Life: Metaphors of Twentieth-Century Biology.* New York: Columbia University Press, 1995.

Kellogg, R. Introduction to *The Sagas of Icelanders.* New York, Penguin, 2000.

Kindleberger, C. P. *Manias, Panics and Crashes: A History of Financial Crises.* New York: Basic Books, 1978.

Kunzig, R. "Blood of the Vikings." *Discover,* December 1998, pp. 90–99.

Lalli, F. "Now Only Clinton Can Stop Congress from Hurting Small Investors Like You." *Money,* December 1995.

Langenbach, J. "Island: Kafkaeskes Gen-Fischen." *Der Standard* (Vienna), September 30–October 1, 2000, p. 37.

Laxness, H. *The Atom Station.* 1948. Sag Harbor, NY: Second Chance Press, 1982.

———. *The Fish Can Sing.* 1957. London: Harvill Press, 2001.

———. *Under the Glacier.* 1968. Reykjavík: Vaka-Helgafell, 1972.

Leonard, S. S. M. "Keiko Discovers What 'Hammer' Time Is All About." Air Force Link, September 11, 1998. www.af.mil/news/Sep1998/n19980910_981375.html (accessed June 18, 2001).

Lerach, W. S. "The Private Securities Litigation Reform Act of 1995—27 Months Later: Securities Class Action Litigation under the Private Securities Litigation Reform Act's Brave New World." *Washington University Law Quarterly* 76.2 (Summer 1998): 597–644.

Licking, E., et al. "Move Over, Dot-Coms. Biotech is Back." *Business Week,* March 26, 2000. www.businessweek.com/2000/00_10/b3671142.htm (accessed March 26, 2000).

Lockhart, D. J., and E. A. Winzeler. "Genomics, Gene Expression and DNA Arrays." *Nature* 405 (June 15, 2000): 827–36.

Luskin, D. "Genome Gnomes Cause Market Mayhem." *Red Herring,* 2000. www .redherring.com (accessed March 16, 2000).

MacPherson, K. "Tapping Iceland's Genetic Jackpot." *Newark (NJ) Star-Ledger,* December 17, 2000, pp. 1, 29–32.

Marcus, G. E. "Critical Cultural Studies as One Power/Knowledge Like, Among, and in Engagement with Others." In *Ethnography through Thick and Thin*, 203–30. Princeton, NJ: Princeton University Press, 1998.

Marcus, G. E., and M. M. J. Michael Fischer. *Anthropology as Cultural Critique: An Experimental Moment in the Human Sciences.* 2nd ed. Chicago: University of Chicago Press, 1996.

Marshall, E. "Gene Prospecting in Remote Populations." *Science* 278 (October 24, 1997): 565.

Maurer, B. *Mutual Life, Limited: Islamic Banking, Alternative Currencies, Lateral Reason.* Princeton, NJ: Princeton University Press, 2005.

McCaffery, R. "The Reason to Avoid Biotech Stocks." *Motley Fool*, April 5, 2001. www.fool.com/news/foth/2001/foth010405.htm (accessed December 30, 2007).

McGarry, D. "Biotech Stocks Push Key Index Up 12%." 2000. www.cbsmarketwatch.com (accessed February 16, 2000).

McPhee, J. "Cooling the Lava." In *The Control of Nature*, 95–179. New York: Farrar, Straus and Giroux, 1989.

Meek, J. "Decode Was Meant to Save Lives . . . Now It's Destroying Them." *Guardian* (Manchester), October 31, 2002. www.guardian.co.uk/science/2002/oct/31/genetics.businessofresearch.

Merz, J. F., G. E. McGee, and P. Sankar. "'Iceland Inc.': On the Ethics of Commercial Population Genomics." *Social Science and Medicine* 58.6 (2004): 1201–9.

Mitchell, P. "UK Launches Ambitious Tissue/Data Bank Project." *Nature Biotechnology* 20 (June 2002): 529.

Muldoon, K. "Keiko May Be Moved Unless He Swims Free; Will He?" *Oregonian*, June 9, 2001.

National Bioethics Advisory Commission. *41st Meeting of the National Bioethics Advisory Commission*, vol. 2. Rockville, MD: National Bioethics Advisory Commission, 2000. http://bioethics.georgetown.edu/nbac/transcripts/june00/6–5-00–2.pdf (accessed December 2007).

Nature Biotechnology. "Accidental Death of a Bubble." *Nature Biotechnology* 18 (May 2000): 469.

———. "Keep the Story Straight." *Nature Biotechnology* 16 (June 1998): 491.

Nature Genetics. "Genome Vikings." *Nature Genetics* 20 (October 1998): 99–101.

Nietzsche, Friedrich. *"The Birth of Tragedy" and "The Genealogy of Morals"* (New York: Doubleday, 1956).

Nordal, J., and V. Kristinsson, eds. *Iceland: The Republic.* Reykjavík: Central Bank of Iceland, 1996.

O'Brien, S. "Fund Manager Sees Biotech Bubble." CBS Market Watch, February 19, 2000. www.cbsmarketwatch.com (accessed February 19, 2000).

Orlean, S. "Where's Willy?" *The New Yorker*, September 23, 2002, pp. 43–48.

Oslund, K. "Protecting Fat Mammals or Carnivorous Humans? Towards an Environmental History of Whales." *Historical Social Research* 29.3 (2004): 63–81.

Pálsson, G. "Human-Environmental Relations: Orientalism, Paternalism, and Communalism," in *Nature and Society: Anthropological Perspectives,* 63–81. London: Routledge, 1996.

Pálsson, G., and P. Rabinow. "The Iceland Controversy: Reflections on the Transnational Market of Civic Virtue." In *Global Assemblages: Technology, Politics, and Ethics as Anthropological Problem,* ed. A. Ong and S. J. Collier, 91–103. London: Blackwell, 2005.

———. "Iceland: The Case of a National Human Genome Project." *Anthropology Today* 15.5 (1999): 14–18.

Pender, K. "Biotech Stocks Make for a Thrill Ride—If You Can Stomach It." *San Francisco Chronicle,* July 4, 2000.

Perino, M. A. "What We Know and Don't Know about the Private Securities Litigation Reform Act of 1995." Testimony before the Subcommittee on Finance and Hazardous Materials of the Committee on Commerce, U.S. House of Representatives, October 21, 1997. Available from Stanford Law School, Securities Class Action Clearinghouse http://securities.stanford.edu/research/reports/19971021.html (accessed July 2, 2000).

Pennisi, E. "Academic Sequencers Challenge Celera in a Sprint to the Finish." *Science* 283 (March 19, 1990): 1822.

Petryna, A., and A. Kleinman, eds. *Global Pharmaceuticals: Ethics, Markets, Practices.* Durham, NC: Duke University Press, 2005.

Philipkoski, K. "Genetics Scandal Inflames Iceland." *Wired,* March 20, 2000. www.wired.com/news/politics/law/news/2000/03/35024 (accessed December 30, 2007).

Preston, R. "The Genome Warrior." *The New Yorker,* June 12, 2000, pp. 66–83.

Risch, N. J. "Searching for Genetic Determinants in the New Millennium." *Nature* 405 (2000): 847–56.

Roberts, L. "NIH Gene Patents, Round 2." *Science* 255 (1992): 912–13.

———. "OSTP to Wade into Gene Patents Quagmire." *Science* 254 (1991): 1104–5.

Roche. "Roche and DeCode Genetics Inc. of Iceland Collaborate in Genetic Disease Research." Roche press release, February 2, 1998. www.roche.com/roche/news/mrel97/e980202b.htm (accessed July 23, 1998).

Ronell, A. "Hitting the Streets: *Ecce Fama.*" In *Finitude's Score: Essays for the End of the Millennium,* 63–81. Lincoln: University of Nebraska Press, 1994.

Rose, H. *The Commodification of Bioinformation: The Icelandic Health Sector Database.* London: The Wellcome Trust, 2001.

———. "An Ethical Dilemma." *Nature* 425 (2003): 123–24.

Rosen, R. A. "The Statutory Safe Harbor for Forward-Looking Statements after Two and a Half Years: Has It Changed the Law? Has It Achieved What Congress Intended?" *Washington University Law Quarterly* 76.2 (Summer 1998): 645–80.

Rotman, B. *Signifying Nothing: The Semiotics of Zero.* New York: St. Martin's Press, 1987.

Seabrook, J. "Why Is the Force Still With Us?" *The New Yorker,* January 6, 1997, pp. 40–53.

Shields, A., M. Fortun, E. Hammonds, R. Rapp, C. Lerman, and P. Sullivan. "The Use of Racial Categories in Genetic Studies of Smoking Behavior: Implications for Reducing Health Disparities." *American Psychologist* 60.1 (2005): 1–27.

Shiller, R. *Irrational Exuberance.* Princeton, NJ: Princeton University Press, 2000.

Sigurdsson, Skúli. "Electric Memories and Progressive Forgetting." In *The Historiography of Contemporary Science and Technology,* ed. T. Söderqvist, 129–49. Amsterdam: Harwood, 1997.

——. "Springtime in Iceland and $200 Million Promises." April 20, 2002. www.raunvis.hi.is/~sksi/e_web.html (accessed July 2005).

——. "Yin-Yang Genetics, or the HSD deCODE Controversy." *New Genetics and Society* 20.2 (2001):103–17.

Slud, M. "Boom Time for Biotech." CNN Money, February 22, 2000. http://money .cnn.com/2000/02/22/companies/biotech (accessed December 30, 2007).

Soros, G. "The Theory of Reflexivity." Remarks to the MIT Department of Economics, World Economy Laboratory Conference, Washington, DC, April 26, 1994. www.geocities.com/ecocorner/intelarea/gs1.html (accessed July 1, 2005).

Specter, M. "Decoding Iceland." *The New Yorker,* January 18, 1999, pp. 40–51.

Strauss, N. "It May Be Small, But Reykjavík Rocks Big Time." *New York Times,* October 31, 2000.

Taylor, M. C. *Nots.* Chicago: University of Chicago Press, 1993.

Terwilliger, J. D., and K. M. Weiss. "Linkage Disequilibrium Mapping of Complex Disease: Fantasy or Reality?" *Current Opinion in Biotechnology* 9.6 (1998): 578–94.

Thieffry, D., and S. Sarkar. "Postgenomics? A Conference at the Max Planck Institute for the History of Science in Berlin." *BioScience* 49.3 (1999): 223–27.

Toobin, J. "The Man Chasing Enron." *The New Yorker,* September 9, 2002, pp. 86–96.

Turner, S. "Dresdner's Biotech Fund Springs Back to Health." WorldlyInvestor.com, 2000. www.worldlyinvestor.com (accessed June 14, 2000).

U.S. Congress. Senate. Committee on Energy and Natural Resources. *Workshop on Human Gene Mapping.* Washington, DC: U.S. Government Printing Office, 1987.

——. Senate. Subcommittee on Energy Research and Development. *The Human Genome Project.* Washington, DC: U.S. Government Printing Office, 1990.

U.S. Securities and Exchange Commission. "Concept Release and Notice of Hearing: Safe Harbor for Forward-Looking Statements." Release Nos. 33–7101, 34–34831, 35–26141, 39–2324, IC-20613. File No. S7–29–94. Washington, DC: U.S. Securities and Exchange Commission, 1994.

Veggeberg, S. "Controversy Mounts Over Gene Patent Policy." *The Scientist,* April 27, 1992, p. 1.

Wallace, R. "Opportunity, Not Exploitation: Valuing the Icelandic Genome." *Drug Discovery Today* 8.8 (1998): 335–57.

Washington Post. "Override the Securities Bill Veto." *Washington Post,* December 22, 1995, A18.

Weinstein, J. N. "Fishing Expeditions." *Science* 282 (October 23, 1999): 628–29.

Weiss, E. J., and J. E. Moser. "Enter Yossarian: How to Resolve the Procedural Catch-22 That the Private Securities Litigation Reform Act Creates." *Washington University Law Quarterly* 76.2 (Summer 1998): 457–507.

Williams, R. "Listen Up, Genomics Day Traders!" TheStreet.com, March 14, 2000. www.thestreet.com (accessed March 14, 2000).

Wilson, J. F., M. E. Weale, A. C. Smith, F. Gratrix, B. Fletcher, M. G. Thomas, N. Bradman, and D. B. Goldstein et al. "Population Genetic Structure of Variable Drug Response." *Nature Genetics* 29 (November 2001): 265–69.

Winickoff, D. E. "Genome and Nation: Iceland's Health Sector Database and Its Legacy." *Innovations,* no. 2 (Spring 2006): 80–105. www.mitpressjournals.org/doi/pdf/10.1162/itgg.2006.1.2.80 (accessed December 2007).

Winickoff, D. E., and R. N. Winickoff. "The Charitable Trust as a Model for Genomic Biobanks." *New England Journal of Medicine* 349.12 (2003): 1180–84.

Winnick, E. "Biotech Stocks Rebound, Genomics Mixed." Medscape, 2000. www.medscape.com (accessed March 20, 2000).

Wolpe, P. R. "Not Just How, but Whether: Revisiting Hans Jonas." *American Journal of Bioethics* 3.4 (2003): vii–viii.

Wong, N. "Judgment Day Is Here for Biotechs." WorldlyInvestor.com, March 20, 2000. www.worldlyinvestor.com (accessed July 20, 2000).

Index

Icelandic personal names are alphabetized by first name, in accordance with Icelandic practice.

Text: 10/13 Galliard
Display: Galliard
Compositor: Integrated Composition Systems
Illustrator: Bill Nelson
Printer and binder: Thomson-Shore, Inc.